About Island Press

Since 1984, the nonprofit organization Island Press has been stimulating, shaping, and communicating ideas that are essential for solving environmental problems worldwide. With more than 1,000 titles in print and some 30 new releases each year, we are the nation's leading publisher on environmental issues. We identify innovative thinkers and emerging trends in the environmental field. We work with world-renowned experts and authors to develop cross-disciplinary solutions to environmental challenges.

Island Press designs and executes educational campaigns in conjunction with our authors to communicate their critical messages in print, in person, and online using the latest technologies, innovative programs, and the media. Our goal is to reach targeted audiences—scientists, policymakers, environmental advocates, urban planners, the media, and concerned citizens—with information that can be used to create the framework for long-term ecological health and human well-being.

Island Press gratefully acknowledges major support of our work by The Agua Fund, The Andrew W. Mellon Foundation, The Bobolink Foundation, The Curtis and Edith Munson Foundation, Forrest C. and Frances H. Lattner Foundation, The JPB Foundation, The Kresge Foundation, The Oram Foundation, Inc., The Overbrook Foundation, The S.D. Bechtel, Jr. Foundation, The Summit Charitable Foundation, Inc., and many other generous supporters.

The opinions expressed in this book are those of the author(s) and do not necessarily reflect the views of our supporters.

THE GRAND FOOD BARGAIN

The Grand Food Bargain

And the Mindless Drive for More

Kevin D. Walker

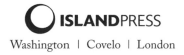

Washington | Covelo | London

Island Press is a trademark of The Center for Resource Economics.

Library of Congress Control Number: 2018959604

All Island Press books are printed on environmentally responsible materials.

Manufactured in the United States of America
10 9 8 7 6 5 4 3 2 1

Keywords: acute illness, antibiotic resistance, CAFOs, chronic diseases,
consumerism, empty calories, environmental resilience, farm bill, finite
resources, food assistance, foodborne outbreaks, food safety, food waste, free
markets, global markets, global warming, GMOs, individual choices, industrial
food production, international trade, laws of nature, malnutrition, market
society, monoculture, monopoly power, natural selection, obesity, fertilizer and
pesticide runoff, pseudoscience, political influence, processed foods, regulatory
capture, resource depletion, SNAP, social norms, societal benefits, stewardship,
supermarkets, sustainability, taxpayer subsidies, vulnerable populations/
communities, unexpected consequences

To those from the past, present, and future who remind us that food is about more than what we decide to eat.

We must think about things as they are, not as they are said to be.
— George Bernard Shaw

The mind of this country, taught to aim at low objects, eats upon itself.
— Ralph Waldo Emerson

Contents

Acronyms

CDC	Centers for Disease Control and Prevention
EPA	United States Environmental Protection Agency
ERS	Economic Research Service
FDA	Food and Drug Administration
FSIS	USDA Food Safety Inspection Service
GAO	Government Accountability Office
IICA	International Institute for Cooperation in Agriculture
MSU	Michigan State University
NAL	National Agricultural Library
NASS	National Agricultural Statistics Service
NIFA	National Institute of Food and Agriculture
NOAA	National Oceanic and Atmospheric Administration
OECD	Organisation for Economic Co-operation and Development
OIG	Office of Inspector General
OMB	Office of Management and Budget
PLoS	Public Library of Science
USDA	United States Department of Agriculture
WHO	World Health Organization

PART I

TAKING STOCK

Chapter 1

The Third Relationship

It is curious how seldom the all-importance of food is recognized.
— George Orwell

On a bright, cloudless morning, a slim Bushman walked away from the security of civilization and into the vast expanse of the Kalahari Desert. Trekking up and down gently rolling hills of shifting sand, he panned the horizon for signs of life. The wet season, marked by sporadic rain showers and lasting just a few weeks, was over. Plants and roots were mostly dormant. Insects had sought shelter in tunnels. Birds were sparse. Fruits and leaves had all but disappeared. Carrying only a short digging stick, he moved in silence, occasionally poking the ground to probe for signs of edible roots or wandering insects.

My friend Paul and I were tagging along. Searching for food in this desolate land on the other side of the world seemed surreal. We did not speak the Bushman's language, nor he ours, so communication was limited to gestures and facial expressions. Training our attention on his every movement, we dutifully followed behind, trying to keep pace while our feet battled the deep desert sand beneath us.

Our chance venture had happened so quickly that we barely had time to grab hats and water bottles, let alone contemplate whether we were putting ourselves in harm's way. Now, surrounded by endless red hills accented by thorn trees and desert bushes, we were ill-prepared should something go awry.

Conspicuously absent were signs of civilization. There were no people moving about, farms growing crops, ranches with fence lines, or wire strung between telephone poles. As I looked across the unending terrain, barren of trails or markers that could guide us back, it dawned on me that my compass was back in camp. Should we become separated from the Bushman, the Sun rising toward the center of the sky would be our only reference. Knowing that our fate rested with someone we had just met less than an hour ago, a heavy feeling descended over me; our lives were in his hands. We needed him, and he did not need anything from us.

Marching along, he stopped occasionally to point at something far off in the distance. Try as we might, our untrained eyes could not detect what he saw so easily. As he motioned, we nodded our heads in acknowledgment, as if this gesture had somehow improved our vision. A bit farther along, he changed direction to move downwind of whatever invisible creature was lurking.

As the morning wore on and the temperature climbed, fatigue settled in. Then, without warning, he quickened his pace. He had picked up signs of an ostrich, that flightless nomadic bird weighing up to three hundred pounds. With tracking skills honed over a lifetime, he guided us past clues that ended at a clump of bushes. Tucked beneath the bushes was a clutch of ostrich eggs, likely deposited by more than one female. Each egg, we would later learn, weighed between three and five pounds.

Before he took a closer look, the Bushman scanned in all directions for signs of nearby life. When threatened, an ostrich's first instinct is to hide or run, its powerful legs reaching speeds up to forty-five miles per hour. But if the bird chooses to fight, one powerful kick from those same legs can easily break the bones of its aggressor.

A mother ostrich, unwilling to surrender her offspring, was not the only threat. Hyenas in search of food could also be within close range. When he was satisfied that we were clear of immediate danger, the Bushman kneeled and peered at each of the half-dozen or so eggs. Pleased with what he had found, he reached in and carefully removed a single egg. Cradling it in his hands, he stepped away, leaving the remaining eggs undisturbed.

The Bushman handled the egg gently, savoring the reward of an age-old primal drive to seek food. In this desolate sea of sand, where scarcity reigned and there was no telling where the next meal would come from, uncovering a treasure trove of protein-rich, energy-dense ostrich eggs marked a rare find and a good day.

Paul and I were already preparing for what would happen next: between the three of us and one daypack, we would tote the remaining eggs back to his fellow Bushmen, also known as the San people. His sudden good fortune would bring welcome smiles from the community. His stature would rise a notch higher.

But when we pointed down at the remaining eggs and gestured our willingness to help carry them, he walked away. A single egg would suffice. His response bewildered me. All living beings, no matter their culture or species, are driven by the quest for food. Passing it up seemed unnatural, and certainly not conducive to survival. There, deep within this African desert, I witnessed something almost unfathomable to a Westerner.

Following our time in Namibia, Paul returned to his career in Minnesota and I resumed my work directing agricultural health and food-safety programs from my headquarters in Costa Rica. One day a package arrived. During our desert trek, Paul had snapped a photo of our guide with his arms behind his back, one hand clenching his digging stick, as he stared out at the red, sandy plains of the Kalahari. Paul had framed the picture and sent it to me where it soon found a new home alongside my computer. Whenever the daily grind of deadlines and meetings took its toll, momentarily gazing at the image helped me restore perspective.

Since then, I have learned more about our Kalahari adventure. Less than 10 percent of ostrich eggs survive the seven-week incubation period. Only 15 percent of hatched chicks reach one year of age. Some seventy eggs are needed to yield a one-year-old ostrich. But if just one egg becomes that single adult, the cycle can continue with an untold number of eggs for decades to come. Ostriches, it turns out, are some of the longest-living animals on Earth, capable of surviving some forty years in the wild.

While this helped explain why the Bushman took only one egg, I still couldn't fully square his decision (or the San people's lifestyle) with what I perceived to be human nature. After all, laying claim to all of the eggs was his reward for making the effort to hunt, especially since he had no assurances of finding food. Also, he would have known that predators like hyenas roamed the desert. If they were to come across that clutch of eggs, their actions would be less magnanimous.

Besides, with no one from his community looking on, he was free to indulge his own appetites. Given his thin frame, he would have likely benefited from extra calories and protein, and he surely would have enjoyed them. Even if he had denied himself personally, he could have generated much goodwill by sharing the eggs with others.

Leaving those eggs behind seemed at odds with what I thought of as the universal approach to food scarcity: always take advantage of having more food on hand whenever possible. Yet the more I stared at that photo, the more I realized that my perspective wasn't universal. It was decidedly Western.

My modern world had brought about such an immense availability of food that past generations of Bushmen would have found hard to even imagine. It had changed how people related to food. But had something else happened along the way? Had an abundance of food changed modern society in ways its people never considered?

Living apart from the rest of the world for more than twenty thousand years, the Bushmen were reminders of how humans first related to food. To meet the need for daily nourishment, they lived nomadic lives, continually hunting and gathering. Their odds of survival ebbed and flowed with the availably of edible plants, roots, nuts, insects, and animals, which in turn depended on a dynamic environment. They had to withstand disease and pestilence, flash floods, severe temperatures, and droughts. Besides the constant uncertainty, little else could be taken for granted.

In the full scope of history, it was not that long ago when my ancestors' path diverged from that of the Bushmen. My early forebears eventually became dissatisfied with the precarious hunter-gatherer life and began to experiment with the environment. Manipulating its cycles of life, they gathered and spread seeds, learning how to propagate edible plants. They domesticated animals. As they harvested the fruits of seeds they had sown, and the meat and milk from animals they had raised, they changed their relationship with food.

This second food relationship—farming—was far from placid, but it offered the first glimpses of stability. Through trial and error, people cultivated and crossbred crops that produced higher yields, fended off pests and disease, and became more resilient to swings in temperature. Literally and figuratively, they put down roots. It took two million years, until 1804, for the human population to surpass one billion people. But as farmers became more proficient, the world's population doubled to two billion people in the next 123 years.

Step back for a moment in time to 1776. A new nation had declared its independence from the British Empire. As America embarked on its own path, two resolutions were brought before the Second Continental Congress that recommended aid for farmers. As Thomas Jefferson later declared, "Agriculture is our wisest pursuit, because it will in the end contribute most to real wealth, good morals, and happiness."

In 1790, the inaugural census reported that 90 percent of the labor force worked in farming. Those numbers would change quickly as the first patent law spurred mechanical innovations in planting, harvesting, processing, and preserving food. When the Civil War began seven decades later, few expected it to last long. But improvements in farming and processing meant more men could remain on the battlefield; fewer were needed back home to grow food. The war raged on for four years.

In the midst of those years of carnage, the die was cast for what would become our third relationship with food. With President Lincoln's signature, land was made freely available to anyone willing to homestead and farm it; states and the federal government established a platform for agriculture education, science, and experimentation; a national department of agriculture was created; and, paving the way to later distribute food across the country, a transcontinental railroad was built.

What Lincoln had set in motion cannot be understated. Though America was still in its infancy, no other nation had started out with such abundant fresh water, rich topsoil, open land, and favorable climate. An engaged citizenry believed in the role of government to improve their lives through laws they had pushed to enact. Almost immediately, the nation's investment in government and science paid dividends through higher levels of food production.

With that abundance, a new welcome reality settled in. Households no longer needed to produce their own food. By 1880, less than half the labor force worked on farms.As workers left the fields for new jobs in America's booming industrial economy, families moved away from rural areas. Instead of a nation of farmers as the founders once envisioned, American society was quickly becoming a new class of food consumers—one that, as time went by, knew less and less about where their food came from.

The third relationship to food had taken root. At its core was the "grand food bargain." As with any bargain, there were two parties. One was a rapidly growing society of consumers who wanted more food with less effort. The other was a rapidly growing industry of food providers whose profits depended on volume. The vehicle that kept the grand food bargain on track was the modern food system. Like most systems, this one operated with a singular purpose—continually turn out more food year after year. Food scarcity, a fact of life for 2.8 million years of human existence, would no longer control the nation.

Indeed, as the nineteenth century came to a close, food *surplus* became a national challenge. The need to find new markets for a glut of American products helped drive the former colony to begin taking its own, controlling five, including Guam and the Philippines, by the end of 1898. As one historian wrote, "Merchants and manufacturers salivated at the prospect of a launching pad for trade with China; magazines and newspapers were full of calculation about the fabulous wealth that awaited them if they could persuade the Chinese to wear cotton clothes, use American kerosene, build with American nails, or begin eating bread and meat instead of rice and vegetables." Whether it was expansion into Asia or, later, protection of US-owned banana plantations in Central America, an abundance of food had become part of American foreign policy—one backed up with military force.

The twentieth century brought even more food. Sixteen years after the Wright Brothers demonstrated their first airplane, aerial crop dusting began. Large warehouses were built to accommodate refrigerated railcars. As prosperity climbed, the portion of household income that consumers spent on food fell.

America's plenty did not go unnoticed in other parts of the world. German imperialists watched in dismay when the United States increased wheat acreage by more than 50 percent in five years to meet Europe's wartime demand. Less than a decade after Germany's defeat in World War I, Adolf Hitler wrote that "Europeans—often without realizing it— take the circumstances of American life as the benchmark for their own lives." Hitler was envious of America's land empire and its food system. Plotting Germany's return to power, he wrote that "to lead a life comparable to that of the American people" required taking the fertile lands of neighboring countries so more food could be produced without disrupting German manufacturing industries.

In fact, World War II marked the only time when food in America had to be rationed. To feed the armed forces, more processed and canned foods were produced and shipped overseas. Fresh fruits and vegetables were still grown domestically, but they were harder to come by in cities as transport vehicles, tires, and gasoline were diverted to support the war effort.

When the war ended, so too did rationing. New policies and programs underwrote loans, funded research, created new markets, and provided insurance that together incentivized greater production. The technology that had been used to build bombs and chemicals was channeled into producing food. Synthetic fertilizers and pesticides, more-powerful farm equipment, animals packed together (some on top of each other) and raised with antibiotics—all contributed to the modern industrialized food system.

For the most part, consumers were content with their grand food bargain. Technology like flash freezing and preservatives helped fill cupboards and refrigerators with food. "TV dinners" and other prepared meals meant less time in the kitchen. The microwave oven, the upshot of an engineer conducting research on radar and discovering that the candy bar in his pocket had melted, allowed meals to cook in record time.

A generation after the war, food rationing had been banished to footnotes in history books. Being surrounded by food was the new normal. Farming had replaced hunting and gathering. The grand food bargain had replaced farming. An abundance of food was taken for granted.

Today, enough calories are churned out per person in the United States to feed two moderately active adult women. Expending effort to cook, prepare, and clean up afterward is now optional, bordering on obsolete. Without giving it much thought, Americans experience convenience and selection that legions of royalty never dreamed about. Anybody can have and eat unlimited portions of whatever food they desire, so long as they bring money.

Take, for example, fresh eggs, found almost any time in any grocery store. The sheer number of cartons, typically stacked high on rolling pallets behind the glass doors of room-sized coolers, suggests their supply is unlimited. The lower the price, the more consumers will buy—including shoppers who didn't come into the store with eggs on their list. All act independently of each other, never asking themselves how their individual actions might affect overall supply.

The fact that the production of eggs depends on a solitary planet governed by laws of nature, with set limits on resources like water and land, has no bearing on the number of eggs each person decides to take with them. Our third relationship to food allows us to ignore anything beyond personal considerations, and certainly anything unpleasant. It is this relationship to food that Paul and I brought to the Kalahari when we encouraged the Bushman to empty the clutch of all its ostrich eggs.

In one way or another, my life has always been linked to the modern food system. I grew up in the shadow of Utah's Wasatch Mountains on a family farm. We raised cattle, grew crops, and tended to fruit orchards, both to sell and to feed ourselves. My earliest memory of farming was climbing onto the metal seat of an old grain binder left to rust in the corner of the farm. Pulled by a team of horses, it cut and bundled wheat stalks into mushroom looking "shocks," which were later fed into a thresher to separate the grain seeds from the chaff.

From stories my uncles told of spending long and hot summer days caked in dust during grain harvest, I knew my life on the same land was much easier. I benefited from a stable of tractors, combines, and specialized farm implements. But even with the machinery, there were plenty of other manual chores waiting to be done, including irrigating fields, hauling hay, picking fruit, cleaning ditch banks, feeding and dehorning cattle. The more sweat I expended, the more vested I became in the results.

While there were years with bumper fruit crops, an extra cutting of hay, or more corn silage than what the silo could hold, what I remember most were the late spring frosts that wiped out a winter of pruning trees. Or the countless hours we spent planting, cultivating, and irrigating alfalfa fields, only to battle an infestation of boll weevil. Or tending cattle, only to find one that would weaken at the knees and go down with disease. Or the time a milk cow choked to death on a bolus of grain despite our efforts to save her. I learned that no matter the number of long days covered in sweat with muscles aching, producing food was always a partnership with forces beyond our control.

I also learned that our farm was steeped in the traditions of the past rather than the trends of the future. When my father and uncles worked the land, farms like ours filled the landscape. But as homes and roads sprouted around us, taxes on farmland started to rival the profits it produced. Cities wanted tax bases that came from urban development, not growing food.

My father foresaw that farming as he had known it was no longer the viable occupation it once was. He pushed me to go to college but did not dissuade me when I chose agriculture as my major. I still had plans to be part of producing food, even though I didn't know where and how I would do it.

In college, I took classes from well-meaning professors who drilled into me the idea that the modern food system was the only way to sustain a fast-growing population and rapidly changing society. Farming was no longer a way of life, they emphasized, but a series of smart business decisions that maximized profit.

Financial success came from consistently ratcheting up productivity to boost revenue while scrubbing costs. Chemicals opened new doors to planting massive fields in a single crop. Antibiotics and hormones did the same for raising meat animals. Those farms poised for prosperity were growing bigger by leveraging debt and participating in government programs. Their size was proof positive of what the future looked like. Being at the vanguard of food production meant adopting the latest technologies in genetics, fertilizers, nutrition, chemicals, and antimicrobials.

As my years of education increased, the feasibility of farming as a profession diminished. Three universities and three degrees later, I rejected overtures to stay in academia and accepted a job with Farmland Industries, then North America's largest farmer-owned cooperative. With its storied history and customer base spread across sixteen states in America's heartland, I felt well positioned. I believed in the company's cooperative mission, liked my department's focus on quantitative analysis, and enjoyed the people I worked with. Though I was no longer farming, I was firmly embedded in the modern food system.

One day I was asked how more nitrogen fertilizer could be sold to farmers. Farmland had the manufacturing facilities to turn out more nitrogen than any other company in North America. So I formulated a large mathematical model to evaluate its production, distribution, and retail capacities. With my supervisor, we analyzed each of the company's 256 markets. Then I programmed the computer to optimize the entire system, from purchasing natural gas to retailing final products. Pouring over the computer printouts, I saw the potential for substantial increases in sales and profitability.

When the fertilizer division began to implement our recommendations, the results did not disappoint. Overall sales and profit margins went up as farmers applied more fertilizer. So did yields and the volume of products flowing through the modern food system. The outcome was almost textbook perfect. Farmland, its farmer-owners, food manufacturers, distributors, retailers, and consumers had all benefited. From a market-economics perspective, society was better off. My reward was a significant year-end bonus.

Though I valued the satisfaction (and compensation) of a job well done, something was gnawing at me. While I was running different scenarios on the computer, colleagues asked how much more nitrogen could be applied before returns pointed downward. Preliminary results suggested there were no immediate limits. In practice, I knew that farmers would apply more and more nitrogen to maximize their profits, even if it resulted in additional fertilizer runoff into streams and waterways. So long as farmers were not held responsible, they could simply ignore the consequences.

Caught up in the zeal to perform well, I fell back on the justification that more food was why the modern food system existed—producing higher yields benefited society, which always trumped adverse side effects. Still, I was uneasy. And rightfully so.

As a gas, nitrogen is all around us. In fact, the element makes up 78 percent of Earth's atmosphere, though not in a form plants can use. In nature, transforming atmospheric nitrogen into a nutrient requires a symbiotic relationship between certain plants and bacteria like rhizobia. But as more synthetic fertilizer is used, the role of nature fades. The outcome is relying more heavily on manufactured nitrogen fertilizer made by drawing down finite reserves of natural gas.

Yet simply short-circuiting nature's nitrogen cycle is not the end of the story. A by-product of synthetic nitrogen is nitrous oxide, which is three hundred times more damaging to an already warming planet than carbon dioxide. Seventy-nine percent of nitrous oxide in the atmosphere comes from agriculture.

Neither is the problem limited to global warming. As hydraulic fracking sweeps across the country, the temporary boost in natural gas supplies lowers its price. Incentives to build more nitrogen manufacturing plants increase, particularly in the Midwest. Thus, when a new three-billion-dollar nitrogen plant was announced, the president of the company sold its importance to the public by saying the added nitrogen would "help farmers raise healthy, profitable crops to feed a growing global population." In other words, the fertilizer plant was necessary to sustain a mindless drive to produce more food.

Not mentioned in the press release was how nitrogen applied in fields adds to the runoff flowing into rivers, lakes, and oceans. Too much nitrogen or phosphorus (another fertilizer) spawns toxic algae blooms and so-called dead zones, habitats where oxygen levels in water are so low that marine life cannot be sustained. The largest dead zone, roughly the size of New Jersey, is found where the Mississippi River flows into the Gulf of Mexico, discharging its runoff from the upper Midwest.

Nitrogen in our water endangers both the landscape and the people who live nearby. Elevated exposures can lead to blue baby syndrome, a life-threatening condition in which the blood cannot distribute oxygen, as well as other afflictions including bladder cancer, thyroid problems, and birth defects.

Health concerns have come to a head in Iowa, the Mecca of corn, soybeans, pork, and egg production, where agriculture is the top contributor of nitrates in water. The Des Moines Board of Water Works sources its drinking supplies from rivers downstream of farms, spending heavily on specialized technology to strip out contaminants. After years of struggling to stay ahead of rising nitrate levels, the water utility sued three northern counties for violating the Clean Water Act. The suit was dismissed by a federal judge who ruled that water quality was governed by the Iowa legislature.

The issue has divided agricultural interests (the state's largest industry) against individual and public health advocates. As the battle has intensified, so has the collateral damage. Legislation was introduced to dismantle the independence of water utilities like the Des Moines Board of Water Works. The editor of the *Storm Lake Times* (the local paper of a small northern Iowa city) won a Pulitzer Prize for calling out powerful agricultural interests. As of this writing, the legislature passed a $282-million bill to improve water quality, though there is no agreement on how any improvements will be measured.

Within a year of winding down my role in the nitrogen initiative, I left Farmland. It was not an easy decision. The company was doing well. My future looked promising. Yet buried in my jumbled thoughts at the time was a bubbling anxiety that I was giving too much credit to human ingenuity and not enough deference to nature and the environment. At some point, my enthusiasm for devising novel models to ratchet up food production had hit a ceiling.

When offered a position in Colorado at the United States Department of Agriculture (USDA), I accepted. Leveraging my previous research in college, I focused on animal diseases that might limit meat and milk production, including bovine spongiform encephalopathy ("mad cow disease"), bovine tuberculosis, and *E. coli* O157:H7.

The charge of the center I directed was to assess emerging issues for policymakers. Pathogens were always the enemy. Each risk assessment we undertook looked at a possible invasion, or if the disease was already established, how it was transmitted and spread. The modern food system, with its constant incentives to increase production, had helped create some of the problems we were addressing. While our work could call attention to the underlying causes, policymakers knew they were on thin ice if they put forward policies that challenged the premise that we must always produce more.

When I moved from USDA to Costa Rica and the International Institute for Cooperation in Agriculture (IICA), I hoped the political constraints to helping countries safeguard their food and protect the health of their plants and animals were behind me. Yet as the years went by, I realized how closely international development was tied to replicating the modern food system. To the extent that they succeeded, these countries would face the same consequences from unprecedented abundance that the United States was experiencing.

When I returned stateside, I landed at Michigan State University. Over the years, my misgivings about the modern food system and its implications continued to build. On a campus of this size, one which benefits from Lincoln's signature and America's third relationship to food, MSU seemed like a good place to channel my observations into a larger context for understanding.

Soon enough, I realized the depth of expertise residing in one place. Whether I had questions on bacteria in soil or malnutrition in infants, there seemed to be someone on campus who could provide answers. MSU was well regarded and had done an admirable job affirming its historical purpose—specialized research and education.

Yet some of the strengths that had served the university so well in the past were limitations when looking forward. In the end, exploring broader linkages across the modern food system proved difficult. Like many universities, its infrastructure and administration prized advancement within narrow fields of specialization. While some faculty welcomed broader exploration, others simply responded to my questions with "not my area of expertise."

One day, the dean of my college wanted to talk. Over the years, we had closely collaborated and many times had traveled together to meetings. We knew each other well. When he suggested that I write a book that would become *The Grand Food Bargain*, I listened without interrupting. Use your background and experience as a food insider, he encouraged.

But I was reluctant. By the time our conversation ended, my mind had already conceived my response. I would search the library and Internet for any number of books to show why another one was not necessary. Then I would show him a sampling of such books so I could move on to another topic.

That other topic is still waiting. Writing this book from a lifetime of food system experience has reinforced for me how heavily Americans are vested in the third relationship to food without asking themselves why. From 90 percent of the labor force in 1790, farmers comprise 1.4 percent today. Because of specialized farming practices, even farmers turn to supermarkets and restaurants, just like everyone else. For the remaining 98.6 percent of the labor force and their families, food now resides on the periphery of life. Cooking and food preparation are falling by the wayside. Today, more money is spent on food eaten outside the home than within.

Most of us do not think about how, throughout 99.99 percent of the time that humans have roamed this planet, food and scarcity always went hand in hand. If the timeline of the human race were reduced to a single day, the grand food bargain began less than five seconds ago. Our current relationship with food is a historic anomaly. From this perspective was born my fascination with the Bushman.

While his ancestors had survived for thousands of years by seeking harmony with a hostile environment, the fate of recent generations was different. When settlers moved in, the Bushmen's relationship with food was scuttled. Common rights to land were abrogated by those who now asserted ownership. Slow-replenishing supplies of underground water were pumped dry. As the fences went up, communities were rounded up, relocated, and made dependent on others. His way of life, once in line with the unpredictability of the Kalahari, would not prevail against societies who embraced a different relationship with food.

We have fashioned a country where being surrounded by unending food now seems normal. When we feel hungry, we open cupboards, look in refrigerators, or stop at any number of nearby restaurants or supermarkets. The implication of being fed by a system rarely enters our minds. Implicitly we place our full trust in it. We assume the modern food system will always be there. We expect it to continually turn out more food, reinforcing our central belief that more is always better.

It is the precariousness of this third relationship to food that sparked this book. Looking back over time, we have seen people's ability to overcome scarcity, but no such ability to erase the ensuing unwanted outcomes. When all we need to know about food is the location of the nearest restaurant or supermarket, it is easy to ignore that unforeseen consequences even exist.

The good news, however, is that our relationship to food is never static. Rediscovering our reliance on forces always present but seldom thought about sets the stage to fashion a new food bargain, one where wants and realities become two sides of the same coin. But before we can get there, we first need to understand how we arrived at this point in the first place.

Four basic elements encompass the grand food bargain. This book examines each, starting with taking stock of our relationship to food in Part I. As we've already begun to explore, when we change food, food changes us. Compared with the past, our relationship with food today is a huge outlier. While the modern food system introduced conveniences, there were never guarantees that being able to take food for granted would last. Dismissing this broader understanding is just one outcome of a modern food system that caters exclusively to individual preferences.

Part II covers the forces that result in having unprecedented food on hand. Five forces—the will to survive, the assumptions behind resources, the norms underpinning governance, the beliefs placed on science, and the values bestowed on markets—fuel the modern food system in its drive to always produce more. Some forces are inherited, some were already present, and some were human inventions. Understanding how each operates, separately and together, is critical to recognizing where the modern food system is headed.

Part III is about unexpected consequences. They include the unforeseen, the unwelcome, and the unrecognized. They range from polluted rivers to acute and chronic disease to global warming. Some are hidden. Others we willfully ignore. Many we presume to control, unsuccessfully.

Part IV is about choice. Heightened awareness is the first step in dismantling well-worn justifications that perpetuate the failings of the modern food system. Only when people recognize how individual decisions culminate in collective results will we chart a new direction. Ultimately, it is consumers—in this case eaters, which means all of us—who can uniquely establish our next relationship with food.

The Grand Food Bargain is about one of our most fundamental relationships, the forces that drive it, the consequences of our actions, and, ultimately, the choices that only we can make. For many of us, choices about food are reduced to decisions made in the supermarket. Pasta or rice? Beef or chicken? Apples or bananas? So to begin our exploration of where everyday choices are leading us, let's start with the humble banana.

Chapter 2

My Food, My Way

Pile it high. Sell it low.
— King Kullen, first supermarket opened in Queens,
New York, 1930

1502: a hurricane-damaged ship is forced to set anchor. Awaiting repairs, its captain ventures into the lush rain forest and exchanges gifts with the native people. Upon his return home, extravagant tales of gold along the "rich coast" set the stage for Spain's claim of what is now Costa Rica.

The voyage was Columbus's last exploration of the New World. In the end, rumors of Costa Rica's wealth were just that: rumors. Five centuries afterward, the most lucrative treasure leaving the country was bananas, originally mass cultivated as a cheap food for workers building a railroad to move coffee produced inland to the coast.

Bananas are the all-time most popular fresh fruit consumed in America—a spectacular achievement considering that almost all bananas are imported. Stocked year-round in grocery stores from coast to coast, their yellow curve appeal is everywhere. Their popularity has made bananas a "loss leader," priced to entice consumers into the store so that they would buy other groceries. Ingeniously packaged by nature, easy to peel with no sticky fingers, void of dribbling juices, bananas are an all-day, anytime snack whose versatility ranges from ice cream sundaes to the stock ingredient in many baby foods.

Under a pleasant blue sky with white pockets of clouds, my two uncles and I were traveling in the northeast region of Costa Rica, some sixty miles from where Columbus first came ashore. Instead of the diverse tropical lowland that greeted Columbus, surrounding us was a monoculture landscape of broad-leaved, adult-height, green banana plants. At the time of our excursion, Costa Rica, roughly the size of West Virginia, was the world's second-largest exporter of bananas.

Following instructions that only lovable Costa Ricans can give, I turned left at the next jog in the two-lane highway, just past the last gas station when leaving town. The dirt lane meandered left and then right as it cut through a working plantation. Snaking in and out among the rows of bananas were tram lines, suspended some six feet in the air by cables and supported by steel arches placed along the ground.

Bananas grow best in humid tropical environments. With a fully ripe bunch weighing 60 to 110 pounds, harvesting bananas is labor intensive. To cope with the heat and humidity, workers arrive in the fields early each morning. My uncles and I watched how, after placing bars of padding between the tiers or "hands" forming each bunch, one worker steadied the bunch on his shoulder, while another wielding a sharp machete sliced through its stem with one fell swoop. Freed from the plant, the bunch was secured to the overhead cable.

On this plantation, human runners transported bunches to a centrally located opening where they were cut up and boxed for shipping. We watched as a runner, outfitted in knee-high rubber boots, bound together a long rack of bunches, then attached the rope to a thick strap around his waist. Taking a deep breath, he lunged forward, fighting for momentum while digging his boots into the loose dirt to gain traction.

Like a train of railcars pulled by a locomotive, the long rack lurched forward, and, once under way, the runner quickened his pace. As he loped through the fields trying not to fall while maintaining momentum, he crossed drainage ditches spanned with single wooden planks. Like most workers on the plantation, he was paid piecework. By the time he arrived at the off-load site, having wound his way back and forth several times across sections of the plantation, he was drenched in sweat. Visibly exhausted, he dropped his waist strap to the ground and bent over panting, trying to catch his breath.

At the off-load, workers with knives took over, reducing each bunch to a number of smaller hands that fell into a trough of water for rinsing. Farther down the line, other workers pruned the hands again, tossing aside any bananas judged unacceptable. As the morning wore on, the piles of discarded bananas grew larger and became a convenient platform for some of the shorter line workers to stand on.

Near the end of the processing line, workers expertly packed rectangular boxes with the curvilinear fruit. As each box was filled, another person checked its weight, adding or subtracting one or two bananas to match the printed weight label on the side. The completed box was then closed, stamped, and loaded into an already cold shipping container whose refrigeration unit hummed in the background.

For my uncles, this was their first trip to Central America and the only time they would visit a working plantation. Fascinated with each phase of the operation, they peppered Eric, the plantation manager, with nonstop questions. As our time with him wound down, I could sense their deep respect for a fellow food producer.

Walking back to my SUV, little was spoken. After a long pause, one brother turned to the other and remarked, "I don't think I can ever look at a banana the same way again."

The planation had triggered old memories of growing up on a farm. The hard labor was a reminder of walking up and down long rows bent over thinning sugar beets. Or loading shocks of wheat onto horse-drawn wagons, then threshing grain under the midday sun, with bodies caked with dust and eyes red from irritation.

Comparisons to physical demands notwithstanding, bananas are dramatically different from beets or wheat. Though bananas appear to come from trees, they are both an herb (the leafy stalk lacks a woody stem) and a fruit (the tiny black specks in the center are remnants of seeds). Thousands of years of experimentation has produced varieties that yield more fruit, but also seeds that have all but disappeared. Bananas can no longer pollinate and reproduce in typical fruit fashion. Propagation relies on tissue cultures or dividing and spreading the root mat.

Such were the beginnings of the most ubiquitous fruit in the world, the Cavendish banana. This particular variety that dominates global trade is essentially a sterile species. Each banana is indistinguishable from the rest—each one could just as easily have come from Asia as from Africa or Latin America. After a single bunch is produced, the treelike stalk is cut down to make room for a hand-picked replacement to take over.

Banana plants are bred to produce more fruit, which results in more-fragile fibrous stalks that can be blown down easily. On the plantation we visited, the sea of green plants was lined with synthetic orange-colored twine wrapped around each stalk and staked to the ground. As the flowers transformed into a bunch, each was enclosed in an insecticide-impregnated blue bag that raised the inside temperature and provided protection against outside chills.

One more fact distinguishes bananas. They are part of an international system that stretches around the world. The temperature-controlled containers we saw being loaded in the middle of a field were trucked to a port in Puerto Limón (near where Columbus once docked his damaged ship) and loaded onto cargo ships with hundreds of similar containers, before docking in US ports on the East Coast a few days after departing Costa Rica.

Wholesale companies would receive the offloaded containers and transport them to giant warehouses. Chambers filled with ethylene gas would turn the still-green bananas to varying degrees of ripeness. The close-to-ripe bananas would be transported to supermarket warehouses, then onto grocery-store receiving docks. Store employees would cart each box to the produce section, open the box, and display its contents for sale. By the time a consumer grabs a hand or two and scurries on to their next purchase, each box has been moved dozens of times, traveled thousands of miles, possibly undergone one or more inspections, and been the responsibility of thousands of people. For the average American, such breadth and complexity is invisible. Each person will consume ten thousand bananas by the age of forty, rarely, if ever, considering the workers' hands that touched them.

At one point during our visit with Eric, we sat in a windowless room while he explained how his planation fit into the larger system. Their bananas went to the United States and ports beyond. Each buyer had their own list of requirements. Failure to meet all of them was grounds for rejecting the entire shipment. At the top of the list were appearance, size, and shape.

Countless bananas were being culled and discarded, he told us, because they were too long, too short, too big in diameter, too much curl, or bore superficial blemishes like scarring. Their appearance had nothing to do with nutrition, taste, quality, or food safety but everything to do with what the system dictated that a banana must be. Over time, consumers had come to believe that every banana should be identical and perfect. The fact that nature doesn't operate this way was immaterial.

Eric worked in a system where competition for contracts was high and profit margins were thin. His operation was smaller than many other plantations, which meant his margins were even thinner—and that amplified his fear of a shipment being rejected. He also worried about workers' pay, turnover, and productivity.

As if that were not enough, Eric faced mechanical breakdowns and the flare-up of pests and diseases like black sigatoka (leaf spots that spread quickly and can reduce yields by 50 percent or more). He was also well aware of the environmental destruction from bananas written into Costa Rica's history, including entire regions so damaged that they could no longer produce bananas at all.

In this system, buyers hold the leverage, he remarked, and are never shy to point out how other plantations are ready and willing to meet their terms. If not in Costa Rica, then Guatemala or Honduras. Becoming part of the banana system was little different from farming corn in rural America. Having invested up front thousands of dollars per hectare before a single banana was produced, Eric had one option: stay on top of costs.

Yes, he told us in response to our questions, he was very concerned about risks to workers' health and threats to the environment. But until the system changed, operating differently was more dream than reality. As I interpreted what he said for my uncles, I wondered how much satisfaction in growing food was being swallowed up by a system that squeezed profits until the plantation teetered on collapse.

The very idea of a *system* has not always existed. In fact, it is relatively new to history. In the sixteenth century, planets such as Venus and Mercury were already known. Unknown, however, was a unifying explanation that tied them and Earth together. Enter Copernicus, who mathematically ordered the planets in relation to the Sun. The following century, Galileo's observations firmed up Copernicus's earlier work and solidified the existence of a *system*, a Greek-derived word meaning a whole concept formed from several parts.

A "solar system" seems obvious today without having to recall how it began as an effort to understand the relationships of nearby planets. But it is worth remembering that such an understanding, especially one without Earth at the center, landed Galileo a conviction of heresy and kept him under house arrest until his death in 1642.

Despite the rough start, the concept of systems has served humans well, as did combining ink with parchment, or etching pictorial stories onto cave walls. Systems helped capture ideas, sort through observations, and refine understanding. This unifying premise accelerated learning. Thus, bodies of water became systems where rainfall runs off land, forming brooks that turn into streams and then tributaries flowing into rivers before emptying into lakes and oceans. The human body became understood as a series of systems that carry oxygen, provide nutrition, fight off disease, create offspring, and much more. Through systems we could tie what we ate to gastrointestinal eruptions. Or relate time to seasonal variations.

Insight into natural systems undoubtedly inspired human-made systems. Adding zero to an arbitrary set of nine numbers led to the base-ten numbering system that paved the way for measuring wealth. Governance was a system that unified informal norms around acceptable behavior, which eventually morphed into a political system called government.

In every possible way, American life is now permeated with systems. Defense systems protect us. Insurance systems shield us from extraordinary risk. Healthcare systems treat illness. Transportation systems provide mobility. Financial systems manage money. Marketing systems advance commerce.

Today, people understand systems by what they do—not by how they work. Their existence is affirmation of our ready willingness to let systems control at least part of our lives. When we take out a loan, our questions center on repayment terms, not the money supply controlled by the Federal Reserve System. When filling our cars with gas, we think about which grade of fuel and its price, not how crude oil residing deep beneath the surface of the Earth became gasoline deposited a few feet away beneath our feet. When we enter a supermarket, our minds are on how food can satisfy immediate wants, not how different pieces and parts of the modern food system are meshed together to make food available.

Systems allow us to dismiss not knowing what we do not know, to paraphrase the Arabic proverb.* The nitrogen model I discussed in chapter 1 represented Farmland's nitrogen system. It contained over three thousand equations. In presenting it to executive management, I covered the results without dwelling on the limitations of systems. Projections of higher returns initially grabbed their interest. When trial implementation proved positive, any remaining doubts turned into optimism.

For me, the experience reinforced my understanding that I should never overlook how systems work. In every system surrounding us, assumptions have been made about how its different components relate to each other. Yet in everyday life, as long as systems perform the way we want them to, no one questions those assumptions. Ignorance can inspire trust and confidence, even when neither is merited.

Human-made systems that affirm what one wants to believe are particularly dicey. While living in Costa Rica, I discovered a new favorite fish called corvina, known as Chilean sea bass in North America.

---

* He who knows not, and knows not that he knows not, is a fool. Shun him.
   He who knows not, and knows that he knows not, is simple. Teach him.
   He who knows, and knows not that he knows, is asleep. Wake him.
   He who knows, and knows that he knows, is wise. Follow him.

With its moist, white flesh, mild flavor, and absence of "fishy" taste, it became my preferred seafood entree at restaurants. Aware that the Earth's oceans are overfished, I quizzed a few chefs and waiters about its origin and sustainability. No need for concern, they told me, corvina came from deep ocean waters in the southern hemisphere. Long considered a trash fish, its supplies were plentiful. Because I always ordered the fillet, I never saw the entire fish. Instead, I pictured lakes back home with healthy bass populations, imagining, self-servingly, that all was well.

A couple of years later, a colleague shared an article warning that the fish was quickly disappearing. Corvina was really the Patagonian toothfish, a species of cod. With its bulging oversized eyes, gray-black skin, protruding jaw, and sharp teeth, this fish was big, ugly, and menacing—not something chefs could easily dress up and display on a platter with fresh garnish. For decades, commercial fisherman and fish buyers had shown little interest in Patagonian toothfish, even at rock-bottom prices. Its name, unattractive image, and deep ocean habitat, which made fishing difficult, had protected the fish from human exploitation.

This all changed when a US fish wholesaler in Chile made it his mission to build a system around it. He started by rebranding the fish as "Chilean sea bass." Targeting North American markets, a few featured chefs discovered its taste, texture, and ease of preparation. Suddenly, this ugly old fish morphed into a new image associated with fine dining. Demand for Chilean sea bass shot up.

Large fishing trawlers outfitted with sophisticated electronics, on-board processing equipment, and freezers recognized opportunity. These ships could ply the frigid southern seas for months at a time, putting out "longlines" containing thousands of individually baited hooks that stretched fifteen miles and more. Catches of ten to twenty tons a day were not uncommon. In a matter of years, ocean stocks fell precipitously. The fishery was unsustainable.

Sometimes referred to as "white gold" for its premium price, the fish became a magnet for illegal fishing, especially in remote southern oceans where deepwater nets were used. Though countries established limits on catch, they were ill-prepared for the onslaught of illegal fishing vessels, vast seas to patrol, and harsh weather conditions. Efforts to rein in catch and protect remaining stocks were easy to skirt.

To stop this and other fisheries from collapsing, the nonprofit Marine Stewardship Council came up with a "certified sustainable" label. For a fee paid to MSC, retailers could display their trademarked label alongside fish being offered for sale. By paying for an extensive audit, fishing vessels could become certified suppliers. Stores went along, hoping to sell more fish. Fisherman signed up, hoping to catch more fish. And some consumers climbed on board, hoping to rely on MSC's pledge that "Choosing seafood with the blue MSC label helps ensure fish for tomorrow."

Not part of this system were a host of biological, environmental, behavioral, regulatory, and legal consequences beyond MSC's control. Despite appearances, labeling seafood in supermarkets like Chilean sea bass as "certified sustainable" came with no guarantee that the fishery was indeed more sustainable. What the label *did* do was reinforce our trust in systems without understanding how they work or how their future viability is being gambled away. As one Patagonian toothfish buyer said, "As long as people are willing to buy, I'm willing to sell."

Returning stateside from Costa Rica after several years away required readjustment. I had lost touch with how summer days in northern latitudes were longer and winter days were shorter. I welcomed the fresh renewal in the transition from winter to spring when brown faded away, new colors appeared, blossoms filled out trees, and birds chirped more earnestly. And I realized how deeply consumption was ingrained in American life. The sheer number of products continually marketed as needing homes, lest one's life be ruined through incompleteness, was overwhelming. Several months would have to pass before the advertisements faded into the background.

Buying food was no different. Walking into a supermarket with its stocked shelves brimming with whatever one could imagine was bedazzling. To ensure that the message of abundance and variety remains fresh, nearly twenty-one thousand new or updated food and beverage products are rolled out each year. These almost exclusively processed foods, designed for personal appeal, dwarfed what I could easily recognize as nutritious fare.

Conveniently located right off the main entrance was the produce section. There they were, almost front and center: Cavendish bananas no different from those I saw being boxed in Costa Rica. It was the same variety dating back decades. Little had changed, each was essentially a clone of the other. The only difference was the sticker affixed to the yellow peel announcing the company and country of origin.

By all accounts, Cavendish bananas are inferior to a variety sold more than a half century ago, the Gros Michel. Known more commonly as Big Mike, they were larger with a creamier texture, fruitier taste, and thicker skin. Big Mikes were so rugged they were shipped as bunches, without needing to be padded, disassembled, and boxed. At port, ships' cargo holds were loaded and unloaded by tossing bunches of bananas like luggage on airplanes. The global banana market had rapidly developed around this single variety.

Then came word of a devastating fungus infecting banana plantations. Called Panama disease because of its origin, the fungus spread with abandon. Unable to contain it, banana companies tried outrunning it by abandoning existing plantations and moving farther away. Wielding enormous political leverage (including the long arm of the United States government), these corporations cleared vast tracts of tropical rain forest to start new plantations.

Despite all their efforts, growing a single variety of bananas still left plantations vulnerable and eventually infected. Fifty years after the fungus was identified, the Big Mike variety was wiped out. With the international market for bananas verging on collapse, companies stumbled onto the Cavendish variety, which appeared to be resistant to Panama disease. Using tissue cultures, mass production was scaled up.

What happened next is worth remembering. Having built an entire system around a single variety only to see it fail, the industry reconstituted the same system using another single variety. Any lessons learned from Panama disease and monoculture food production soon faded away.

In the late 1960s, an outbreak with similarities to Panama disease started appearing in Cavendish bananas in Taiwan. Since losing the Big Mike and landing on the Cavendish, the banana industry had shown little interest in developing alternative varieties. The new fungus was named "tropical race 4" and was later genetically linked to Panama disease. TR4 discolors the plant's foliage and chokes off its water supply, leaving the plant to die from dehydration. Transmitted through soil and water, TR4 has since spread to other parts of Asia, the Middle East, Africa, and Australia.

In the Americas, the region that supplies some 80 percent of bananas traded worldwide, the question is not *if* TR4 will show up but *when*. Like Panama disease, TR4 has proven to be unstoppable. And though a search for a replacement banana variety is under way, traditional breeding methods are time- and labor-intensive. Specks of seed must be extracted, then carefully nurtured in test tubes where only a fraction germinate. A new plant requires about two years before it bears fruit. Thousands must be cross-bred and evaluated to find one that can be plugged into the existing system.

The banana is just one example of how the food system continually promises more, while at the same time throttling back the natural variety of what supermarkets offer and consumers eat. Of the estimated 250,000–300,000 edible plant species in the world, only 150 to 200 have been adopted by humans. Of those, only a small fraction make it to the produce section.* Each variety on display in a modern supermarket has been bred and selected for uniformity, appearance, transportability, shelf life, ease of handling, volume, and profitability. Missing are traits like genetic diversity to withstand environmental vulnerability.

What else is missing? Look at the typical supermarket tomato. Rather than flavor, this tomato was bred for color, appearance, and transportability. For mass-produced carrots, the deciding factors have been uniformity and size (so-called baby carrots, which they are not), even though full-size carrots pack more flavor. The common potato, the number-one vegetable consumed, is stripped of most of its nutrition (by peeling away the skin), making it a cheap medium to deliver fats (oils, butter, sour cream) and sugars (ketchup).

So here is the irony. Our food system trains us to want more in the way of *volume*, while offering less in terms of *nutrition*. Health-wise,

---

* Following the common layout of foods offered in modern supermarkets, "produce" in this book refers to unprocessed fresh fruits, vegetables, and nuts.

fruits and vegetables are the most important part of our diet. Loaded with fiber and antioxidants, they constitute the one food group no one needs to limit. Yet despite such benefits, they make up less than 9 percent of total calories consumed.

The produce section has some of the highest margins and revenue per square foot of retail space. Yet compared with the rest of the store, the space allocated is small. Why? Could it be the lack of variety, flavor, and taste? Or maybe consumers are resigned to accepting what the food system offers up?

The remainder of the supermarket doubles as a laboratory where companies conceive and test new ways to move greater volumes of food. One result, the chronic oversupply of food, has altered the way people perceive of calories. Prior to the grand food bargain, calories were a good thing. Eating more calories meant more energy to accomplish more work, particularly farm work. No longer. Nowadays, calories are to be shunned, hidden from view as much as possible. Awash in calories, food providers resort to more nuanced ways to peddle food.

Meat is one example. Loaded with calories, terrestrial meat—beef, poultry, pork, and lamb—is consumed in greater quantities in America than in any other country. Compared with Mexico, more than two pounds more per person per week. Compared with Canada, almost one pound more per week.

The meat industry follows a simple strategy—high volume from largely three kinds of meat controlled through a handful of multinational companies that own or take control of most meat animals. To increase profitability, low-wage workers now slaughter and fabricate the meat; feed is subsidized via government agricultural policies; environmental regulations meet strong resistance; and opposing food safety regulations is a routine part of doing business.

Often decried as the poster child of "industrial food" gone awry, the meat sector has kept up its end of the grand food bargain by consistently finding ways to move more volume. At one time, ground beef came from the day's production of low-valued cuts of meat and fat trimmings. Today, ground beef comes from bovine animals nationwide and various parts of the world. Separate two-thousand-pound "combo bins" are filled with fat from feedlot steers, lean meat from culled dairy cows, and imported scrap trimmings. The bins are mixed, ground, shipped, remixed, and reground based on market opportunities. The typical meat patty can contain bits of multiple cows from different countries.

To squeeze out more meat, a few companies have developed technology that harvests bits of meat embedded in fat. Heating and centrifuging fat trimmings, then treating the mixture with ammonia or citric acid, creates a beef slurry. Meat listed as "pure ground beef" on the ingredient label can be as much as 15 percent added slurry.

The meat sector prefers to call the slurry "lean finely textured beef." When ABC News reported on it, they quoted a USDA microbiologist who did not consider the slurry to be ground beef at all, instead dubbing it "pink slime." A defamation lawsuit was filed by one of the companies against ABC News. Terms of the settlement were not disclosed. Yet the case illustrates just how important carefully chosen words and labels are to selling food.

In the dairy section of the modern supermarket, a major rebranding is under way. Advertisements of celebrities and athletes with white mustaches have fallen out of favor, especially among younger people who drink less milk. While sales of cottage cheese and milk are declining, competition from alternative beverages is heating up. Saving the day, along with butter and cheese, is the spectacular growth in yogurt sales.

Food producers are riding a wave of excitement about probiotics, promising that the fermentation process used to make yogurt will boost your immune system, reduce symptoms of lactose intolerance, and improve gastrointestinal health. Probiotics, meaning "for life," are part of an exciting frontier to understand our microbiome, the community of microbes that live on and in us. Yet what is currently known about probiotics added to foods pales in comparison to what is not known, including their role and efficacy.

What food providers do know is that invoking health claims sells more food—a practice that dates back to when micronutrients were first being identified. Adding probiotics to yogurt has been money in the bank. Producers have chosen varieties that are easy to grow yet survive processing and packaging; their inclusion is a minor cost of production. Some are proprietary, some are mixed, some a single strain, yet all become part of carefully worded and unprovable promises. In 2007, the European Union instructed companies to provide the evidence behind their claims. Its scientific advisory group subsequently reviewed and rejected all of them.

Whether or not such claims are true, total milk production in the United States over a decade went up by 16 percent, while the number of milk cows grew by only 2 percent. The deviation points to another key feature of the modern food system. Each year, the average cow is expected to be more productive or else is cut from the herd. On paper, a Holstein (black and white) cow can live twenty years before succumbing to old age. In practice, 35 to 40 percent of typical modern dairy herds turn over each year as cows die or are culled and sent to slaughter. In a system plagued by excess production, this is survival of the fittest. Cows compete with each other while replacements are groomed to take their place when one falters. Under the grand food bargain, dairy farms survive by treating cows as machines and by scrutinizing costs—a process not dissimilar to growing bananas.

Even bread, the "staff of life," has been stripped down and dressed up to move more loaves. Wheat flour starts from seeds, whose role is to propagate the next generation of life. The seed's outer shell is nutrient-rich layers of bran loaded with fiber. Inside, the embryo or "germ" is encased by tissue called the "endosperm" that nourishes new life with proteins and starches until photosynthesis kicks in. Our ancestors ate all of the seed. Their bodies thrived on it. Our DNA traces back to them.

An early breakthrough of the modern food system was new grain-milling technology that removed the bran and germ but kept the endosperm. Calories went up (flour was more concentrated), nutrients went down, fiber disappeared, and a bleaching agent was added. In return, shelf life increased and flour boasted a consistent white appearance that masked impurities and a slightly yellowish tint. But then deficiency diseases like pellagra and beriberi due to missing nutrients started appearing, evidence of how digestive systems had assimilated all of the seed. The government responded by requiring certain nutrients (but not fiber) be added back in.

So why not return to using the entire seed? Because consumers and producers alike have grown accustomed to the taste and convenience of white flour. People prefer its softer texture, how easily it bakes, and how tastily it pairs with everything from fruit preserves and peanut butter to lunch meat. Today, grain products made of mostly white flour make up 22 percent of all calories consumed.

No matter how much bread we eat, the unending challenge is how to sell more. The latest strategy is to tout the very parts of the seed that have been largely removed. Fair warning: labels like "multi-grain," "made with whole grains," "contains whole grains," "made with whole wheat," "100% wheat," "cracked wheat," "bran wheat," "7 grains," "12 grains," and "24 grains" are all code for "contains white flour."

Once again, carefully chosen words are crucial to selling more. In describing flour, "refined" does not mean that impurities are removed but rather that the grain is stripped of fiber and nutrients. "Enriched" does not mean that the flour has been somehow improved but rather that some (but not all) nutrients were added back in, though not necessarily at the original levels. Producers rarely include the substantive fiber needed to slow the absorption of sugars, aid healthy digestion, curb weight gain, and reduce the risk of heart disease.

Dressing up inexpensive ingredients to appear wholesome and nutritious is one of the food system's most tried-and-true strategies. The only label that ensures that bread contains the entire seed and all its fiber is, wait for the drum roll, *100% whole wheat*. Alas, even then, 100 percent whole wheat does not preclude the addition of sugars, fats, and salt.

If ever a statue were to be erected to the modern food system, the center aisles of today's supermarket would be the inspiration. This is the territory of processed food, a place where nutrition is the underdog competing against cheap calories for shelf space. Here boundaries blur between what is and isn't food. Here certainty gives way to opacity.

Highly processed ingredients are a food manufacturer's best friend. They enable high-volume, low-cost manufacturing. Seasonality, availability, spoilage, and quality are easily managed. Taste, texture, color, and flavor are created using artificial flavorings, colorings, emulsifiers, and thickeners. Shelf life and food safety are satisfied with preservatives, temperature control, and packaging. Some ingredients like salt, which is abundant and cheap, bring enormous added value for little additional cost. As a preservative and flavor enhancer, salt makes it possible to substitute more processed ingredients for less whole food.

If all that consumers asked of food were readily available calories, then manufactured foods would easily fit the bill. But instead, we pursue an oxymoron: heavily processed foods that are tastier, easier to clean up, and have a longer shelf life than whole foods, yet are still somehow wholesome. Creating this illusion is critical to a product's success. Catchy phrases and bold labels are tested. Packaging is redesigned. New conveniences are added. Not surprisingly, the majority of information consumers receive about food comes from the food industry itself. Marion Nestle, who has written extensively for years about food policy and practices, puts the phenomenon succinctly: "The more extravagant the health claims, the more extravagant the price."

That aphorism can be extended: The more extravagant the preparation, the more extravagant the price. The in-store prepared foods section is our final stop. Aware that people spend the majority of their food budgets on meals and snacks away from home, supermarkets are now competing with restaurants. To be profitable, they turn to centralized kitchens and bakeries to scale up cooking and prepare sauces, breads, salads, and soups. They rely on mass-produced ingredients to bolster taste while tempering costs. Their approach mirrors what regional and national restaurants have done for years.

For consumers, the trade-off for meals prepared outside the home is more calories at a higher cost. Services like processing, packaging, transportation, retail space, utilities, labor, advertising, preparation, service, and cleanup are all part of the bill. Of every dollar we spend to eat, as little as seven cents goes toward actual food.

The sticker price of food introduces one more global system hidden in the checkout aisle of the supermarket: market economics. Before food companies surrender their products to consumers, this mother of all human-made systems is called into action. The Englishman credited with enlightening America on how market economics could benefit the country was Adam Smith. In his seminal book, *The Wealth of Nations*, Smith wrote that when individuals act in their own self-interest, societies attain greater prosperity. His book was published in 1776—opportune timing to grab the attention of a nation of farmers and guide them forward.

Smith's teachings laid out the way societies could move beyond subsistence living. When workers specialize in particular tasks, he noted, their productivity increases. Higher levels of productivity multiplied across countless households and businesses result in the availability of more goods and services as well as rising levels of income. More people can buy and consume nonessential products like imported spices, better cuts of meats, and fashionable clothes. Higher standards of living can be attained. Smith regarded as self-evident his understanding that the ultimate goal of a market economy was to maximize the country's wealth, conveniently measured in terms of the total amount of goods and services produced.

What set Smith's ideas apart, at a time when basic subsistence and government-imposed practices favored society's elite, was his thesis that the pursuit of self-interest by the masses had the unplanned benefit of greater overall national wealth. Each person, Smith wrote, "is led by an invisible hand to promote an end which was no part of his intention." In short, a market economy blesses selfishness as the gateway to altruistic outcomes.

Of course, coupling individual self-interest with benevolent outcomes was premised on certain qualifiers worth remembering as we explore the grand food bargain and the modern food system. The first is increasing reliance on markets functioning effectively. Smith believed that markets were self-correcting. Competition would hold supply and demand in check. Too much surplus and prices would fall, whereby businesses would pursue other options. Too little availability and prices would rise, whereby businesses would produce more. In actuality, what comprises competition and competitive conditions becomes critically important as to how markets perform over time, as we'll see in chapter 7.

The other important qualifier to keep in mind is that market economics is a human-created system, a societal invention founded on what people are willing to value and are capable of measuring. Market economics has no divine authorship. It was never a third tablet left on Mount Sinai and later picked up by Adam Smith. The "hand" Smith describes may have been invisible, but its origin was not. Market economics did not invalidate the need for government nor replace laws of nature or geophysical realities. Though markets can play an important role in the modern food system, they are not omnipotent. While Smith acknowledged the known limitations of his time, in the modern era, society's unquestioned reliance on markets has increased.

So how has market economics fared from our brief glimpse of the modern food system? Over time, the portion of income spent on food has declined. More than twice the number of calories a moderately active adult woman needs to function are readily available. The Cavendish banana is now the number-one fruit consumed.

But market economics did not save the Big Mike from extinction, or arrest the global spread of the TR4 fungus. It accelerated the loss of the Patagonian toothfish fishery rather than protect it. In meat, it promoted protein while soft-pedaling fat. In dairy, it helped yogurt become a top breakfast food even when (or especially when) yogurt is loaded with added sugars or fat. For processed foods, it rewarded health claims that blurred nutritional content and homogenized consensus of science. In prepared foods, it reinforced the consuming of more calories despite a national epidemic of overconsumption.

Alas, markets are not a forever-infallible guide in our relationship with food. Like other human-made systems, they are based on assumptions and values that change over time. Not questioning the premises that markets are built upon can lull us into believing that being awash in food is ideal, serves America well, and will never let society down.

To be clear, markets do play an important role in the food system. But to overstate their power is to understate the influence of other forces. In part II of this book, we'll cover in more detail the five primary forces that together set the course of the modern food system.

The evening of our day trip to the banana plantation, my uncles and I sat down for a dinner that included plantains, another member of the banana family. Their familiar shape and size provided the perfect segue for me to ask what stood out from the earlier visit. Both of my uncles had been farmers, remembered when food was rationed during World War II, and served in the Merchant Marines and the Army.

The ready availability of bananas in the store, they remarked, did not capture how systems change everything. For a few hours they had experienced a region that provided fruit that Americans took for granted. They had seen how people's lives revolved around a single crop and how low prices did not address environmental and individual health risks. Accustomed to eating bananas without giving much thought as to why each one looked and tasted the same, they had never considered what happens when nature fails to produce the perfect fruit.

Since then, one uncle has passed away and the other turned ninety. In celebration, my wife and I traveled to Seattle to visit. If average consumption patterns are a reliable guide, he was closing in on twenty-three thousand bananas. Age had limited his mobility, but not his mind. So I asked if he still remembered visiting the banana plantation in Costa Rica. "Very much so," was his response. When I inquired if he still looked at bananas differently, without hesitation he replied, "I still do."

PART II

FORCES DRIVING MORE

Chapter 3

More Is Never Enough

Each morning on the plains of Africa, a gazelle awakens, knowing it must outrun the
fastest lion or be killed. At the same time, a lion wakes up, knowing it must outrun
the slowest gazelle or starve to death. So whether you are a lion or gazelle does not
matter. When the Sun comes up in the morning, start running.

—African Proverb

On a weekend reprieve from work, Pablo and I traveled down a washboard dirt road so straight it narrowed before vanishing into the horizon. We were in South Africa, near Botswana's border. Staring back at us was a brown monotone landscape of desert bushes, rock outcroppings, and plateaus. Such drab, uninspiring scenery was not what I had hoped for, given the region's importance in human history. For anyone who ever lived in the last eight thousand generations, this continent was home—this was where the human race began.

Journeying this far merited contemplation of long-ago history, but the immediate future took priority. Within an hour we would arrive at a game park reserve and stay overnight. Pablo had made arrangements for a guided safari deep within the park's boundaries so that we could observe, up close, wild animals within their natural habitat.

Running parallel to the dusty road was the park's ten-foot-high electrified fence, built to keep wild animals in and people out. As practice for the safari, I tried staring through the fence, hoping to preview what awaited us. But except for a single giraffe's head I saw nibbling a thorny acacia tree, there were no animals to be seen.

Our afternoon arrival provided just enough time to drop off our bags, meet our guide, and climb aboard the bench seats of a modified pickup with its unprotected sides and open top. First stop, after several miles of winding trails that doubled as roads, was a watering hole. This was the time of day when animals gathered to drink, our guide told us. As we approached, he reminded us to talk softly and not to make any sudden moves. This was no zoo, he emphasized—keeping your wits about you was your best protection.

Eyeing a herd of female elephants with their calves, he approached slowly, before shutting off the engine and letting the truck coast. Just as it stopped, the alpha elephant lifted her head, swung her trunk toward us, and began ambling in our direction. As the rest of the herd fell in behind her, our guide issued a second subdued caution— stay calm!

Remaining still and silent as the herd marched our way, we quickly jettisoned any lingering doubts as to whose territory we were in. Looking up at the alpha's massive head and girth, I knew that she could easily upend our vehicle with us in it. A few footsteps later, she was close enough to smell. Then, as if playing a game of chicken, she veered left and kept moving, the rest of the herd in tow. Despite their number and size, they soon blended into the background and disappeared into the desert landscape.

Relieved, we ventured on to new habitat. With the Sun continuing its descent, we came across a group of assembling impalas. Then, as if on silent cue, they moved as one beyond the dirt road and into the bush. The few stragglers dawdling behind quickly caught up, and before long, they too were gone from sight. Banding together offered protection against carnivores prowling the night, our guide remarked.

Driving further, we observed wild dogs cordoned off by another fence. Seeing us approach, they momentarily flashed their teeth in our direction and growled, then resumed their ravaging of a small animal, demonstrating how effortlessly their powerful jaws could tear flesh from bone. As we watched them snuff out any remaining signs of life, the truck's two-way radio started squawking. Another guide had spotted a pride of lions settling down and shared the coordinates with us. A few minutes later, we were within view of the pride. While the younger cubs jostled with each other, the adults remained vigilant.

Moving in closer, our guide shut off the engine and coasted to a stop. All afternoon he had followed the same routine. I estimated our distance to the pride at two, maybe three adult lion bounds. Without warning, one of the lions lying on her side suddenly rose up on her front paws and stared our way, prompting other lions to follow suit. I tensed up. The farm mechanic in me thought about the expected life of the truck's starter motor. Did the guide have a backup plan if the solenoid failed and the engine did not start?

This was not my first venture into the African wild. Several years earlier, in Tanzania's Serengeti, three friends and I awoke well before daybreak and headed out on an early morning safari. Our guide, driving a similarly outfitted truck, parked on a hill overlooking a large watering hole. It was an ideal vantage point for watching wildebeests, impalas, and zebras appear from different directions and approach the water to drink. As the Sun's light cracked over the horizon, our guide pointed farther up the slope from where we were parked to a female lion lying down. As we looked at her, she stood up and began walking our way.

Believing the lion would walk past us and descend closer to the watering hole, the guide did not move the truck. But this lion had other plans. She moved closer and then steered a direct course toward us. As she approached, the guide slid one hand inside the scabbard resting on the hood of the truck and onto the handle of his rifle. Two of us were in the direct line of sight between him and the lion. The hair on the back of our necks stood up—if the lion did not get us, the gun would.

As she drew closer, we froze and remained absolutely still. Now standing alongside the rear quarter-panel of the truck, she looked in the direction of the watering hole and then lay down, her spine abutting the sidewall of the rear tire, her head panning the animals below. One wrong move on our part, and an effortless three-foot leap with no obstructions, was all that separated her from us. If she was after fresh meat, we were an easy takedown.

Over the next several minutes we barely breathed. Some say that when voluntary control is ripped away and the possibility of death is at one's doorstep, time slows down. For me, the next few minutes seemed an eternity, but eventually the lion stood up and walked way, glancing back at us while ambling down the slope. Feeling more secure, we let out a sigh of relief and calmed ourselves with nervous laughter.

Later that evening, as flames from the fire licked the night sky, the conversation turned back to our earlier encounter. We had started the day as passive observers of wildlife. Then a lion reordered our priorities, involuntarily putting us in touch with the raw fear of death. Our lives back in the States had rendered conscious thoughts about survival unnecessary, even obsolete. Yet thousands of miles away from home, in unfamiliar territory, subconscious survival instincts had sprung into action. When it appeared we might be part of the food supply of wild animals, the desire to live took command.

The experience was a stark reminder that all people are products of their environment. This oft-used phrase usually refers to home and community. Yet we had just witnessed how the environment extends back thousands of generations to relatives we had never known. Go back far enough in time, and our existence intersects with ancestors whose biggest challenge was surviving each day. Just as in the African proverb, each morning they started out running, not because they needed the exercise but rather because they wanted to live. That will to live was passed down from one generation to the next until it reached us.

Back in South Africa, watching the lion rise up on her front legs had reminded me of the Serengeti. Her one move had reinforced how my environment encompassed geographies outside of the Americas and time horizons beyond my lifetime. Fear of wild animals and preventing my own death could be traced back to inheriting my progenitors' will to live. Without that past, there would not be a present or the possibility of a future.

As the lions relaxed and fixed their gazes elsewhere, I did too, watching the sunset turn to night. During the drive back, with the truck's headlights undressing the bushes and trees from their cover of darkness, our guide talked of rare sightings of leopards stealthily moving about. Over dinner, he shared more stories of close encounters. While listening, it was hard not to wonder what life was like without modern-day protections like guns, secure lodging, fences, and locks.

After dinner, as we walked from the lodge along the lighted path to our cabins, I looked up at the stars shining in full splendor. Living in central Michigan with its typically overcast skies, I had forgotten how beautiful stars could be. The desert's clear night sky and new moon immediately took hold of me and didn't let go.

Bidding Pablo goodnight, I stopped long enough at my cabin to grab a jacket and flashlight. To take full advantage of this opportunity, I walked along a worn trail away from the lodge and into the darkness. A night of solitude was indulging my fascination with celestial planets. As the lights from the lodge dimmed and the cool desert sky fell over me, I was swept up by stars seemingly close enough that I could reach out and touch them.

Looking skyward to the spectacular view, I noticed my breathing was shallower. I was alone, no one knew I was here, yet I did not feel alone. While unafraid of the dark, I felt apprehension take hold. I rationalized that this was simply an overreaction to an afternoon of watching wild animals and hearing the associated stories. Encountering an enchanted evening like this was rare. I turned off my flashlight and tried to focus on the night sky, searching for the Southern Cross, observing an occasional shooting star, and making up constellations of Greek gods, warriors, and chariots of my own choosing.

Though I wanted to soak up the galaxies, I was interrupted by a faint rustling of bushes in the distance. The "rule" for confronting creatures in the night—green eyes are herbivores while red eyes are carnivores—played with my mind. I switched on my flashlight and pointed it toward the noises, half hoping to see green eyes. Instead, I saw nothing. Perhaps it was the wind, I said to myself, though I felt no breeze on my face. The rustling came and went but the anxiety remained.

Unable to will away the uneasiness, I gave in. This was an unfamiliar environment. What I sensed existed for a reason. Being alone in the dark made me an easy target, a rich source of food with plenty of meat and fat. Not acknowledging what was happening worked against me. I was not, after all, the only creature around with a desire to live. If there were carnivores lurking about, then being here was about survival, not recreation. The brilliance of the night sky would have to wait for some other evening. Turning my flashlight on, I tipped my hat toward the rustling bushes and walked toward the security of my cabin.

The human race has literally been bred to survive. The uniqueness of each person's DNA builds genetic variation into the overall population. Some of those variations introduced traits that made survival *harder* for future generations; their descendants eventually went extinct. Others brought traits that made survival easier for future generations, which explains our being around today.

Lest people feel too privileged, we should remember that humans are just one of an estimated 8.7 million species, all following the same script. Being bred for survival bestows opportunity for continued survival but not immunity from extinction. Whether or not we live depends in large measure on pressures created by our environment. Our living on a planet spinning at 1,000 miles per hour while hurling through space at nearly 67,000 miles per hour is one example. The outcome is mild-to-extreme variations in climate and weather—and, subsequently, survival.

Also worth remembering is that the need for food is universal for all species, not just ourselves. If food were easy to come by, survival would be easier . . . at least until the number of living beings exceeded the planet's capacity to support them. To keep Earth from becoming a barren wasteland, each species in need of food is itself a source of food. This basic circle of life is why survival is tied to competition, and why access to food is never guaranteed.

Perhaps one day, future generations will discover a planet, tucked away in some far corner of the universe, that perpetuates life differently. But for earthlings of all kinds, the only two options available are finding ways to adapt, or going extinct. Barbaric as it sounds, eat-or-be-eaten is how life on this planet rolls.

This makes staying alive a never-ending test to determine winners and losers. The winners are granted survival so they can continue competing. The losers go extinct and are soon forgotten—a fate that has befallen more than 99 percent of species that have ever roamed the planet.

After four-plus billion years of genetic mutations, life on Earth has become an almost unfathomable diversity of species, traits, and behaviors tailored to survival. Those species with the longest track records are the smallest or microscopic ones. Yet even their proven ability to adapt and populate has been held in check by other species.

Aphids, for example, are tiny, sap-sucking insects that naturally clone themselves to produce other females. Drop a few aphids into a vegetable patch and within days millions are present. Yet aphids have not overrun the planet, because those seeking food are also food themselves. Ladybugs, those seemingly sweet polka-dotted insects, coevolved alongside aphids, targeting them as their food source.

Other species evolved differently. Honeybees and flowers maintain a symbiotic relationship that allows both to survive. Viruses and harmful bacteria have adopted a more devious approach, attacking their hosts, seizing control of cells and repelling antibodies. Some species boost their chances of survival by providing food at the very start of life. Many seeds, for example, contain the nutrients a new sprout needs until it can convert the Sun's rays into energy.

As humans, we have zero ability to populate as quickly as microscopic organisms or convert energy like plants. Instead, we have evolved a host of other traits: walking on two legs to move faster and to better spot distant threats; opposable thumbs to help us climb, use tools, and grip food; an instant dislike for bitter-tasting plants to protect us from ingesting harmful toxins; a preference for sweets, meats, and fats because they are dense with calories; and the ability to store excess energy for when food is scarce. These traits, refined across thousands of generations, are present at birth. They exist to secure food in an insecure world. Yet are they enough?

If I'm standing alone in a game park in Africa in the dark of night, my answer would be no. Human traits do not include a gazelle's lightning-fast reflexes and ability to run some forty miles per hour.

Nor can they compete with a lion's sharp claws and nighttime vision. Unlike microscopic organisms, which have survived for 3.5 billion years, humans do not have a long genetic record. In fact, our species is quite recent, only coming on the scene some 200,000 years ago.

So with nonstop environmental pressures, how have humans managed to survive? Three behaviors forever remapped the way humans interacted with the environment and other species. The resulting benefits were immense, but so also were the vulnerabilities.

Starting the ball rolling was fire. Fire changed everything. As it killed pathogens and cooked food, it unlocked nutrition bound up in the cellulose of plants, as well as the tissues and bones of animals. Illness and death diminished. The amount (and likely the kind) of nutrients the human body could absorb shot up 50–95 percent, paving the way for brain size to increase and the number of neurons to rise dramatically. Enormous advances in cognitive reasoning followed, along with greater ability to regulate complex bodily functions. Today's humans have a smaller, more efficient digestive system, and a brain almost seven times larger than mammals of similar mass. At just 2 percent of body weight, the brain uses a quarter of the energy consumed from food.

As fire killed pathogens and improved nutrition, it also made our ancestors' lives easier. Fire kept people warm, scared away predators at night, allowed hunters to flush out and corner potential game, and even made chewing and digestion less of an effort by softening up meat and plants alike. While cooking changed humans physiologically, harnessing the energy of fire changed societies, eventually creating modern economies powered by burning fossil fuels.

Fire also set the stage for the second behavior that separates humans from other animals: language. As people coordinated hunts of larger animals, attracted mates, lived in communities, and avoided predators and marauders, complex communication became indispensable for survival. Development of precise forms of language and expression accelerated discovery and became the foundation for science and technology.

Language, in turn, set up the third behavior: collective memory. Thanks to memory, experiences were no longer forgotten when people died. Instead, insights about how to find food while withstanding environmental pressures were passed along. The stories of long-deceased generations could now live on.

Fire, language, and memory markedly improved the odds of human survival. Yet life was still tenuous. Competition for food was constant. The environment remained unpredictable. So in the quest for food, humans migrated northward and outward over land and by sea to other continents and islands. As their numbers ebbed and flowed, other species of humans unable to survive went extinct. Only one remained—*Homo sapiens*. Every person on Earth today is one of their descendants.

Fast forward tens of thousands of years to when hunting and gathering had faded away, and humans were staking their future on farming. The Europeans who came to America, long after Native Americans had already arrived, were coming to farm some of the richest land on the planet. Yet tying their survival to farming was far from guaranteed. From the land and the environment came hard lessons in how to turn virgin soil without breaking plows, how to withstand torrential flooding, how to tolerate blistering summer heat, and how to endure seasons of deep snow.

Not until being handed a picture of snow falling on Cabot, Vermont, did I think much about the challenges colonial farmers faced when confronting environmental pressures. The sight of snow blanketing buildings and leafless trees was not out of the ordinary for a cold winter's day in December or January. But the caption written below the image riveted my attention—July 4, 1816.

That year began much like any other in New England with cold January weather and plenty of snow. Spring arrived a bit early, but temperatures were still within normal ranges. In mid-April, a late snow blanketed the region, but by the end of the month, thermometers had climbed to the low 80s.

As farmers planted their crops and vegetables, hopes ran high for a good year with bountiful harvests. Then came May and abrupt changes to the climate that nobody had anticipated. Just as seedlings were poking through the ground, trying to capture the Sun's warming rays, fog was settling across the region. Gray skies were blocking the sunlight and temperatures were falling. By June, as the cold ruptured the cell walls of plants, newly planted fields intended to provide next year's food were failing.

For a moment, imagine that you were a farmer living in New England. Two weeks before the summer solstice, snow was again coming down. Before it ended, eighteen inches covered the fields, burying beneath it your efforts of the last four months. Your entire world was turned upside down. Farming had never been easy. You always hoped for nature's cooperation, but there were never assurances it would always come.

If you had started too soon in the spring and temperatures had dropped below freezing, newly planted crops and vegetables would not have survived. If there had been too much rain in the fields, saturating the ground, your now-waterlogged seeds from last year's harvest would not have germinated. Yet if you waited too long, and planted late in the spring, an early autumn frost would have shortened the season and reduced the harvests by possibly more. In good years, you cashed in your extra for more meat or flour, maybe a few extra chickens. In bad years, you drew on what was left over from the last harvest and you and your neighbors helped each other out.

Across New England, theories about what had happened ran wild. Some said the extensive tracts of forests were preventing the sunlight from reaching the ground. Others asserted the reverse; destroying the forests had allowed cold winds to sweep across open areas, which generated great quantities of ice that melted and lowered ambient temperatures. But the most fervent explanations attributed the climatic shift to sunspots, or simply to divine will—direct communication from God to his people.

Over the next year food was scarce. Homesteads survived by sacrificing livestock and rationing what was left in root cellars. New Englanders learned that around the world other communities and families were likewise barely coping. Those hardest hit lived in the northern latitudes. In Europe, the peace that followed Napoleon's defeat at Waterloo was cut short by riots that broke out when wheat yields plummeted and bread disappeared. In northern China, rice crops failed and water buffalo died. Extreme monsoons and flooding in India dispersed cholera all the way from the Bengal region to Moscow.

What had baffled New Englanders was eventually explained by Earth's geology. The event had started deep beneath the planet's crust, where temperatures reach 2,200 degrees Fahrenheit. The constant heat churns molten lava, its energy forcing tectonic plates to collide and push upward. Like steam in a giant pressure cooker with no relief valve, the energy continues to build upward. On April 10, 1815, on Sumbawa, a far-away island in Indonesia, the pent-up pressure exploded skyward. The volcanic eruption of Mount Tambora contained the force "equivalent to sixty thousand Hiroshima-sized atom bombs."

Tambora's eruption radically altered the Earth's climate. Fine sulfur particles traveled beyond the troposphere (where clouds and weather happen) into a cloudless layer known as the stratosphere. News of the volcano had reached New England, but colonists did not connect the event to their predicament until late the following year. Only when gravity forced enough particles back to the ground in Europe did the pieces of the puzzle fall into place. The suspended volcanic particulates had acted as a filter, keeping the Sun's rays from reaching the Earth's surface, causing winter to return, and bringing farming to an abrupt halt.

In America at the time, agriculture was the principal livelihood for 80 percent of the country's workforce. Most people and their neighbors had descended from generations of farmers, growing up with stories of scarcity. They watched their parents go through times when all that sustained them was an iron will and a lack of alternatives. They learned from their parents' experiences, yet still chose to follow in their footsteps. Farming, after all, was what fed their families.

Yet as they watched the temperatures fall and winter return, events that contradicted all understandings of seasons and weather, the thought occurred that this might be the end. No matter how early they began each day, nor how hard they ran, it was not enough. With an unpredictable and sometimes hostile environment always looming, there could never be enough food.

When New Englanders learned the reason why the climate had changed, all breathed a sigh of relief. The year was dubbed "Eighteen Hundred and Froze to Death." The phenomenon became part of their collective memory of environmental forces that could bring farming to a halt. When spring arrived and crops were planted the following year, their sense of vulnerability was still fresh. The best medicine was producing as much food as possible, or as farmers would say: "Make hay while the Sun shines."

Two years later and farther west, grasshoppers were destroying the crops farmers had planted in Minnesota's Red River Valley. Off and on during the nineteenth century, insects ravaged fields from Minnesota to Texas, the Midwest to California. One farmer described a particular invasion as being so thick with locusts it resembled "hell from above." Another remarked that the bugs destroyed "everything but the mortgage." The largest swarm ever recorded appeared in 1875, reportedly 1,800 miles long and 110 miles wide.

While locusts were highly feared, they were not alone in wreaking havoc. Fungi appeared in fruit orchards. Boll weevil showed up in cotton fields (purportedly from across the Rio Grande). Chinch bugs and wheat rust descended across wheat fields. And screwworm (fly larvae that feed on living flesh), foot-and-mouth disease, and hog cholera invaded animal herds.

These biological invasions were different from the Tambora "winter." This time, farmers themselves had helped create the unwanted adversaries. As people spread westward and settled down, they set up farmsteads in close proximity with each other, grew the same crops, and raised the same animals. Undercutting the diversity of nature, with its competitive checks and balances on food, favored those species that adapted more opportunistically.

Farmers fought back. Non-crop plants became *weeds*, which were lumped together with rodents, fungi, insects, etc., and labeled *pests*. New pesticides were tried. And protracted eradication campaigns were carried out, which pushed foot-and-mouth, hog cholera, and screwworm beyond United States borders.

In the quest to conquer food scarcity through an abundance of crops and animals, efficiency has become king. Seven of every ten acres planted are devoted to just three crops—corn, soybeans, and wheat. Cattle, hogs, and poultry provide 92 percent of all meat consumed. Some fifty thousand pesticides have been used on American farms. Eighty percent of all antibiotics consumed are in agriculture. The majority of food sold comes from a small proportion of farms that specialize in one or two enterprises such as raising hogs or growing wheat.

So how do fire, language, and memory figure into our modern food system? We use mastery of fire in everything from the production of fertilizers and pesticides, to internal-combustion engines in tractors and harvesters, to trucks and refrigerated trailers destined for retail outlets. Language facilitates the development of new technologies and higher yields. But collective memory, accumulated over generations to remind us that survival and the environment are inextricably bound, has become antiquated.

Taking the place of memory was money. For a nation of non-farmers, the rows of vegetables, orchards of fruit, and fields of wheat, once understood as beholden to environmental pressures, were replaced by supermarket aisles of harvested and processed food. Food availability was no longer linked to weather and climate, the absence of pests, or the presence of other species. If one wanted more food, the solution was bringing more money. Our new connection to food could not have been more straightforward—nor further removed from the realities of nature.

While equating money with access to food is most evident in the United States, similar outlooks have taken root in other countries. Working overseas, I often wondered how and why countries prioritized agriculture and food differently, especially neighboring countries where climate, resources, and cultures were similar. Take, for example, Venezuela and Colombia.

The last time I was in Venezuela, agriculture accounted for around 5 percent of total goods and services produced each year, nearly four times less at the time than Colombia. Its cultivable land supported one-third the number of people. Its population was 40 percent smaller.

Along with my two daughters, I traveled from the country's petroleum capital, Maracaibo, to the mountainous city of San Cristóbal. Along the route, evidence of oil was everywhere. Pipelines ran adjacent to roads, then darted off in different directions like enormous strands of spaghetti. Signs of unintended seepage along the ground were common. Gasoline was half the price of bottled water. Oil was so cheap that rather than rebuild worn-out engines, roadside stands sold bottles of motor oil poured from large oil drums.

In San Cristóbal, we spent an afternoon with a family who were close friends with my daughter Melissa. The father, Daniel, owner of a small business, was engaging and well read. As we talked about professions, cultures, and interests, I shared my observations about the differences in agriculture and food in Venezuela and Colombia, and I asked him for his insights.

He referred back to a time, decades ago, when farming and food were central to the lives of Venezuelans. Back then, he noted, the country shared much in common with Colombia, before each chose a different path to prosperity. A fast-growing industrialized world wanted oil, and Venezuela was sitting atop plentiful reserves, easily accessible. Extracting and selling oil became the country's future. The easy money it brought in changed the way people lived; standards of living increased.

With such ample petroleum reserves so readily available, the government was less concerned with promoting farming and domestic food production. To bring in additional revenue, more crude oil was pumped out of the ground and additional money flowed in. Whether Venezuelans produced their own food or imported it from other countries, access to food was easy. So while Colombia kept its eye on domestic food production, Venezuela's attention turned elsewhere.

As a country, Venezuela was at the beginning of the end, Daniel remarked. Remaining petroleum reserves were less accessible. Extraction costs were increasing while prices were softening. Profits flowing back into the economy were declining. Rather than face new realities, the government stayed the course, which explained why oil products domestically were so inexpensive. Venezuelans had grown accustomed to cheap oil. Like consumers anywhere, he added, they liked it that way.

Daniel was not optimistic that the country would remember when producing food was central to how people lived. Domestic prosperity sustained by extracting crude oil had pushed all that aside. The only solution people could see was higher-paying jobs to buy more food and lead better lives. He feared that because the economy had relied on petroleum for so many years that Venezuelans no longer retained any historical memory. And now they faced an uncertain future. "Oil has been our curse," he concluded.

This was 2001. In the succeeding years, the downward spiral Daniel foresaw accelerated and worsened. At the center of protests and riots was the lack of food. For people of ordinary means, buying staples like rice, beans, and cooking oil meant queuing at state-run supermarkets before dawn, in the hope the shelves would not be empty when they reached the front of the line hours later. Food shortages became so chronic that the government handed over control of the food supply to the military; the country's food ministry, in fact, was headed by an army general.

To boost food supplies, the government encouraged people to grow gardens and raise chickens, even though more than four of every five Venezuelans live in cities. Many had no experience growing food. Those who did lacked suitable soil, seeds, or access to feed for raising poultry.

Today, as the shortages persist, more people are scavenging through garbage thrown out by society's privileged. For those with money, a black market offering food is thriving. Food trafficking, controlling who can bring in food, seeds, or feed from outside the country, or what local merchants receive from outside suppliers, is big business, and is now dominated by the military. As one retired general put it, "The military is in charge of food management now, and they're not going to just take that on without getting their cut."

Food shortages opened new ways to profit from scarcity and help the government retain power. To fight back, the people routinely call for nationwide stoppages, further damaging the economy. Early one morning under the cover of darkness, protestors risked being arrested while setting up barricades. When asked why they had resorted to such risky and drastic measures, one answered, "We want liberty. We want democracy. We want everyone to have access to food."

As Venezuela's food crisis deepens, more and more lives are shattered and the recovery becomes progressively more painful. Meanwhile, inept government officials, a corrupt military, and merchants exploit hunger and malnutrition to reap windfall profits. A monthly handout of heavily subsidized basic food staples for the poorest Venezuelans helps keep the existing government in power. With quadruple-digit inflation, Venezuela's economy resembles an out-of-control forest fire that leaves behind a burnt landscape in shambles.

Desperate to extinguish the flames, Venezuelan experts blame the failure of markets—as if restoring markets can somehow turn back the clock. And media reports focus on the drama of the day, not on the country's decades-long history of relying on petroleum while neglecting their own food production.

Venezuela's tragedy is a reminder that you can't eat money. The false equivalency between cash and access to food does not disabuse our innate fear of hunger. Venezuelans, in their dire circumstances, are involuntarily reacquainting themselves with evolutionary genetics. In the end, this genetic drive for sustenance and survival may one day rescue the country from imploding and restore access to food.

While Venezuela's economy has been in free fall (shrinking 16 percent in 2017), Colombia's economy has become the thirty-ninth-largest in the world, placing it in the top fifth of the world's national economies. (Venezuela's economy, meanwhile, because of the nation's sorry state of affairs, and despite its immense oil reserves, is not included in the world's top two hundred economies by the World Bank.) In the last half century, its population nearly tripled. In the last quarter century, national income rose by 600 percent. As the economy became more diversified, agriculture's financial contribution to overall growth declined.

Nonetheless, livestock production still dominates land usage, and agriculture still benefits from vast natural resources. Agricultural research spending has recently increased by one-third. Over a quarter century, the availability of fruits and vegetables has more than doubled, and the level of undernourishment has fallen by close to one-half.

Yet Colombia is not without its challenges. Refugees have flooded in from Venezuela. Its shared borders with other countries jeopardize earlier progress made to control animal diseases. Curtailing cocaine production is a perpetual challenge. And the accord that ended the longest-running insurgency in Latin America is in jeopardy. But the country exports more agricultural and food products than it imports, and its tradition of wide-ranging support for domestic food production is well ingrained.

Although not as obvious in countries where food is plentiful, the role of genetics to control scarcity through the quest for more food never relents. At the core of America's obesity epidemic is individual DNA hardwired with the imperative to overcome food scarcity. In anticipation of having to live through lean times, whenever possible, we are genetically programmed to pack away excess calories in the form of fat. No matter what others may tell us about health and well-being, our DNA regards this buffer of excess weight as a matter of life and death.

Equating access to food with money seduces us into ignoring that we are always bound to the natural environment. When we sit down to enjoy a steak, we rarely think of the cow it came from, much less how environmental pressures were overcome to raise the animal full-term before it was slaughtered. As our collective memory fades, and we lose sight of how such realities affect food production, always wanting more defines who we are. Always producing more reinforces it.

Of the five forces that fuel the modern food system, this one—our belief that more is never enough—is the most important. Yet its implications go unquestioned, even as it accelerates the inevitable face-off with nature. While I was growing up, news reports on how many people one farmer fed, which I translated into how much land one person could farm, always intrigued me. I began assuming that larger farms—by virtue of producing more food—benefited society the most. The eventual implications stemming from such an outlook seemed less important.

On occasion, I helped another farmer cultivate his fallowed land to control weed growth. His property bordered the mountains and was the largest contiguous piece of land I ever worked. Completing the entire field took three days—plenty of time to hear the rumble of the tractor's diesel engine, feel the summer heat rise in the morning, and watch the Sun descend across the skyline in late afternoon. As I crisscrossed back and forth, I sometimes daydreamed about whether my ancestors would have been amazed were they to see such a large expanse of land worked by just one person. From their era came the definition of an acre: the amount of land that could be plowed in one day with a yoke of oxen and a single plow. What took them an entire day, I accomplished in a matter of minutes.

Other fantasies to pass the time came from a collection of stories I received one Christmas. One written by Leo Tolstoy featured Pahom, an ambitious peasant who amasses large plots of land that make him wealthy. Not satisfied with his riches and wanting more, he hears of a faraway village where, for one thousand rubles, all the land he could circumambulate in one day would be his.

Excited at his prospects and with his servant in tow, he seeks out the village elder. Yes, it is true, the old man says, with one condition: if by sundown, he has not returned to the exact spot from where he began, he will forfeit the one thousand rubles. At sunrise the following morning, Pahom heads down the hill from the village at a brisk pace, pausing occasionally to survey what will soon be his. Each new hill he crests reveals more lush land than the previous one, enticing Pahom to walk farther. At noon, with the Sun directly overhead, he looks back but is unable to spot the hill with the elder and his servant awaiting his return.

With half of the day already past, Pahom turns and works his way back to the starting point. But by late afternoon he is tired. His feet are cut and bruised, his throat is parched. Off in the distance, he can see the hill where he started—but the Sun is descending quickly. Though exhausted, he walks faster, then starts running. As he ascends the last hill, his lungs burn and his heart pounds. He cries out in pain but keeps going.

Just as the Sun is dipping below the horizon, Pahom reaches the top and falls forward, his hand landing on the spot from where he began. Well done, says the elder—but Pahom is dead. His servant picks up his spade and digs a grave, six feet from head to heel—the exact amount of land one man needs.

Sitting on the tractor, looking over such a large field, I often wondered how much land would be enough, if I were presented the same bargain. Knowing what befell Pahom, would I be content walking around a field this size, or would I feel remorse returning before sunset without having tried for more? As I entertained possible scenarios, my tendency was always to push for more and not be content with less. As I neared completion at the bottom of the field, I would peer off in the distance to where I had begun. At that moment, being able to accomplish more brought a sense of satisfaction, leaving me convinced that the ability to farm more was always a good thing. Alas, understanding the pursuit of more in the context of our inherent drive for survival and the larger environment around us would take me years to fully grasp.

Whether we awake and start running like the gazelle and the lion or believe that money equals food, we are still bound to the environment. When always wanting more dominates our outlook, always *having* more becomes the solution for never seeing the value in living with less. The more that food is valued based on abundance, the less food can remind us of our reliance on other species, nature, and the environment. When this happens, the memory of how our ancestors once survived, while perhaps still interesting, no longer seems relevant.

Without memory, we live naively in the present. We believe we can always have more. We assume that resources like land and water will always provide more. Yet all our resources come from a single planet. By definition, they are limited. As we will see in the next chapter, ready access to resources stokes our belief in an infinite supply of finite resources.

Chapter 4

An Infinite Supply of Finite Resources

Our civilization runs by burning the remains of humble creatures who inhabited the Earth hundreds of millions of years before the first humans came on the scene.

— Carl Sagan

O n a crisp and breezy October morning, with school canceled due to a teachers' conference, I slept later than usual. My father had left for the day, forgetting to leave behind his customary list of tasks to be completed before his return. Attending to my chores, I fed the cattle from a large mound of loose hay accumulated over the summer. Not wanting to remind my mother I would be home all day (and risk prompting her to generate a list of tasks), I lingered in the barnyard, then climbed atop the haystack.

On three sides of the stack were corrals with open-faced roofs where our cattle and two horses were kept. To protect the hay from the elements, we always built the haystack higher instead of wider, reducing the surface area exposed to snow and rain. Building higher was only possible because our baler spit out wire-tied bales compressed like bricks, each weighing at least eighty-five pounds. When the last bales of hay of the summer were added, the entire stack was capped with two rows of baled straw plus a thick layer of loose straw as added protection.

Atop the stack, I peered over the front edge, wondering if I could jump far enough to land on the loose hay. And, assuming I succeeded, would the pile of hay be sufficient to cushion my fall? While contemplating whether jumping was a test in courage or an exercise in stupidity, I smelled smoke and heard crackling noises. Turning around, I instantly realized that our entire haystack was on fire.

Unbeknown to me, my younger brother had discovered matches. To avoid detection, he hid against the backside of the haystack before striking the first match. A quick study, he soon learned how fire plus curiosity could set a massive haystack ablaze. As the hay started to burn, the fall breeze fanned the flames upward. When the fire crested the top of the haystack, the layers of dry straw became the perfect accelerant. In a matter of seconds, my escape route was blocked. With the flames licking at my heels, I jumped.

As soon as my mother realized what was happening, she called the volunteer fire department a few miles away. Fighting disbelief, we released the animals into the adjoining fields. By the time the fire truck drove up the lane, flames and dark smoke were billowing skyward. Immediately calling for backup, the firefighters directed their hoses at the surrounding structures. Within the hour, fire trucks from three more towns arrived, followed by a Forest Service tanker truck and two bulldozers.

Because our farm was situated on higher ground near the foothills, black smoke filling the sky could be seen from miles away. Onlookers near and far showed up. A few asked how they could help. Most were transfixed by the unfolding destruction. One farmer, who was also the local mayor, drove up on his tractor pulling a water-filled tank-sprayer equipped with a large fan to spray pesticides on apple trees. He wanted to help, and this was all he could think of. As the number of spectators grew, I overheard one shout to another that the farmer who lived here should charge admission and would likely recover his loss.

When word of the fire reached my father, he sped home only to find there was little he could do. Efforts to contain the blaze carried on for hours. As I watched the flames devour the hay, waves of emotion swept over me. Food to feed cattle, our milk cows, and horses was gone. With winter around the corner, the season to grow hay had passed. Watching months of hard work and sweat-filled days vanish in smoke was hard for me to fathom, let alone accept.

When the flames subsided, bulldozers pushed the still smoldering broken bales onto the adjacent field, destroying sections of concrete ditch and fencing along the way. One of the barns was charred but none of the structures had been destroyed. No one was seriously injured. As the flames died out, onlookers lost interest, returned to their vehicles, and drove away. Firefighters gathered up hoses, talked with my father, then headed back to their fire stations. Broken bales of hay, pushed into the field, would smolder for weeks.

As dusk set in, I stared at muddy bulldozer tracks and ground that oozed water with each step. My parents, who never discussed financial matters in front of their kids, said little. It didn't matter. All of us knew that the road back would be arduous. Fire had consumed the food that was meant for the cattle. Their sale would have kept the farm going over the next four seasons. The fire had robbed our farm of revenue while leaving intact all of its costs.

What was gone forever extended beyond bales of hay and lost income. The sense of accomplishment from having endured hot summer days had also vanished. Of my siblings, I was the only one afflicted with allergies; baling hay kicked up clouds of dust that made my eyes burn and brought on sneezing fits. None of it changed the fact that each bale had to be loaded and stacked on the wagon, then unloaded and stacked once again. Moving the bales to the barnyard came down to brute determination. When hay-hauling time came around, the Sun seemed to move twice as slowly across the sky.

Each year, a new haystack was started. With each load, the one drawing the short straw got the more demanding and difficult job of placing the bales that became the new stack. By the end of the summer, the results showed. A poorly constructed haystack made it harder for me to break the stack down and feed cattle over the following year.

At the beginning of summer, with lingering memories of fighting precariously built haystacks in the ice and snow of winter, I voluntarily took on the job of building the new stack the entire summer. With each load of hay, I meticulously crisscrossed the bales for maximum rigidity and made sure that as the haystack went higher, it remained level and plumb. At summer's end, as I set the final bale in its place, I was worn out yet I felt content. The finished haystack, standing true and tall, was a hard-earned accomplishment—something I not so humbly pointed out to anyone within earshot.

After the fire, each family member dealt with the loss differently. For me, the long days and sometimes nights of hard work had been for naught. All the extra effort I'd put forth with nothing to show for it would take time to get over.

Despite the tragedy, what had happened that year set the stage for new insight. Previously, I thought of farming as a means of fulfilling consumer wants. Farms existed to satisfy their sensory pleasures: thick, marbled cuts of T-bone steak; ripe, juicy tomatoes; succulent, deep-red cherries; freshly picked ears of bright yellow sweet corn. Each offered taste and flavor, appearance and color, textures, aromas, even sounds. Farmers produced foods to please food shoppers.

The fire allowed me to see food and farming in a new light. Farming was the business of combining different kinds of energy, then transforming that energy into sustenance people wanted to eat. On our operation, it began with the Sun's rays that plants converted into chemical energy before animals transformed that plant energy into muscle and fat. There were other forms of energy involved as well. Kinetic energy brought water to irrigate plants. Farm machinery came from mechanical energy. Fossil energy powered tractors and equipment. And physical energy sowed and then harvested plants, built haystacks, and fed animals.

While food is prized for its sensory appeal, its true value is the energy it provides, with minerals, nutrients, and fiber as added bonuses. Seeing food through this lens, one realizes that life-sustaining sustenance is not possible without the Sun. Also that plants are never indispensable (so far as humans are concerned), and that farming is really the business of energy.

Prior to farming, energy embedded in food was outside human control. Breeding new plants, enslaving other humans, deploying draft animals, building water wheels, forging moldboard plows, and combining fossilized plants (coal) with water to produce steam (and a new measure for energy called horsepower) were all incremental steps to channeling energy into making more food.

Eighteen months before the Civil War began, a new source of energy would burst on the scene—crude oil. From crude oil came refined liquid energy that, when combined with fire, changed civilization by orders of magnitude never before seen in human history. Petroleum products carried exponentially more energy punch than wood or coal, without the bulk or weight, and could be transported and stored relatively easily.

Liquid energy's origin dated back to when sea levels were higher, the Earth's climate was warmer, and all of the planet's dry land lay on one supercontinent. The formation of liquid energy required millions of years along with other inconceivable geological events. First, organic matter had to be buried faster than it could decay. Next, the matter had to be deep enough, but not too deep, so it would cook slowly and its organic molecules would not burn off. Finally, an impermeable layer had to form and seal in this liquefied substance. Liquid energy was precious—and it was limited.

In the nineteenth century, pictures of crude oil gushing out of the ground gave the illusion of just the opposite—an unlimited supply. In 1919, the energy equivalent of one barrel invested in extracting oil returned a thousand barrels. The net energy unleashed on markets (999 barrels), was akin to strapping the economy to a rocket ship. Crude oil was labeled "black gold." Its refined products soon powered factories, manufactured steel, generated electricity, built new infrastructure, and produced America's food.

Refined crude oil (along with natural gas as a by-product) remapped how societies operated and how people lived. It became irreplaceable on the front lines of battlefields. Served as justification for waging war. Filled store aisles with consumer products. Provided medical supplies and drugs. Transported mothers to hospitals to give life, and dug their graves when they died.

Oil's footprint in food production had no parallel. Diesel- and gasoline-powered internal combustion engines in tractors and harvesters became the centerpieces of agriculture, and natural gas became the feedstock for manufacturing synthetic ammonia under high heat and pressure to produce nitrogen fertilizer. Liquid energy powered the manufacture of pesticides and chemicals, drilled high-output wells for water before generating the electricity to pump the water to the surface and distribute it on fields. Liquid energy built the highways, railways, and waterways, then fueled the trucks, trains, and ships that became the backbone of the modern food system. Soon enough, a network of oil tankers, refineries, storage tanks, and filling stations would make liquid energy appear as infinitely available.

As dependence on oil intensified, this illusion of an infinite supply carried over to other resources. Scarce water was suddenly made to seem abundant by drilling wells and pumping groundwater. Marginal land was converted into intensive crop production by using synthetic chemicals and fertilizer. With so much open space available nationwide, few were concerned with guarding prime farmland from development.

~

The richness of the soil, and the vast quantity of lands, have deceived many.
— Alexander Hewatt, 1779

I grew up watching farmland get divided into roads, sectioned into building plots, covered over with concrete, and planted with lawns. As farmers aged and the value of farmland for development soared, selling out to anxious buyers was just a matter of time.

Despite the Dead End sign where the lane to our house turned off the main road, strangers in search of opportunity ventured up the lane, parked in the driveway, and knocked at the front door. Preferring to let my father handle it, my mother dispatched them toward the barnyard where my father was working.

After a bit of searching, they would find him in the middle of a task, often holding a wrench or grease gun. Like most farms, ours never lacked for things that had to be done. Though pressed for time, my father would invariably stop working and talk. After a few pleasantries about the weather or the latest local happenings, the emboldened visitors broached their question—would he part with just an acre or two so they might build a home?

Before answering, he would look down at the ground, then kick up a bit of dirt with his steel-toed boot. "I haven't quite figured out how to grow crops and raise animals without farmland," he would answer.

Then he would pause and deliver the same message I had heard before: "I plan to hold on to the land, not for what you might be willing to pay, but for what the land can provide." With that explanation, the strangers would walk dejectedly back to their car. As they drove away, he would remind me, "You know, they're not making any more farmland. Once it's sold, it's gone for good."

I had watched him turn down buyers enough times that, a few years later, I was caught off guard when he sold several acres of prime farmland. The year previous, he had shattered his leg in an accident and spent the next nine months housebound, unable to farm. During the long recovery, a physician visited occasionally. Just as with others, the conversation eventually turned to wanting to buy farmland. In the near future, the story went, he would build a home, stable a few animals, and grow some hay.

With the understanding that, if the doctor changed his mind, my father would have first rights to buy the land back, they came to an agreement. My father believed a person was as good as his word, and the deal was consummated with a handshake. Money was exchanged and title transferred. While it was not my place to question his actions, I nonetheless wondered whether the accident and cabin fever had influenced his decision.

Soon thereafter, a fence appeared, marking the boundary between the physician's new property and our farm. In a manner of weeks, once prime farmland was producing weeds. The realization set in that the new owner was not interested in building a home and growing hay. Every so often, a hired man showed up with his tractor and rotary brush cutter to knock down the weeds; but the owner no longer came around. When my father resumed farming and worked the adjacent fields, he had plenty of time to look over what had once been productive farmland for growing food.

Whatever he thought, he chose not to share it with me. The seasons passed and life went on, until one day he was diagnosed with advanced kidney cancer. Four months later he passed away.

The week following his burial, before a headstone was placed at his gravesite, posts were sunk into the ground at the entrance to the sold field. A large sign was erected. Land he once farmed to grow wheat, barley, and alfalfa was put up for sale. The asking price was not based on what the land could provide, but rather on the profits to be earned after it was converted into streets and building sites.

When he sold the land, my father didn't anticipate a future subdivision, and street access was limited. Undeterred, the new buyers took my mother to court, where a judge ordered additional land be surrendered for roads. Because it was just farmland, compensation was set at one dollar.

People commonly refer to land as "dirt" before spending small fortunes to cover it over with everything from asphalt to ornamental plants. Dirt is what irritates eyes on windy days, sticks to clothes, muddies cars after rain showers, turns pristine streams brown. Dirt often seems like an annoyance, with little redemptive value.

Yet dirt is Earth's protective skin. Teeming with microscopic organisms, dirt is the membrane between a geological world of inert rocks and minerals, and a biological world chock-full of life. Dirt plus life becomes soil. Within a handful of rich soil are billions of living creatures busily breaking down minerals in rocks and decomposing organic matter. Without any fanfare, soil supplies plants with nutrients, filters away impurities to provide clean water, sequesters carbon, and remediates waste and pollution.

The United States has some 22,000 different soil types. The best for growing food is a mix of silt, clay, and sand, which offers excellent drainage, circulation of air, and access to nutrients. To locate such soil, simply follow the ancient glaciers that started in the Arctic and descended through Canada. What they left in their wake became the better portion of the Great Plains as well as parts of the Southeast and Northwest.

These vintage soils were protected by perennial grasses. Roots extending three to seventeen feet belowground, along with flat gradients or gently rolling hills, minimized erosion from wind and rain. Meanwhile, deep underground, weathering rocks were releasing minerals and new soil was forming. As time went by, a natural balance evolved between loss from erosion and new formation.

Early settlers venturing across vast expanses of grass-covered plains had no idea that America was home to some of the world's finest soils.

Time-tested by nature, this land could withstand extended periods of drought, heavy rains, and strong winds. In the absence of people, the soils could thrive indefinitely.

But people saw farming as the path to prosperity, and they needed land. So for more than a century, Congress floundered about trying to distribute it. What resulted was a patchwork of ill-conceived laws and inadequate oversight. Land was given away for free, sold at a fraction of its value, or offered on credit with repayment terms that were easy to exploit.

An unprecedented abundance of land presented vexing challenges. Politicians lacked the motivation to prioritize its usage. Early colonists followed the least expensive farming practices. Erosion was common. Crops were grown without adding back nutrients. Boosting soil fertility required more time and effort than simply abandoning existing fields, moving farther inland, and acquiring more land.

This haphazard approach to managing the nation's land was not without critics. George Washington called it "as unproductive to the practitioners as it is ruinous to the landholders." Concluding that improving the soil was next to impossible on large estates, Washington ultimately divided his land into smaller tracts with specific instructions on how to promote soil improvements.

Noting how Europeans valued and treated farmland differently, Jefferson wrote, "The indifferent state of [agriculture] among us does not proceed from a want of knowledge merely; it is from our having such quantities of land to waste as we please." Tobacco and corn were two crops ruinous to soil. Yet they were highly profitable. When the United States Capitol opened for business in 1800, its white marble columns were adorned with carvings of corncobs and tobacco flowers and leaves. A half century later, little had changed. Landscape architect Andrew Jackson Downing, who proposed Central Park in New York City, decried what was happening as "a miserable system of farming pursued by eight-tenths of all farmers."

The illusion of endless land was bolstered by some rather fortuitous transactions. The British capitulated their claim to America by placing a higher priority on defending their Caribbean (sugar) empire. The French nearly doubled the size of the United States when Napoleon abandoned plans for a western empire (in Haiti) and sold off the Louisiana Territory, using the fifteen million dollars he received to finance conquests in Europe. The Spanish sold Florida for five million dollars. The United States and Great Britain amicably divided the northwestern part of the United States and Canada. Texas and the Southwest were seized from Mexico. And Alaska was bought from Russia for less than two cents per acre, bumping up the size of the United States an additional one-fifth.

As settlers moved westward, their utilitarian mindset descended on the Great Plains, home to the nation's richest soils. The steel plow defeated the deep root resistance put up by prairie grass. Mechanized grain harvesters incentivized farmers to expand their operations. Two years after World War I, the number of tractors on farms had tripled to almost a quarter of a million. Prairie land was quickly being plowed under and planted.

In the 1930s, when severe levels of soil erosion became too widespread to be ignored, most farmers were adamant that nature was to blame, not farming practices. In the end, farmers were rewarded financially through taxpayer-funded programs to change how they farmed. In the mid-1980s, government conservation programs began paying farmers to plant erodible land with trees and vegetation under ten- to fifteen-year contracts.

In recent years, as prices at the farm went up, substantial amounts of land put into conservation were brought back into production—their owners determining that higher profits were more important than reducing erosion. But not all farmers value land the same way. Some have stopped plowing in favor of less invasive no-till practices. Others bolt on additional tires or use tractors with tracks to reduce compaction. Some contour their fields and install underground drainage tile to carry away excess water.

While such farming techniques are important, they are not universal. Overall, they have not reversed the impacts of modern farming practices. As Professor David Montgomery points out, "Few places [in the world] produce soil fast enough to sustain industrial agriculture over human time scales, let alone over geologic time." The United States is not one of them, where soil is being depleted eighteen times faster than nature can build it back.

While unmitigated intensive farming practices degrade the land, commercial development removes farmland completely from any consideration of future food production. Beginning early in America's history, the richest farmland with access to fresh water corresponded with the places where populations chose to live and subsequently develop.

Such trends have not changed. Developers are eager to snap up farmland near populated areas. Municipalities are after higher property tax revenue, invoking legal tools such as eminent domain if need be. In just two decades, 1992–2012, some thirty-one million acres of farmland were lost to development, on par with losing the entire state of New York or most of Iowa. At nearly three acres per minute, the equivalent of 3,200 football fields each day are being lost to nonagricultural uses.

Seeing America's prime farmland as a national heritage formed over millions of years and worth protecting to ensure food availability has never been part of the national psyche. Land is foremost about acquiring wealth, controlled by those willing to pay the most, irrespective of its connection to food.

When my father chose to sell prime farmland, he did not set out to validate how society regards farmland. Yet that was what happened. A country possessing some of the world's most prized soil made it easy to overlook land as an irreplaceable resource for sustaining life.

Every so often when I visit family, I am reminded how once-productive farmland became an elite subdivision. Within it are homes exceeding a million dollars in value. When "developed" in this way, the *soil* that once grew food now holds zero value. In the minds of the developers and buyers, there is little difference between dirt and soil.

~

We never know the worth of water till the well is dry.
—Thomas Fuller

In 1994, over a period of a hundred days, a mass genocide killed more than 800,000 people in Rwanda. Its heinous brutality shocked the world. Years later, an international criminal tribunal was convened in

Arusha, Tanzania. My friend Ricardo made arrangements for four of us to interview the court's justices in person. For the better part of the day, we listened while trying to comprehend why such acts were carried out. By the time we left, we were emotionally spent.

Early the next morning, we arrived at a home on the outskirts of Arusha. In this more humble and serene setting, we talked with a woman whose mission was to improve the lives of other women. In addition to traditional household chores of cooking and cleaning, she told us, women shouldered the primary responsibility for cultivating crops and herding livestock.

Their lives were filled with hard labor, and many endured constant illness and hunger. They also suffered in silence from abuse—often inflicted by loved ones. Few opportunities existed for basic education, let alone upward advancement in society. As our host shared her personal experiences and those of others, we found ourselves once again subdued in thought, struggling to make sense of continuing hardships with no relief.

As the morning drew to a close and we prepared to leave, I asked her this: if she could accomplish one thing, what would it be? I expected her response to circle back to an earlier topic. Perhaps greater educational opportunities, more human rights awareness, targeted nutrition programs, easier access to basic health care, or micro-credit loans for women. Instead, she paused for a long moment, looked at us, and then said, "Make water more easily accessible."

Her answer struck at the core of a universal need, one we had never had to think about. In America, you turn on the tap and water flows out. It hadn't occurred to us that lack of water could surpass other more-pressing problems.

From that moment on, as we resumed our journey in Tanzania's rural countryside, we were acutely aware of just how much women's lives revolved around water. From the moment they awoke until they lay down to sleep, thoughts about how to manage water carefully were never far away. Each new day was subsumed with finding, carrying (in vessels precariously balanced on their heads), storing, and dispensing water—not just for drinking and cooking but washing, nourishing plants, and quenching the thirst of animals.

I should have known better. On our operation, farming and irrigation were like conjoined twins. Each year, as winter turned to spring, the two canals bordering our land filled with water. The largest of the two, which we called "the big canal," could fill an Olympic-size swimming pool in 160 seconds. Its width and depth varied with the contours of the foothills it followed.

In wintertime, I sometimes climbed down its sides and looked up as if I had descended into the bowels of an oceangoing tanker. In summertime, I occasionally jumped in at the end of a long hot day, but I was always leery of being swept too far and having to struggle to climb out. Its volume and size had gained my respect.

The canals were not the only reminders of water. Twenty-five miles away was the reservoir that filled both canals. High in the mountains were white-capped peaks, signs of melting snow turning to water before flowing downstream into rivers, lakes, and municipal storage tanks. Pipelines brought that water into residences and commercial buildings. Fire hydrants appeared beside main roads. Homes and schools were plumbed with spigots and water fountains. Because water was available on demand, there was no need to think about it.

In school, teachers covered the water cycle, from evaporation to condensation in the atmosphere, precipitation through rain and snow, collection through rivers and lakes, then repeat. Because we were part of the arid West, to nudge the hydrologic cycle along, we counted on Congress to finance the construction of massive dams, aqueducts, and canals.

Buried in these dams were the bodies of workers who helped build them, my teacher told the class one day. Then she showed a black-and-white reel-to-reel film of gigantic dams being constructed across the West. Once they started pouring concrete, the narrator said, they could not stop without weakening the structure. For an impressionable kid, it made sense that workers could die this way.

In films and pictures, the sheer size and massive amounts of water gushing out of their bypass tunnels reinforced the grandeur of dams like Hoover, Glen Canyon, and Grand Coulee. The structures and enormous lakes that filled in behind were legacies to the engineers, hydrologists, geologists, and workers like those who dangled hundreds of feet above the ground while pressing jackhammers against rock ledges. Closer to home, my grandmother told me stories of how my grandfather and others helped carve out the big canal.

Through these stories, one could see how the arid West was made habitable. How flooding was controlled, drought alleviated, crops irrigated, electricity generated, new towns created, and recreation expanded. Through ingenuity, America had triumphed by converting what were limited supplies of water into an on-demand resource.

The presumption that we could control water started early. Along America's frontier, people believed that farming actually created more rain. As the settlers pushed past the 100th meridian, a line that bisects North Dakota, runs southward, and marks the change from humid to semi-arid plains, farmers noticed an increase in rainfall as more land was plowed. A few scientists and government officials provided support for the idea that the climate was indeed changing. Respected journalists like Horace Greeley endorsed and broadcast the news. What began as mythology among farmers morphed into a widely accepted view that "rain follows the plow."

Congress, cognizant that too little rain would deter western settlement, passed the Timber Culture Act in 1873, granting homesteaders an additional 160 acres, provided 40 acres were planted in trees so as to alter the climate with more rain.

Both myths were later refuted, but the quest to command water continued. When diverting surface water was not feasible, digging a deep hole and calling on divine intervention was the next best option. If water appeared, a windmill was built. When word spread of what would be revealed as one of the world's largest aquifers, stretching across portions of eight states, Model T's were hooked up to centrifugal pumps to bring its water to the surface.

Roosevelt's New Deal brought electricity to rural areas and eventually large-capacity wells. From new technology came high-lift turbine pumps, center-pivot irrigation systems, industrial engines, and cheap natural gas. Wells more than a half mile deep and capable of filling thirty-two bathtubs per minute were drilled. The amount of water extracted each year from this High Plains Aquifer System was estimated at several trillions of gallons.

Meanwhile, more dams were built and more water was diverted. Most notable was the Colorado River basin with its iconic Grand Canyon. To divide the water spoils, seven states within the basin entered into compacts and allocated surface water based on assumptions of annual streamflow. Twenty-nine major dams and accompanying reservoirs went up, as well as enormous pumping stations and hundreds of miles of aqueducts and canals.

But the apportionments were based on flawed assumptions. The water rights granted on paper far exceeded the physical water available. Mexico and Native Americans were conveniently left out. Water that would normally flow to the Gulf of California was diverted for other uses. Today, forty-four of every one hundred acres now irrigated with Colorado River water lie outside the basin's natural topography. In addition, one in six gallons stored in reservoirs is lost to evaporation.

The practice of allocating a percentage of total water to upper-basin states created incentives to hoard water upstream. In lower-basin states, water allotments converted water into a marketable commodity that was sold, traded, or banked. In regions like California's Imperial Valley, otherwise nonarable land was brought into production. Massive produce farms became so reliant on Colorado River water that any rain fall disrupted tightly established production schedules for planting and harvesting. Power plants were constructed and massive amounts of fossil fuels were burned to pump water up and over thousands of feet of elevation to supply cities and cropland, some of it used for growing cotton in Arizona.

Infighting among states and legal challenges to overturn court decisions have been ongoing for decades. As scarcity and global warming loom more ominously, states have schemed to protect their own interests. Over a recent fifteen-year time span, the Colorado River's average streamflow has fallen by almost one gallon for every five gallons of water discharged, when compared with the previous ninety-four years. As much as one-half of the decline is due to unprecedented temperatures, which are expected to become more extreme.

All this futility stems from an assumption of an unending supply, which helps explain why the United States *never* established a unified approach to using water. In the East, surface-water laws were based on proximity to rivers or lakes. In the West, surface rights were based on who used the water first, regardless of proximity. For groundwater, the framework for state laws and court decisions assumed that water flowed through underground rivers or percolated through the ground. Either way, the amount available was presumed to be inexhaustible.

This approach could not have been more scientifically wrong. Instead of images of underground streams and cavern-like lakes, a more apt metaphor is a sponge of varying thicknesses. By pressing a straw to the sponge, water can be sucked out. How much water can be withdrawn depends on the size, pressure, and number of straws. How quickly it recharges provides clues to the water's origin.

For the High Plains Aquifer System, its slow recharge rate suggests the water is from the last ice age. Extracting this "fossil" water has parallels to extracting crude oil. As early as 1940, its overall level began plummeting and has declined ever since. By 2010, an estimated 30 percent was drained, a volume roughly equivalent to Lake Erie. Despite a rapid decline, the pumps continue to draw more of the water. Over the next four decades, almost 70 percent will be drained.

So why does America persist in pursuing failing strategies? Old thinking dies hard. I cannot look at massive dams without thinking about men entombed alive, even though I later learned that this was never true. Texas, the second-most-important agricultural state, has seven thousand dams, more than any other state. Its population is expected to grow by 80 percent in the next half century. Groundwater from the High Plains and Gulf Coast aquifers is diminishing. The state's primary solution: build more reservoirs.

Nationally, agriculture uses some 80 percent of ground and surface water. In many western states, it's over 90 percent. In the wake of California's latest drought, new laws portending a more sustainable approach were enacted. Yet the self-imposed deadline is not until the year 2040.

To change, California must overcome a jumble of Roman, Spanish, English, and indigenous systems spanning from infrastructure to rights of usage. Over decades, surface-water rights were *over*allocated by five times the annual runoff available. Groundwater is not regulated—the state has no way to track remaining reserves. When surface water was rationed, the number of newly drilled wells exploded. As one newspaper headline put it, "The California Drought Isn't Over, It Just Went Underground."

Seizing opportunity from California's plight, Nebraska agribusiness leaders launched a campaign to attract California dairy farmers. To the question "Why move to Nebraska?" the spokeswoman recruiting California dairy farmers said, "We have ample clean water because we live above an underground lake called the aquifer."

Whether water comes from above or below ground, the total amount is fixed. When aquifers containing fossil water are drained, we lose access to this resource. When water is polluted with toxins, its ability to promote life is forfeited. "All the water there will be, is." Though that fact is irrefutable, we exhibit more faith in our existing laws and infrastructure than the laws of nature.

In years past, when I returned to the old farmstead, I walked along the big canal road and looked at the water. I was drawn by its unwavering volume as it serpentined along the foothills. The canal had occasionally taken human life, but it had also given life on a grander scale.

As the valley's population grew, subdivisions filled in what was once farmland. At some point, homeowners complained of living near such a large unsecured open channel of water. Fences were installed and access restricted, but these were not foolproof. Periodically, the big canal still claimed another life.

One fall, a century after it was built, the big canal was drained for the last time. Over winter, steel pipe was laid in, welded together, and backfilled with dirt. On top, an asphalt path for walking, running, and biking was laid down. The headgates that diverted water to irrigate our crops were gone. The cement ditches running along the top of our fields were destroyed during the pipeline's construction.

Not long ago, my daughters and I walked along the path, directly on top of what was once the big canal. Pointing toward the spots where the headgates were opened and water flowed into our ditches, I tried to recreate what they would never see. These fields, I told them, were where I walked up and down with shovel in hand, adjusting its flow, clearing away obstacles. Most of the time I was by myself, except for the occasional truck and driver or rider on horseback traveling along the canal's access road, waving or shouting words of encouragement.

As we walked, I explained how water had made the land more productive, which in turn fed more people but also attracted newcomers to the valley. Their interest in the land was not to provide food, but rather a home. The water they needed came from a tap.

As we walked slowly while talking, runners and bicyclists detoured around us. The path they were on wound through different subdivisions. Any connection to the big canal and how it brought life to the valley had disappeared. Its water was out of sight and out of mind.

~

The waste of plenty is the resource of scarcity.
—Thomas Love Peacock

Appearances can be deceiving. Size-wise, Brazil is larger than the continental United States. The fact that it looks smaller on some maps is due to early cartographers who scaled the world to favor the northern hemisphere, the hot market for selling maps.

In Brazil sugarcane is king. In the 1970s, when global oil prices quadrupled, Brazil adopted a strategy of phasing out dependence on crude oil by producing biofuel from sugarcane. Over time, its vast quantities of land and ideal growing climate made Brazil the world's largest sugarcane producer. I and others from IICA had been invited to see how sugarcane becomes biofuel.

Though forewarned of unending landscapes of sugarcane, we found ourselves staring at mile after mile of towering green stalks on both sides of the road, with nothing but more fields all the way to the horizon. After two hours of traveling past the same vistas, we arrived at a field being harvested. The latest technology was everywhere. Caravans of combine harvesters painted the familiar tractor-green were zipping along rows, cutting the plants near the base, stripping away the leaves, chopping the cane into sections, and hurling the cut sections into trailers pulled by tractors, all in perfect choreography.

Meanwhile, trucks hitched to loaded triple trailers were headed to the nearby biofuels plant. The off-loaded cane was washed before a series of revolving knives and presses separated the juice from the plant's fibrous matter, called *bagasse*. The juice was further refined into biofuel, while the bagasse was burned. From the plant's boilers generating electricity, to the trucks and tractors working the fields, energy from sugarcane powered it all. For each barrel of energy consumed to produce biofuel, eight barrels of energy were returned.

Cars and light-duty pickups were flex-fuel equipped, able to operate on biofuel and gasoline. As Brazil's economy and population grew, so also did the amount of land planted in sugarcane. When I quizzed our Brazilian expert about how the country planned for even greater demand, his formula was simple: more land, more mechanization, and more biofuel plants. The strategy for liquid energy relied on advances in technology, a favorable growing environment, and deploying more land.

In 2005, the United States launched its own biofuel initiative. The Energy Policy Act came with a pledge to reduce dependence on foreign oil and expand production of so-called renewable fuels. Henceforward, set volumes of biofuels would be blended with gasoline. With a ratio of energy out to energy in of 8:1, sugarcane was the ideal feedstock.

But America lacked the climate for widespread sugarcane production. Biofuels made from cellulose like wood, grasses, and crop residues had a ratio of 5:1, but were not yet commercially scalable. Any ratio less than 3:1 required subsidies to cover the added costs of blending and distributing the finished product to filling stations. The United States had plenty of corn that could be made into biofuel, but for every one barrel of energy used to produce corn biofuel, between 0.87 to 1.27 barrels were returned.

Still, with biofuels now mandated, the only way to comply was to use corn. The easiest way to cover the subsidies was obligating consumers to pay them directly, each time they bought fuel. When challenged, both political parties defended the law as a bridge until cellulosic technology could catch up. More than two decades later, the promise of cellulosic biofuels has yet to materialize. Of the 17.9 *billion* gallons of biofuels produced in 2016, only 4.3 *million* gallons were classed as cellulosic—almost all came from landfill gas.

Subsidizing biofuel production further enshrined the preeminence of corn in America. For 1,500 miles from Pennsylvania into Colorado, corn dominates the landscape. Many times over the years, I have traveled across Nebraska and into eastern Colorado. Each time I have watched as land once planted in wheat or soybeans was replaced with corn. Just as dramatic was the increase in center-pivot irrigation, drawing its water from the High Plains Aquifer System (known in Nebraska as the Ogallala Aquifer).

On a recent trip, I turned off I-80 and headed southwest into Colorado, where corn has likewise replaced wheat and sugar beets. In a large field I spotted a massive center pivot. Instead of water flowing through its spray heads, the water gushed out the far end, as if a fire hydrant had been uncapped, turned on, and then abandoned. The image of fossil water washing away the soil on a hot summer afternoon stuck in my mind.

What started as a promise to reduce dependence on foreign oil and expand renewable energy had ended with society paying farmers to grow more corn. Close to 90 percent would be exported, ground into animal feed, or distilled into biofuel. What was left was destined for industrial use or food products like sweeteners, oil, starch, and beverages.

With subsidies incentivizing more corn production, additional land was planted. Heavy doses of synthetic fertilizers manufactured from natural gas were applied. And more fossil water was pumped out of the ground to achieve optimal yields.

Without consumers picking up the tab, the energy produced from corn biofuel was not financially viable. In 2011, the National Academies detailed how biofuel from corn had not lived up to promises. Yet the report made no difference. Corn's control over cropland increased. Like the handful of banks who ruled Wall Street and intimidated Washington, corn ruled over the nation's land, water, and fossil energy. Corn was agriculture's version of "too big to fail."

The promise of moving the country toward energy independence was never sincere. Politicians were no more committed to it than Bernie Madoff was to looking after his clients. So long as the United States buys and sells oil on the global market, energy independence does not exist, period. Instead, we degrade existing soils and exhaust fossil water to produce so-called renewable corn biofuel while exporting finite reserves of crude oil. In December 2015, Congress repealed a forty-year ban on exporting crude oil to other countries. By 2017, the United States was exporting 1.1 million barrels of oil a day.

America's track record of recognizing and then stewarding finite resources has not been good. Rather than confront reality, our modus operandi for overcoming scarcity in one resource is to *cannibalize* another finite resource. Hydrofracking for oil and natural gas is a current example. The method requires immense quantities of water. While some water can be recycled, its toxicity to land, along with the absence of any guarantee that underground water will not be contaminated, is pushed aside. Proposals to desalinize ocean water provide a further example of the narrowness of our thinking. The desalinization process itself is known to be highly energy-intensive, and that's without even considering the matter of how to transport water inland to where fertile soil is located.

Land to grow food is in a precarious state. The warnings from Washington and Jefferson of ruinous land practices have gone unheeded. Relying on fossil energy to compensate for soil nutrients has pushed more food production onto marginal lands, allowing an estimated one-half of soil loss to go unnoticed.

Belief in an unlimited supply of finite resources is the second driving force behind the modern food system. The 8.7 million miles of roads, enough to wrap around the world 350 times, gave unbridled access to farmland. The 3.5 million miles of rivers and 75,000 large dams ("large" meaning six feet or higher) provided plenty of water. And the network of 2.5 million miles of petroleum, gas transmission, and distribution pipelines assured on-demand availability of liquid energy. We have built an infrastructure and a lifestyle that presume that finite resources are always infinitely available.

Not long ago, ExxonMobil ran an ad campaign under the banner "Energy Lives Here." In a series of television commercials, viewers saw just how much finite energy was part of everyday life. One commercial traced natural gas from the drilling rig to an egg being boiled in the comfort of a home. The ad's central message: "You don't need to think about the energy that makes our lives possible, because we do."

There are no independent means for verifying how much fossil energy remains. The government's Energy Information Agency relies on self-reporting. Their latest forecasts only extend "for the next twenty-five years." Our best indicator is looking back to how much oil has been consumed.

Most crude oil still comes from legacy oil fields. Of the largest oil fields, all but two were discovered prior to 1970. While new discoveries are common, the estimated reserves are much smaller than in the past. From recorded data, more than 50 percent of all petroleum ever used was consumed in the last twenty-five years. Had the 2008 recession not occurred, the percentage would have been higher.

Alas, campaigns like ExxonMobil's are treacherous. Whether we think about it or not, the reality is that the world contains a finite supply of resources—oil, land, and water are limited. No matter what any company or government promises, there are no free lunches.

Chapter 5

Expecting More, Committing Less

If men were angels, no government would be necessary.
— James Madison

No sooner did the last fire truck pull out of the gate and head down the lane than a new and unwelcome reality took over. For the time being, temporary patches were affixed to the damaged structures. Cattle were rounded up and herded back into corrals for the evening. And remnants of hay bales were salvaged and loaded onto the hay wagon. I was fully aware that my father was grappling with what lay ahead. As we attended to the chores, few words were exchanged between us. Inwardly, I was struggling with the loss and palpable silence.

All around, the smell of fire lingered. Smoke from smoldering hay hung low against the evening sky. Images of the men and machines who had battled the blaze could still be seen. Where the haystack once stood, there was now a soggy bog of mud and soaked hay from thousands of gallons of water. In the months ahead, fences would need to be repaired, and sections of concrete ditch, destroyed by the bulldozers, would need to be reformed and poured before the big canal filled with water the following spring.

As the Sun dipped lower on the horizon, two trucks rumbled up the lane and into the barnyard. Their fronts nosed upward as they were stacked high with hay, the hay's weight compressing their suspensions, flattening the leaf springs, and threatening to blow out the rear tires without warning.

The driver of the lead truck stopped just inside the gate, stepped outside his vehicle and walked toward my father. He remarked that he had been out of town all day, but when he returned, he'd heard something about a little excitement at our place. It so happened, he told my father, that he had more hay than he knew what to do with. Maybe my father could take it off his hands.

In our community, most farms were now part-time operations, putting up just enough hay in the summer to feed livestock and horses the following winter and spring. My father knew this farmer; having too much hay on hand was more pretense than fact. So he responded by saying that there was indeed a small fire, but the excitement was just an attempt to entertain the neighbors. He appreciated the offer but assured the man that no hay was needed.

While he was talking, the second farmer had gotten out of his truck and joined the conversation. Looking around at the mud, the charred structures, and the ghost of a haystack, he remarked that it appeared to have been more than just a little excitement. He repeated the same line of having extra hay and asked my father where they should stack it. Faced with too much evidence to refute, my father changed his approach and offered to buy both loads. He barely got the words out of his mouth before both interrupted; they had not come here to sell hay—and they were not leaving until both trucks were unloaded. Then, as if to tamp down any further resistance, one added that all this standing around and talking was only wasting good sunlight.

It was clear that my father was not going to get his way. So all of us went to work unloading the hay until both trucks were empty and the last bales were stacked. As we brushed the hay leaves off our clothes, my father tried to thank them only to be cut off once again—no need to say anything, they responded, he would have done the same for them. The farmers' unsentimental generosity was kind, but not extraordinary. It was simply how people in our community responded to each other in moments like this. While the fire would later become a lasting lesson connecting energy and food, the evening's events taught me why social norms were so important to governance.

Decades later, I witnessed a similar phenomenon in the mountains outside Cuzco, Peru. My friend Jeanice and her Peruvian husband, Mario, had arranged for a small group to spend time in an indigenous community and experience their culture and customs. The villagers who invited us in were Incan descendants, whose mighty empire once extended from central Chile and northwest Argentina to southern Colombia.

Inca history is commonly told through stories of immense treasures of gold and precious metals. Spanish conquistadores later plundered these riches and the people. For these descendants, signs of past wealth had long since disappeared. All that remained was a life marked by agrarian subsistence. During our stay we spent time in their small abodes, participated in family rituals, and shared meals made from potatoes, corn, and, on one special occasion, guinea pigs.

The importance of guinea pigs in Inca culture dates back centuries. When the Spanish invaded, Jesuit priests conscripted Inca labor to build (on top of the foundation of an Inca palace) what is now Cuzco's most famous colonial cathedral. When its exterior was nearly complete, Incan artists painted the cathedral's interior murals, including a reproduction of Leonardo da Vinci's *The Last Supper*. Featured prominently on the table, about to be eaten by Christ and his disciples, were guinea pigs.

Back in the village, the same fate awaited the local guinea pigs. Though they scampered freely around dirt floors of homes and were treated as household pets, with limited protein available each would one day be featured in the family meal.

Although we were at twelve thousand feet in elevation, the village was pitched against the side of an even higher mountain. Rocks were plentiful, but other essentials for living were in short supply. Water to grow food came from snowpack higher up. Each spring, as part of an annual ritual, everyone in the community trekked up steep mountain passes until reaching the snow's base. Together, the villagers cleared away debris and retrenched a channel bringing the water downhill to the community.

One afternoon, I soldiered partway up the mountainside and picked out a spot to watch the sunset. Alone with my thoughts, I reflected on how the community seemed to thrive in such stark conditions.

Food was not abundant, nor did it offer much variation in diet. Wood for cooking was scarce. The climate was generally cold. Water was precious, and land to grow crops was limited. Yet despite these everyday limitations, the people seemed to radiate contentment.

As I stared at the vistas below, a villager descended the trail from higher up, sat down beside me, and asked if I was injured or required assistance to walk back to camp. I was fine, I responded, before commenting on the villagers' agility. They climbed steep trails as if the mountains had disappeared and they were casually strolling along perfectly flat land. They did this at altitudes two miles above sea level, where oxygen was noticeably thinner. Listening to my observation he smiled back at me, no doubt wondering why I was such a weakling!

As we talked, I asked him about his village and how it was organized. When he brought up the mayor, I asked if this position was considered the most important role in the community. Oh no, he said, that distinction fell to the watermaster, the person who oversaw how much water each villager received to irrigate individual plots of land planted in either corn or potatoes.

With my Western background, I automatically presumed that the watermaster had the difficult job of mediating who received more water and who ended up with less. So I asked him how the watermaster arbitrated such tough decisions. There was no conflict, he said—in fact, it was quite easy. At harvest, those who produced potatoes traded with those who produced corn. In his case, he grew potatoes while his neighbor grew corn. The more water the neighbor had, the more corn there would be to trade for his potatoes. "I want him to have as much water as he needs," he told me.

Thinking that maybe this was just an extension of a barter economy, I asked him what happened if someone in the community became ill or was injured, and could not work. He responded that people helped out until the person was able to resume.

His comments drew me back to the support my family received following the fire. But there was another insight embedded in his answer: through the behavior of each person, the village as a whole had established a form of community health insurance. When people were unable to work, their loss rippled throughout the community. Getting them back on their feet was in everyone's best interest. Those helping out were safeguarding their own coverage, should they one day require care from others.

The same applied to food. The entire community helped to bring water to the village, reinforcing the truth that having sufficient water for all started with the behavior of each one. Their shared commitment encouraged each person to produce as much food as possible with the water provided. Accepting personal responsibility for shared interests maximized everyone's well-being. Governance, it seemed, came down to all for one and one for all.

I thoroughly enjoyed my time with this indigenous community. But their lives seemed to have little bearing on modern Western society, so I filed the experience under the heading of nostalgic anecdotes and moved on. My world was far more sophisticated. In the United States, informal norms had been replaced by formal governments with elected officials passing laws and bureaucrats implementing those laws through regulations. This was how acceptable behavior was now being prescribed and executed.

Then, a few years ago, I came across the work of Elinor Ostrom. Unlike me, she had not succumbed to thinking that our modes of self-government were a *fait accompli*.

Ostrom was born poor in southern California. Her jobless father had left her mother. Her clothes came from second-hand stores. Rather than accept despair as her lot in life, she channeled her ambitions toward shared interests, knitting scarves for troops and rejecting materialistic goals like owning a fine home or an expensive car.

At a time when sexism was pervasive in graduate schools, she pursued a doctorate degree, studying the conflict over water in the Southwest. Overcoming gender stereotypes, she eventually landed a faculty position. Ostrom was particularly keen on how communities managed scarce resources like fresh water, arable land, pastures, forests, and fisheries—basic essentials for food and security. She devoted years of fieldwork in countries around the world.

Then, as now, most economists were guided by Adam Smith, believing that self-interested pursuits automatically benefited society. But some theorists had pushed back, including ecologist Garrett Hardin, who in 1968 wrote a seminal article titled "The Tragedy of the Commons," in which he argued that scarce resources shared by the community were soon exhausted without government regulations.

While scholars were debating theories of what ought to be, Ostrom and her colleagues embedded themselves in communities from Switzerland to Nepal, observing and documenting their behavior. What they uncovered were communities who managed scarce resources through informal norms. Resource use was tied to resource upkeep. What applied to one, applied to all. Behaviors like cheating were not tolerated. Participation in community tasks was a requirement. Individuals accepted responsibility for the overall results.

Ostrom's work highlighted the power of informal self-government. While the results were compelling, her qualitative approach did not receive the scientific accolades of more theoretical treatises and quantitative analyses. That was, until 2009, when Elinor Ostrom became the first woman to share the Nobel Prize in Economics for her "analysis of the role of economic governance, especially at the commons." True to form, her prize money went toward scholarships. Regrettably, in June 2012 Elinor Ostrom passed away.

Her studies in Nepal had parallels to the indigenous community in Peru. The Nepalese farmers whom Ostrom observed also made do with limited supplies of irrigation water. Each year they cleaned and rebuilt crude earthen canals held together with mud, stone, branches, and tree trunks. When the snow melted and the water flowed, they divided the water between them, following long-standing community norms.

For those looking in, how these farming communities governed themselves was not readily apparent or even germane. What they observed were primitive canals badly in need of drastic improvements. So with the best of intentions, these outside observers secured money to build a modern irrigation system complete with cement-lined canals and metal headgates.

For the United States Agency for International Development (USAID) and Nepal's government, the initiative promised to be a winner on all fronts. Their feasibility assessment foretold of crop yields shooting up, food production increasing, family incomes rising and communities dramatically better off. With financing secured and plans completed, the government and its contractors proceeded to replace five antiquated canals in a farming region outside Kathmandu.

For the builders of the new canals, the project presented technical challenges in topography, adequate grade for water flow, and materials logistics. Preoccupied with execution, farmers were not asked about their experiences dealing with landslides and local soil conditions.

After the canals were built, a water-users group was formed. The local farmers who had managed the old canals for decades were initially excluded. Local norms that had governed the old canals were ignored. When the new canals were put into service, promises made at the outset began to crumble: water deliveries were unreliable; only two of the five villages were receiving adequate water supplies; and sections of the new canals were often blocked with mud. Instead of higher yields, total yields declined, especially along the tail ends of the canals.

The project was envisioned to showcase how technology could solve long-standing challenges. Earthen ditches bleed a lot of water, and cement-lined canals eliminate such loss. But the emphasis on technology obscured and ultimately undermined the community's social norms. Individuals no longer needed to focus on shared interests— and so they didn't. The benefits of high-tech expertise and external capital had looked good on paper but never proved themselves on the ground.

In America, people relied on traditional social norms to produce food for more than two and a half centuries. This was a time in America's history of more hunger, more-frequent crop failures, and less knowledge of nature and the environment.

Appeals for the federal government to do more began before the country declared its independence. In 1776, proposals for a federal department of agriculture already existed. If a case were to be made for the federal government to do more, the birth of a new nation was the ideal moment and opportunity.

Most elected officials had farming backgrounds. Agriculture dominated the economy. Its importance to national employment and exports was unquestioned. Members of the "Agricultural Society" were continually petitioning Congress for support. George Washington, in his last annual message to Congress, wanted help for farmers in the "spirit of discovery and improvement." Yet beyond instructing the Army Signal Service to provide farmers with weather reports, Congress did little.

Not until 1825 was a congressional committee on agriculture and forestry even created. Fourteen years passed before one thousand dollars was appropriated to collect statistics, distribute seeds, and conduct investigations. Two years afterward, the first crop reports were issued, only to be discontinued less than a decade later. Going into the 1860s, the nation's platform for agriculture centered on overseas consuls collecting and sending seeds to be distributed, taxing select agricultural imports, and adding cursory farming statistics to the Patent Office's annual summary.

Notwithstanding the absence of federal intervention, new breeds of animals and crops like rice, sugarcane, corn, cotton, and tobacco were established. A few states opened schools of agriculture. Labor-saving machinery like the flour mill, cotton gin, steel plow, reaper, threshing machine, and corn planter were introduced. Seeds touted to be resistant to insects were rolled out. Canning and refrigeration were established.

Eighteen sixty-two is when the tide changed. The government was giving away land. The United States Department of Agriculture (USDA) was established. All states were granted land to build colleges of agriculture. In the decades that followed, federal and state governments began funding research and widely disseminating the results to farmers and rural communities. A federal financial system for agriculture was established, enabling farmers to take out operating loans, buy new equipment, and purchase additional land.

In the 1930s, when the economy faltered and farm income plummeted, Congress arranged direct financial aid. The first section of the 1933 Agricultural Adjustment Act (the inaugural Farm Bill) was titled "Declaration of Emergency." It was an acknowledgment that many farmers were heavily in debt and needed to be bailed out by the federal government.

Five years later, the 1938 Farm Bill was designated as *permanent* law, setting the mold for ongoing subsidies and protections. Thereafter, crafting a new farm bill was automatically part of the congressional docket every five years—or until Congress chose to remove the permanent designation.

Early farm bills, sold to the public by promising more food with less uncertainty, were designed to stabilize food prices and increase farm income. Eight decades later, new farm bills are still being enacted despite average farm income long ago surpassing non-farm income and continuing food surplus. Each new bill is an increasingly costly grab bag of subsidies and protections, which invariably attracts more interest groups and lobbying. Other than loose connections to agriculture, no coherent policy direction exists. Meanwhile, the option to remove the permanent designation sits on the congressional shelf collecting dust.

Food-production subsidies are not confined to farm bills. The Renewable Fuel Standard encourages farmers to grow corn for ethanol, with subsidies paid for by consumers at the gas pump. The Clean Water Act exempts most farms from regulations banning chemicals, fertilizers, or animal wastes that run off fields and into shared public bodies of water. Disaster relief is provided for what the government considers extreme climatic events, natural disasters, or disease outbreaks. Export promotion, targeted food aid to countries, and federal funding for irrigation projects are other examples of ongoing subsidies.

Subsidies, debt, size, and specialization define how the majority of food in America is produced. Over time, the number of farms and size of farms have moved in opposite directions. Today, nearly 90 percent of agriculture sales comes from 12 percent of all farms. Over a decade, corn received 30 percent of farm subsidies; five crops (corn, wheat, soybeans, rice, and cotton) received two-thirds. Subsidizing major crops has also benefited concentrated animal feeding operations that rely on milling cheap grains into animal feed.

To administer wide-reaching subsidies and protections, government programs assume that each farmer acts in their own self-interest. To secure a loan, bankers likewise presume that farmers will maximize income by enrolling in government programs. Like most economists, regulators and bankers describe this emphasis on self-interest as simply "rational behavior."

The problem with acting "rationally" is the ensuing rejection of informal norms, with individuals no longer accepting responsibility for the overall consequences. Letting others underwrite the costs of growing corn or raising hogs through subsidies is just good business. Polluting a stream or pumping methane into the air no longer carries personal consequences. Helping uphold a sense of community is secondary. Business relationships with others are purely transactional.

Unsurprisingly, every so often—especially after social media reports of abuse—the public rails against government subsidies and spending. In the modern food system, much of that ire is directed at the United States Department of Agriculture. As one who has worked for USDA, I can report that being on the inside was both insightful and sometimes frustrating.

Coming straight from Farmland Industries, I soon realized how much I underestimated bureaucratic rigmarole. My new director, who also came from industry, offered some advice. You will find two types of people who work for the government, he told me as I came on board: those who are doing something and those who are trying to stop those who are doing something.

I worked with both. The "stoppers" ranged from administrative gatekeepers to political appointees. They drained enthusiasm and productivity. Fortunately, the majority of those I worked with were consummate professionals, able to rise above the bureaucratic grind, often arriving early and leaving late to complete the task at hand.

Although I was based in Colorado, I spent significant time in Washington, DC, where I learned about the vast number of programs within USDA. For every program, one or more interest groups were lobbying Congress for additional funding or protection from budget cuts. When budgets were generous, obliging each group was easy. When budgets were tight, programs without well-connected lobbyists were often the first casualties.

USDA is part of Lincoln's legacy. In his last annual message to Congress, Lincoln commended the department for advancing "a great and vital interest," writing, "It is precisely the people's Department, in which they feel more directly concerned than in any other." USDA leveraged the people's goodwill to build the only department headquarters actually located *on* the National Mall. Only a last-minute intervention by President Theodore Roosevelt kept the headquarters from being built smack in the middle.

Notwithstanding USDA's politically correct mission statement, there are programs within the department working at cross purposes. One program administers subsidies that favor diets steeped in calories from processed grains, sugar, and fat—while another provides dietary guidelines that promote a healthy diet from nutritious food. To straddle the divide, words like *nutrition* are featured instead of *calories*. In recent farm bills, provisions that provide easier access to diets rich in subsidized calories are titled "Nutrition Assistance Programs."

Some contend that USDA has run amuck. But this "people's department" takes its marching orders from presidents and Congress, both of which leverage USDA programs to amass political capital. People commonly believe that lobbyists pursue senators and representatives with enticements of campaign contributions. But the reality is more sinister—members of Congress have become telemarketers "dialing for dollars." Soliciting money is their top priority, not just to finance campaigns but to gain stature with party leaders.

Part of the payoff from fundraising is being appointed to committees offering greater exposure. Among the favorites is the Committee on Agriculture with its wide array of interest groups vying for inclusion within omnibus farm bills. These committees (in both the House and the Senate) can debate why permanent legislation for agriculture is still needed . . . or they can deliberate about which interest groups deserve funding. The result is always the latter. No matter which groups find their interests rewarded in the final bill, politicians adeptly use the language of shared interests—"the American people," "family farms," "affordable food," "consumers everywhere"—to justify their votes.

Special interests and politicians do not stop with the buying and selling of influence. Another common practice is to install their people in senior staff positions on House or Senate committees where legislation is written. Yet another is executive service appointments, by the party in power, in departments like USDA or the Food and Drug Administration (FDA). High-level political appointees, sandwiched between elected politicians and career employees, wield significant sway to set new agendas or derail existing programs. Among all federal departments and agencies, USDA has the fourth-highest number of political slots, with 220 such positions—only nine fewer than the Department of Defense. Lastly, businesses and trade associations serve as gatekeepers by vetting nominations requiring congressional approval. Lincoln may have believed that USDA was all about the people's agenda, but its most senior managers now come from mainstream agribusiness.

So what has become of norms that reminded businesses and politicians that individual actions affect the greater society? In recent decades, businesses have grown fond of saying that their duty is to shareholders, which is a clever way of rejecting responsibility for the consequences of single-minded self-interest. As Harvard business strategy and competitiveness professor Michael Porter has written, "How else could companies overlook the well-being of their customers, the depletion of natural resources vital to their businesses, the viability of key suppliers, or the economic distress of the communities in which they produce and sell?"

In fairness to food producers, accepting responsibility for the public interest is a hard sell when government programs and legislation cater so prominently to self-interest. With the original farm bill objectives of higher farm income and stable food prices squarely behind us, politicians have time and again pledged to pare back future subsidies and protections in the face of rising federal deficits.

Thus, the 1996 Farm Bill, labeled the "Freedom to Farm Bill," was sold as weaning farm production off federal subsidies. Recipients of direct payments were now prohibited from planting fruits and vegetables, but otherwise these farmers could plant any crop they wanted—or no crops at all. Landowners would still receive federal payments, but this was supposed to be a temporary measure that would give farmers time and money to adjust to market prices when government subsidies ended, and to ready their operations to compete with producers worldwide. Optimism at the time ran high. The mantra of many farmers regarding the new approach was "Bring it on."

Congress did, and for four years direct payments were made no matter what grains were grown or not grown. Then market prices fell and emergency and loan-deficiency payouts were once again parceled out, in addition to the direct payments. In the two succeeding farm bills, the once-temporary direct payments continued.

As the 2014 Farm Bill was being written, federal deficits were at record highs and public sentiment was boiling over. Wealthy absentee landowners living in New York City, Washington, DC, Atlanta, and other cities, it turned out, had been receiving millions of dollars in direct payments dating back to 1996. Under intense public scrutiny, politicians promised that such payments would be stopped.

But Congress had already put in place a plan to maneuver around public outrage. To make it easier for congressional members to defend their actions with constituents back home, food assistance for low-income households had been rolled into farm bill legislation four decades earlier. After two years of lobbying by more than six hundred organizations (from Fortune 500 companies in banking and oil to nonprofits working to end global hunger) that collectively spent more than a half billion dollars, the new farm bill was ready.

The 1933 Farm Bill was 24 pages. The 2014 Farm Bill came in at 609 pages. The estimated cost to taxpayers was $489 billion, or $800 million per page. Financial assistance for low-income households accounted for 80 percent (a topic to be taken up in chapter 11). But direct payments did not totally disappear. As if borrowing a page from the past, the bill's authors labeled the remaining direct payments "transition assistance." But in this latest twist to a long history of twists, new types and levels of subsidized insurance were offered to farmers at unprecedented levels.

Offering insurance to farmers was nothing new, but coverage had been limited to select crops like wheat and extreme weather events such as hail. Because many farmers had been unwilling to pay for insurance, the government was subsidizing their payments under the rationale that underwriting premiums was less costly to taxpayers than federal bailouts following a weather-related catastrophe.

Overseeing insurance has not proven to be the government's strong suit. At one time, for every one dollar sent to farmers, insurance companies were receiving an additional dollar. Taxpayers were better off giving farmers free insurance. The private insurance companies the government uses were making a killing; from 1996 to 2015, their average rate of return on retained premiums (how reinsurance rates are negotiated) was 18 percent.

The 2014 farm bill broadened the scope of insurance coverage to include more kinds of farms and more types of losses. USDA was instructed to devise ways to boost insurance coverage on farm revenue and entire operations. Insurance policies were authorized for 130 products, including fruits and vegetables, nursery stock, pasture, and rangeland. In structuring policies, no payout caps were to apply. And to avoid the embarrassing public outcry from the media disclosing payments, the bill specifically prohibited the release of information at the individual level. At the time of this writing, the 2018 farm bill, awaiting reconciliation between the House and Senate versions, promises to deliver more of the same.

Offering subsidized insurance was good for farmers—but for taxpayers, not so much. On average, the government pays 62 percent of the farmer's premiums. It also picks up the administrative and operating costs, plus the underwriting expenses. Since implementation of the 2014 Farm Bill, many farmers figured out how to be compensated twice for the same crop loss. The cost of this "double-dipping" is passed on to taxpayers.

So what has happened to the social norms that once governed farming, especially given that facing uncertainty is as old as farming itself? Every farmer knows that nature is capable of serving up bumper harvests or no harvests at all. They also know that they can better or worsen their chances by how they choose to farm.

On multiple occasions, I walked with my father through our orchards the day after a late-spring frost. Randomly plucking and peeling open blossoms, he looked closely at the color of the ovary. Green brought a sigh of relief. Black meant most, if not all, of the fruit crop for the year had been lost.

Some springs our fortunes were even brighter. Favorable temperatures at just the right time delivered a spectacular display of blossoms. Weeks later, the budding fruit was so thick it had to be thinned to keep branches from breaking and provide room for the new fruit to grow. Whether the trees were barren or loaded with fruit, the orchard still needed attention. Reward or loss, this was the reality of farming, which he understood well and offset by raising other crops and animals.

Sam, a family friend who lived a few miles away, had a different approach. His farm was exclusively apple orchards. Each spring he automatically worried when temperatures crept upward too early in the year. To ward off frost, he placed smudge pots (oil-burning containers and flues) throughout his orchards. When temperatures dropped too quickly, he walked the orchards at night, lighting his pots.

At times, Sam worried so much that my parents worried about Sam. Sometimes, despite his best efforts, he lost the entire harvest due to a hard late-spring frost. A new crop of apples or not, his orchards needed to be maintained. To keep the farm, Sam's wife worked as the secretary of the local public school.

Farmers know that planting endless fields of the same crop reduces the checks and balances inherent in nature, while amplifying the odds for widespread pest infestations. They also know that packing too many chickens, hogs, and cows in close confinement increases the likelihood of disease outbreaks. The decisions they make set up risks and rewards. If they elect government subsidized insurance, some of the costs from taking risks are passed on to taxpayers, while they keep all the rewards when things work in their favor. When things don't go their way, consumers end up paying twice: once through higher store prices if widespread losses cause supplies to fall, and again though higher taxes to subsidize the insurance. As one farmer in Iowa said about subsidies, "I don't know that I need to be subsidized for doing the right thing. I just want us to stop subsidizing the wrong things."

When Congress passed the 2014 Farm Bill, the White House announced that the bill would be signed at Michigan State University. An advance team was dispatched to identify just the right farm-looking building, which underwent slight demolition so farm equipment could be moved inside and staged as props. Attendance, by invitation only, included federal, state, and local politicians, university administrators, farmers, token faculty and students, and an entourage of news media.

Watching the webcast from my office a country block away, I expected to hear familiar phrases from the past such how "the Farm Bill benefits

American consumers is apparent in every trip to a grocery, where costs of the highest-quality foods are among the lowest in the world." Instead, President Obama doled out accolades to politicians, university officials, trade associations, and farmers. Consumers were never mentioned in his official remarks, even though a nation of consumers was footing the bill. In later press releases, some politicians said that the new farm bill saved taxpayers money, while never explaining their distorted rationale. Others deferred to the standard line that the bill was "a win for farmers and consumers."

Prior to the president coming, I quizzed people in the local community about their knowledge of the bill. The general response was that it dealt with agriculture, but otherwise they had little idea what it contained. When I mentioned the estimated cost, they shrugged their shoulders as if resigned to a government out of control.

Two years after the bill was signed, Congress's own budget office bumped up the cost projections for the insurance provisions an additional 60 percent. The final tally will not be known for years, but it doesn't really matter. The way permanent legislation works, lobbyists and politicians were already contemplating the next round of subsidies and protections, along with perfunctory promises that the new bill will be better than the last and a win–win for everyone.

"If angels were to govern men, neither external nor internal controls on government would be necessary," wrote James Madison. Yet it was in the absence of angels that people came together to form a new nation. Through democratic elections, individuals were chosen to represent the nation and uphold the rule of law. From such a beginning came public roads, bridges, and waterways, national defense, public education, hospitals and research, and greater food availability than at any time in the history of the world.

Reminders of this public spirit are still with us. In 2017, wildfires ripped through parts of Oklahoma, Kansas, and Texas, destroying crops and leaving thousands of animals dead. In response, farmers in Michigan's Upper Peninsula rallied to send as many as forty-five semi-trucks of hay and other supplies because, as one farmer said, "it's the right thing to do."

On a recent trip out West, I detoured to spend time with my college advisor and his wife in Ames, Iowa. Some of the deepest topsoil in America is in Iowa. As I traveled secondary roads meandering up and down rolling hills, I observed the grip that subsidies and debt have on modern farms. Most of the land was planted in corn. To squeeze out as many bushels as possible, crops were planted right up to the drainage ditches bordering each field.

Yet every so often, I came across a field where the farmer maintained a buffer zone between the ditch and the corn. It's a pretty good guess that these are the farmers most likely to plant cover crops like clover over the winter. Buffer zones and cover crops help protect the soil from erosion and reduce chemicals and fertilizer from running off fields and into ditches, eventually ending up in rivers that supply drinking water downstream to communities. Planting cover crops is not rational behavior, at least as represented by the Farm Bill and public policy. Yet here were select Iowa farmers still guided by a norm saying that individuals have a responsibility for the shared interests of the larger community.

Growing up, I sometimes asked a few local farmers whether farming was still worth it. They would smile then repeat the well-worn line that the secret to making one million dollars from farming was to start out with two. These were also the farmers who would drop what they were doing to help out one another—even when it set them back financially.

I can still remember when a farmer was crushed to death after his tractor rolled on top of him while he was turning hay on a steep hillside. Because the accident happened on the hill's backside, not visible from the road, his body was not discovered until hours later. He was survived by a wife and young children. Late that night, news of the accident reached other farmers, including my father.

Because we were behind schedule putting up our own hay, cut alfalfa waiting to be baled was drying quickly. If the leaves became too dry, many would fall to the ground when baling, lowering the hay's protein content. Unaware of the accident, I was awakened early the next morning and told to get ready. I assumed I would be baling our hay while the morning dew lingered on the field. Instead, I was dispatched to the farm where the accident had happened with instructions to not make the same mistake. My job was to get the hay baled so other farmers could haul it, and the bereaved family would not have to worry about it. No matter what we were doing, the norms of the community took priority.

If America has learned anything since 2017, it is that norms still matter. The Constitution contains some rules, but it can never fully guide the behavior necessary to govern a nation. Bridging the divide between, on the one hand, the Constitution and the laws it inspires, and, on the other hand, how people actually live are unwritten norms. One of the most important is mutual toleration, an acceptance that rivals can be equally patriotic and can govern legitimately. Another is forbearance—practicing restraint in the exercise of power, knowing majorities can become minorities.

James Madison wrote that "Governors must arm themselves with the power which knowledge gives," which leads to the question at hand: What kind of governance are we willing to accept? Will we pay enough attention to ensure that it promotes the interests of all people? If we do, the contribution of food to shared interests will come into sharper focus. People will be emboldened to call out self-serving agendas. Businesses will have a harder time claiming sole allegiance to shareholders. We will stop pursuing specialized privileges at the expense of sacrificing broader rights. The pay-to-play politics will give way to informed voters, who will recognize that along with rights come responsibility and personal accountability.

When this happens, the original purpose of governance will be renewed. Norms will be more than what can be legally skirted. Facts will be more than personal opinions. And science will be more than individual beliefs. Because as we will explore in the next chapter, science is not something we pick and choose, as if offered on a dessert tray *à la carte*—science is the closest thing society has to divining true north.

Chapter 6

Science *à la Carte*

It is not just the people who work in the laboratories who do the science, but everyone who takes part in sponsoring, producing, justifying, or making use of scientific knowledge.
— Robert E. Kohler, 1990

At 19,019 miles, winding through seventeen different countries, the Pan American Highway holds the Guinness Book of World Record as the longest motorable road in the world. As it turns south from Prudhoe Bay, Alaska, to Ushuaia, Argentina, the road passes through arctic tundra, boreal forests, prairies, arid deserts, and mountains. In Costa Rica, the highway climbs to almost eleven thousand feet before traversing the "Summit of Death." Undeterred, it continues across rivers and dense tropical jungle before abruptly stopping deep in the Darién province of Panama. From here, the only way south is by water or air, until starting up again in Colombia.

Darién is also where the United States and Panama established a blockade to prevent foot-and-mouth disease from escaping northward out of South America, into Central America and possibly North America. This highly contagious virus infects cattle, pigs, sheep, and goats. It travels easily on air currents or through contact with other animals, clothing, and equipment. When it is detected in a previously disease-free country, other nations have imposed severe trade restrictions that can last for years. In the past, because of the disease's high financial burden to commerce, countries like Great Britain contained outbreaks by drawing wide circles around infected territories and then carrying out massive campaigns to eradicate and burn all susceptible animals inside this outbreak zone.

With only a few months under my belt at USDA, I was asked to be part of the review team evaluating this bilateral foot-and-mouth disease prevention program. After meeting up in Panama City, our team headed out on a smooth two-lane highway destined for the mud-soaked roads and waterways deep within Darién's jungle. A half hour after starting, the paved blacktop surface abruptly ended and the earthen rut-filled road began. Jutting rocks, along with mud holes, tested our driver's ability to goose the accelerator at just the right moment to keep the truck moving without further damaging its already battered suspension.

As we drove farther, the remote jungle enveloped us. Why urbanites stayed away from this forbidding landscape was readily apparent. From Stephen, the program's co-director from Panama, I learned that Darién was where United States special forces trained before deployment to Vietnam. In more recent years, the province had become a tool for managing recalcitrant Panamanian government employees: as a last resort, select insubordinate workers were transferred to posts deep within the jungle. Scarcely any lasted more than a few weeks before quitting, Stephen told me.

For several hours, the road seemed to delight in bouncing us up and down or side to side in an unending test of endurance. With each bend in the road, I would survey the next set of mud holes patiently waiting their turn to have at us. As the day was ending, we arrived at a rustic house where we would stay the night, using the last bit of light to eat a simple dinner of rice, beans, plantains, and small pieces of chicken. With little to do in darkness before an early departure the following morning, we bedded down for the evening.

To catch the outgoing tide, at 3:00 a.m. we awoke and dressed by flashlight, walked to the river, and boarded a small, US-military-surplus boat. As the current pulled us through the water in darkness, remnants of moonlight peaked through the tree canopies. Guided mainly by memory, our local driver snaked the boat around sunken logs and low-hanging branches. The other faint silhouettes on the water, the driver informed me, were likely crocodiles.

By midday, we had arrived at our base and stored our gear. Later we boarded canoes and then ventured up smaller river arteries. The thick vegetation acted like curtains that nature had drawn around us, blocking civilization out and locking us in. Gone were signs of people bustling about stores and businesses, the noise of busy streets, edifices with corrugated roofs, concrete walls, and glass windows. This was a world cut off from civilization.

Yet every so often, as our canoes rounded a bend in the river's artery, a thatched roof poking up near the bank came into view. Beneath the roof was a simple platform perched on stilts reaching a few feet above ground. For the indigenous family who lived there, the structure's open sides and its floors suspended with ropes from the tops of poles offered minimal protection from heavy rains and winds. In the open space underneath the floor, a few chickens pecked at the ground, while a pig, sometimes two, rooted in the dirt. Off to one side was a small plot of land growing cassava, plantains, and bananas.

Periodically, we would stop and talk, listening for stories of infected animals in the area, looking for signs of disease. This remote area acted as a buffer zone. Because pigs were particularly susceptible to foot-and-mouth, they served as sentinels. If evidence of infection in any pigs were to be discovered, their low numbers made it easier to take action and arrest further spread.

At one stop, as two others in our team conversed with the residents, I walked about and tried to take in such unfamiliar surroundings. The absence of food, the remoteness from any towns, and the residents' simple existence were all powerful reminders of how life existed for thousands of generations. The small number of dwellings, scattered across long stretches of river, bore witness to the limited food that such an environment offered up for each household and their animals to live on.

Subsistence dominated their lives. Growing food, let alone sufficient food, was not easy. Before any tubers or plantains could be harvested, a patch of land needed to be cleared of its thick green foliage only to reveal a cruel irony—the soil beneath these dense tropical canopies lacked essential nutrients for plant growth. Right from the start, yields would be low. After a few growing seasons, with the soil further depleted, yields would drop even more. At some point, they had no choice but to abandon the plot, move on, and start over.

Reinforcing our sense of how food was scarce, even the pigs and chickens were undersized. Most of their energy was expended scavenging about for roots, rotten vegetables, or scraps of food that fell through the suspended platform the family occupied. Since the household couldn't subsist on such scrawny creatures for all their protein, they supplemented their diet with fish from the river.

As we followed the river deeper into the bowels of the jungle, it became clear that formal education wasn't much of an option. The people's future seemed locked into subsistence. As I thought about their circumstances compared with mine, geography notwithstanding, the primary difference came down to science—the same science I took for granted.

Before I was born, my ancestors had already hitched their future to science. There was no turning back. As their beneficiary, I don't need to live near arable land or bodies of fresh water. I don't have to structure my life around seasons for growing food. The delicate balance of sunshine, temperature, and rainfall that separates subsistence and hunger from prosperity and plenty can be ignored. There is no need to dirty my hands harvesting tubers or scavenging fruit. I can block out knowledge of how animals are killed and then eviscerated. Even learning how to cook and prepare food that is free of pathogens and parasites is now optional.

Thanks in part to science, it is easy to forget that abundance of food even exists. You and I can be as knowledgeable or ill-informed as we choose, while still reaping the benefits of science and the surpluses that science makes possible. Each of us can choose to write off the past or take the present for granted. Though science is built on knowledge, its benefits still extend to those who openly reject such knowledge. There is, however, one fact about science that merits remembering—this exchange between you, the reader, and me, the author, would not have occurred without science. Why? Our parents and innumerable generations before them would not have been born.

In the history of humankind, more than two million years elapsed before an evolving human race eclipsed one billion people. When agriculture emerged ten thousand years ago, there were roughly six million people. Not until the nineteenth century did the world's population pass the one billion mark. When it did, for many in Europe, optimism turned to fear. "The power of population is indefinitely greater than the power in the earth to produce subsistence for men," Thomas Robert Malthus had written in 1798, enshrining for himself a place in history by shortchanging the power of science.

Owing to an earlier scientific discovery, the nineteenth century ushered in a booming trade in seabird excrement, called *guano*, shipped from the coasts of Peru to Europe. Applying guano to grains like wheat boosted yields. Coupled with new plant varieties, this natural fertilizer launched a new era of food productivity. European concerns were put to rest. By 1927, one hundred and twenty three years later after reaching one billion, the number of people on Earth surpassed two billion.

Fast-forward three decades to the 1960s. The world's population surpassed the three billion mark, yet some 50 percent of these people did not have enough to eat. The US President's Science Advisory Committee reported that the food shortfall was "so great that a massive, long-range innovative effort, unprecedented in human history, will be required to master it."

Despite the ominous warning, Western governments did little to help. So the Rockefeller Foundation hired a scientist named Norman Borlaug and shipped him off to Mexico. Using science, he and his colleagues crossed strains of different wheat varieties until landing on one that produced both high yields and resistance to disease.

Mexico's newfound self-sufficiency in crop science was replicated across Latin America and then Asia. Not stopping with wheat, scientists developed new varieties of rice. Other technologies that were also adopted or advanced included synthetic fertilizers, liquid fossil energy, irrigation from groundwater, modern mechanization, and marketing infrastructures.

In one generation, the amount of food in so-called developing countries doubled. Global population swelled by 60 percent. The daily supply of calories increased by one-quarter. For his role in launching "the Green Revolution," Borlaug was awarded the Nobel Peace Prize.

By January 1970, the world's population had reached 3.7 billion people. A Stanford biology professor named Paul Ehrlich appeared on *The Tonight Show* with Johnny Carson. Channeling Malthus's earlier outlook, Ehrlich was promoting his blockbuster book, *The Population Bomb*, and talking about the impending doom awaiting hundreds of millions of people who "are going to starve to death."

In Urbana, Illinois, a business professor and economist at the University of Illinois named Julian Simon watched Ehrlich and stewed. He believed that science and technology would overcome any global shortages from population growth, but he lacked the acclaim to promote his views.

So Simon baited Ehrlich with a thousand-dollar wager on whether the future prices of any five industrial metals over ten years would rise or fall. For Ehrlich, higher prices would affirm resource scarcity brought on by population growth. For Simon, lower prices would validate how science and technology remediates population growth. When the bet was settled, the world's population had increased another eight hundred million people, while the prices of all five metals had fallen. Simon, it appeared, had shown that science would save humanity. But by then, fewer people were paying attention to how science worked, or the fact that the wager had more to do with vanity than with actual science.

Since then not much has changed. If anything, we have become even more accustomed to the miracles of science, no longer caring about the technology as long as the results work in our favor. When the latest one billion people were added to the planet in just thirteen years, modern societies rolled on uninterested and unfazed.

America's embrace of science did not happen spontaneously. For science and technology to succeed, a supporting platform was necessary. Enter Justin Morrill. A successful self-educated merchant, legislator, and gentleman farmer from Vermont, Morrill was more motivated by advancing experimental horticulture than actual farming.

In 1857, Morrill stood before his colleagues in Congress and made his case that falling yields in crops like wheat and potatoes stemmed from deficient agricultural knowledge and skills. The United States had ninety-five times more land than England, he pointed out before adding that America was importing over $100 million in agricultural products while Europe was investing in agricultural colleges.

America needed to learn from European scientific advances, Morrill argued, but Congress had a responsibility to establish science in America by helping each state build an agricultural college. Financing could come from the sale of public land.

His proposal was welcomed by many and rejected by others. One senator from Minnesota decried, "We want no fancy farmers; we want no fancy mechanics." Southern legislators were mostly opposed. One called it "one of the most monstrous, iniquitous, and dangerous measures which have ever been submitted to Congress." Said another, the proposal was "an unconstitutional robbing of the Treasury for the purpose of bribing the States." Not all farmers were on board, either. Some had deep concerns that their sons might leave farming. As one said, "All I want my boys to know is the Bible and figgers."

It took two years before Morrill won over enough supporters. No sooner did Congress pass his proposed Land-Grant Act than President Buchanan vetoed it. Among his reasons, the bill encouraged states to be reliant on the federal government for their systems of education whereby "the character of both Governments will be greatly deteriorated."

Morrill persisted and in 1861 Congress approved a revised version that President Lincoln signed the following year. Colleges of agriculture in each state were just the beginning. A second land-grant bill targeting former Confederate states was eventually added. Additional laws were enacted to provide funding, set up state experiment stations for laboratory and field trials, and build an outreach network to transfer the results to farmers and rural communities nationwide.

What Morrill launched became a four-legged platform for the advancement of science. The first leg was public financing. Funding research through the government rather than corporations or private interests would, at least theoretically, eliminate any strings or ulterior agendas.

The second leg was the expectation of science. New innovations are the offspring of fundamental or basic research. Before livestock farmers could deploy new vaccines, research was needed to establish how animals contracted disease. Before grain farmers could benefit from fungal-resistant seed varieties, scientists had to understand how fungi spread through crop fields. Since taxpayers were picking up the tab, it was only fitting that basic research should be disseminated publicly in order to enlighten society.

Next was upholding the "scientific method." From our ancestors asking themselves why some grasses contained more seeds or some trees bore more fruit emerged the process of gathering evidence, documenting findings, and submitting the results to be peer-reviewed by other experts. This stepwise approach, universally accepted worldwide, is at the core of sound science. As Carl Sagan aptly pointed out, "The method of science, as stodgy and grumpy as it may seem, is far more important than the findings of science."

The last leg dealt with the results. The objective of science was to provide unbiased findings using available evidence. When the findings were used in a nonpartisan fashion, they served to improve deliberations and enhance policy decisions. The role of science was not to prescribe policy, but rather to inform society and its representatives setting public policy so that better decisions could follow.

To carry out research, universities divided broad domains of science into colleges. Each college was further subdivided into departments. And each department recruited scientists to work in narrow fields of study. This approach helped create scientific communities that eventually extended worldwide. With each scientist both publishing and peer-reviewing the work of others, contributions built on past research were shared openly with the public and became stepping stones to advance future research.

In this manner, we learned that diseases were caused by infectious organisms or the toxins they produced. What became known as germ theory freed societies from the erroneous belief that malaria ("bad air" in Italian) emanated from swamp fumes. Sometimes accumulating new evidence took decades, or even longer. The discovery of vitamins and their role in some food-related diseases, for example, started in the early nineteenth century but was not complete until the mid-twentieth century.

As the building blocks of basic research were put in place, new technologies were developed. Chemicals were manufactured already attuned to the biology of insects and plants. Nutrients were designed to spur growth and fortify foods. And vaccines were developed that arrested disease. But the benefits did not stop there. From basic research also emerged the ability to build a massive global food system and then shrink it down into your favorite supermarket or local restaurant. Turbines were built and powered by steam and water to generate electricity for processing food. Hydrocarbons were extracted from uninhabitable environments and refined into fuel for transporting food. Rubber was synthesized and made into tires that moved refrigerated semi-trucks loaded with food across the country to where you live.

Between 1860 and 1940, America's population boomed by over 110 million. Prior to World War II, federal expenditures for research flowed almost exclusively into food and agricultural production. And up to the 1950s, states steadily increased their research contributions to almost three dollars for every one dollar of federal support.

The *platform* for science would be decades in the making, but once established, its benefits to carrying out science were soon evident. American food production became the envy of the world. Food shortages were no longer a regular part of life; Americans had more to eat than ever before. But when America entered World War II, the federal government's easy flow of money for food and agricultural research came to an abrupt halt. To aid the war effort, federal funding was diverted into wartime technology like radar, the atomic bomb, and penicillin. Overseeing the funding disbursement was Vannevar Bush, an electrical engineer who understood well both politicians and scientists. As the war was winding down, President Roosevelt commissioned Bush to distill wartime lessons into future federal support for science. Less than two weeks before the atomic bomb was dropped over Hiroshima, Japan, Bush released his report, *Science—The Endless Frontier.*

To appease scientists and politicians, and to gain their support, Bush finessed the meaning of "basic research." For scientists, *basic research* still referred to the "purest realms of science." Such research was driven by curiosity and undertaken to unlock the unknown, and was "performed without thoughts of practical ends." But for politicians, basic research meant uncovering "practical applications" that furthered "industrial development." Basic research was driven by tangible outcomes like making money. Speaking of agriculture, Bush cited "the control of our insect enemies" and the "cure of livestock diseases," examples that blurred the distinction between research that advanced knowledge with no immediate payoff, on the one hand, and on the other hand, research that was "embedded in commercial possibility."

Issued at the tail end of the war, the report bolstered public support for funding in health, defense, and other sectors of the economy. Congress signed off on expanding research funding—provided there were identifiable benefits to society. Unlike the period before World War II, research funding was no longer the domain of food and agriculture. The success in boosting America's food and fiber production had ironically helped shift research funding toward other priorities.

Within five years, the National Science Foundation was created. Over two decades, government supported research increased by more than a factor of ten. Funding provided to other federal agencies soon leapfrogged funding apportioned to USDA as well as state and land-grant universities. By 2011, USDA received less than 2 percent of total federal research and development funds.

In December 1980, in the midst of a stagnant economy, Congress passed the Bayh-Dole Act. The intention, along with future legislation that tied up loose ends, was to jump-start economic growth by using "the patent system to promote the utilization of inventions arising from federally supported research or development." Prior to the Bayh-Dole Act, any discoveries from taxpayer-funded research belonged to the public. With the new laws in place, taxpayers still anted up the research dollars, but institutions like universities now owned the discoveries, including any intellectual property rights. Free to negotiate licensing agreements, institutions could pocket any and all royalties or revenues earned.

In 2002, *The Economist* called the Bayh-Dole Act "possibly the most inspired piece of legislation passed in America over the past half-century." Three years later, the same publication offered a more somber outlook, pointing out the unintended consequences that "makes American academic institutions behave more like businesses than neutral arbiters of truth."

Whatever policy makers intended with the Bayh-Dole Act, the *platform* for science to support food production had been significantly altered. Public funding was more limited and competitive. Federal programs had been launched to accelerate licensing, startup ventures, and patent applications. The pendulum for science had swung decidedly toward research that promised rewards with "measurable societal impacts." Funding for (basic) research that lacked identifiable payoffs and unknown timelines had become more difficult to secure.

When I was a graduate student, pendulum swings in research funding were not on my radar. But returning to academia two decades later, I couldn't help but notice the pressure on faculty to secure external research funding. Within a year of returning, I was invited to speak at Iowa State University on trends I saw that were reshaping food. As part of my visit, I met with faculty across several departments, including a professor who oversaw a research laboratory.

As part of exploring our common interests, he gave me a brief rundown of research under way in his lab. When I probed as to which research topics brought the most personal satisfaction, he said that while they all served a purpose, none reminded him of why he had become a scientist in the first place. Intrigued, I asked him why. After all, he was a tenured professor and seemingly well positioned to pursue his own path.

He shared with me that his passion for science was rooted in exploring the unknown. As a student, he had been enchanted with understanding nature. A few professors recognized his interest and encouraged him to pursue graduate school. Early in his career as a new university scientist, life was good. He brought in research funding to supplement what the university provided and collaborated with colleagues near and far. By reading peer-reviewed journals he stayed current on the advances of others and likewise contributed his own findings for review and publication. He fit the mold of stereotypical scientists outfitted in white lab coats peering over their experiments and lost in thought while trying to break the code that would lead to the next discovery.

Rising through the university ranks came through publishing and securing research grants. He eventually earned his own laboratory and hired others to work with him. But along the way, he also began to realize how the platform for science was changing. Securing grants was becoming harder—particularly federal funding, which university administrators prized above all other support because it paid more university overhead, and any discoveries could be turned into future royalties.

"I'm a subcontractor," he stated bluntly. The university provided him with a title and floor space. His job was to find money. On the other side of that door, he said as he motioned toward the laboratory, were individuals who relied on him for employment. Pursuing the frontiers of science was no longer the first priority. Competition for federal funding was fierce. The time required to prepare a single proposal was substantial. The odds of receiving funding were low. To meet his payroll, his laboratory carried out an array of diagnostics and small studies that businesses were willing to pay for. It was not what he planned on when he became a scientist, but it paid the bills.

His experience is far from unique. In public research institutions today, following the money is the norm not the exception. The number-one challenge for university investigators is securing funding, and each year is harder than the last. In 2013, $454 billion was spent on research and development by all sectors of the United States economy. Of that amount, 0.6 percent ($2.8 billion) was spent by the federal government directly on food and agriculture. As a stark indication of how government priorities have changed, each week the same government spends $1.9 billion for programs created by the 2014 Farm Bill.

The decline in funding food and agricultural research is part of society's larger withdrawal from public universities. From the nineteenth century until the mid-1970s, state expenditures on higher education trended upward. Though college graduates reaped benefits from public investments, states also recognized the benefits accrued through new businesses, added innovation, more taxes, less criminal conduct, strengthened public service, renewed civic participation, greater engagement, etc.

In the looming uncertainty of the late 1970s, Americans dealt with a sluggish, poorly performing economy by voting for tax cuts that inevitably weakened public institutions and infrastructures. Grabbing what you could at the moment seemed more prudent than planning for the future. With less revenue, it was simply a matter of time before legislators began cutting state education.

As state expenditures were being whittled back, university administrators nationwide covered the resulting deficits by raising student tuitions. From 1978 to 2012, college tuition and fees skyrocketed 1,120 percent, more than double the rise in medical care expenses, and more than four times the consumer price index. In 1988, average tuition exceeded state (and sometimes local) per-student appropriations in only two states. By 2016, this was true in more than half of all states. At Michigan State University in 2001, state appropriations covered some 183 days of operations; by 2017, that number had fallen to about 75 days. In the 2016–17 school year, almost 71 percent of the general operating budget was coming from tuition dollars. (The general operating budget runs the university, excluding expenses such as athletics, dining halls, and dormitories.)

For both research and education, universities are in a bind—and this is particularly true for land-grant universities with strong ties to food and agriculture. Their business is offering specialized knowledge imparted by highly trained experts in narrow disciplinary fields. It is the same business model dating back to the nineteenth century, when the platform for science was founded on assumptions that society valued scientific knowledge enough to provide ongoing financial support.

For almost two generations, public benefits for higher education and science have been in retreat. Those guided by different priorities and backed up with the financial means and political clout have succeeded in changing the platform for science. States have pared back their commitment. Tuitions are increasing to cover operating deficits; students are taking on more debt financed with decades-long loan obligations, and universities still cling to ever-narrowing fields of expertise.

Looking back, it's clear that narrow expertise was pivotal in achieving unprecedented production and availability of food. The subsistence agriculture that I witnessed in the Darién jungle (a kind of agriculture, incidentally, that does not exist in the United States) is a tribute to scientists who peeled away slices of nature and the environment, then set out to decipher how they worked. What they discovered became the building blocks of knowledge that benefited all of society and ratcheted up our standards of living.

But looking ahead, the modern food system's most foreboding challenges trace back to previous advances in specialized fields of science and technology. The system still clings to this independent mode of research, with its few roadmaps and incentives to collaborate, despite mounting and more-ominous challenges that cut across narrow fields of expertise. Specialized expertise alone, for example, does not address the *connections* among rising rates of obesity, exhaustion of fossil waters, escalating nitrous oxide in the atmosphere, noxious weeds immune to legacy pesticides, growing antibiotic resistance—all the result of how the modern food system operates and how society now lives.

My initial foray into such challenges at Michigan State benefited from collaboration with Scott Winterstein, who was the interim director of the Food Safety and Toxicology Center, where my office was located. Whenever I dropped by and peppered him with questions, he responded with thoughtful insights. In addition, he was a walking who's-who directory on this fifty-thousand-student campus, where plenty of expertise in food certainly exists despite being compartmentalized in different departments and colleges.

In our casual conversations we began to envision collaborative research *across* diverse disciplines rather than *within* narrow fields of study. Joining forces with David Frayer from the business school and Rick Foster from the college of agriculture, we reached out to various faculty. With support of a grant from the W. K. Kellogg Foundation and Ricardo Salvador, we articulated a core set of challenges and their intersections, which we displayed on a wall-size graphic titled "The Global Food Platform."

For a year and a half, we convened periodic informal gatherings for further exploration. To push our horizons, we invited individuals outside academia, including a former US congressman, urban leaders from Detroit, and multinational companies. At one event, I counted five college deans present. We also met separately with the university president and the provost.

Each time we met, the discussions were marked with out-of-the-box exchanges and questions. The possibilities for nontraditional collaborative research seemed within reach. Yet, in the end, as a group, we were unable to turn the corner from talk to concrete actions. With each promising discussion, the same question always surfaced: "Where will the money for research come from?" Behind the question were faculty members who reported to different colleges and departments. Each administrative unit had its own incentives, though all shared one common performance imperative—find more external funding.

The most expedient way to find external money was working the existing networks of narrow expertise. Establishing the Global Food Platform would take time to raise awareness, build new networks and connections, and show proof of concept. Barring a sizable donation from a wealthy benefactor, we were unable to overcome the university's funding and incentive structure. Reluctantly, we eventually pulled the plug.

Perhaps in an earlier era and on a different platform for science, building a diverse interdisciplinary research approach might have worked. But as the platform for science changed, so also did the pressure to deliver immediate rewards that satisfied each discipline and its administrator.

As Scott later said to me, "It certainly seems that everyone sees the need to organize differently, but only if their discipline is at the center." Having advanced through the ranks and served as department chairman, he knew the problems inherent in the current reward system. "Faculty are passionate, in some cases fanatical, about today's challenges," he said, "yet they understand fully that 'publish or perish' is not just some pithy warning used to scare new professors."

It's no great surprise that research results that benefit the funder are common. Even if the studies appear in peer-reviewed journals, there are no guarantees that the researchers were not guided (whether explicitly or more subtly) in the study design, or sent their findings to donors before submitting them for publication. At times, as pointed out by Marion Nestle, the science has nothing to do with advancing knowledge, but serves to push certain marketing messages or mislead regulatory scientists.

Public-private partnerships have become more popular, yet they bring their own challenges. At Michigan State, I supported efforts to strengthen alliances with industry. At one meeting with several large multinational agribusiness and food companies present, their candid critique was that universities were lethargic. I and others, including my college dean, took this assessment as a challenge. Over the next several years, we collaborated with several of the largest food companies in the world on what we hoped would be joint initiatives. While we enjoyed our interaction, we met strong resistance to initiatives not offering immediate and marketable benefits to their companies.

Our experience parallels overall funding trends and priorities. From 1948 to 2013, agricultural production increased 169 percent. The basic research that set up major agricultural innovations in breeding, nutrition, pest management, machinery, etc. was publicly funded. The low-hanging research fruit that followed—new hybrid seeds, chemicals, vaccines, nutrition, farm equipment, etc.—was commandeered by the private sector. Why? Because it was profitable. In 2013, more than three-quarters of the $16.2 billion spent on food and agricultural research came from private sources.

Slashing investments in public research would be easier to justify if society were not facing problems of an exponential magnitude, such as pesticide and antibiotic resistance, global warming, and worldwide declining productivity gains in major crops including wheat, corn, soybeans, and rice. But we are—and weakening the platform for science that funds the research to provide society options for moving ahead is simply shortsighted.

Just as funding and expectations have been shifted, the same is happening with the third leg of the platform for science, the scientific method. The practice of gathering evidence, analyzing and documenting findings, then submitting the results to be reviewed by other subject experts is irreplaceable. Yet the trend to undermine the scientific method with pseudoscience persists. The most well-documented examples include the denial of human-induced global warming, acid rain, the ozone hole, and the health effects of smoking. Even the revered and long-deceased scientist-writer Rachel Carson has been under attack by revisionists.

The most effective practitioners of pseudoscience are scientists well acquainted with how the scientific method works. Like company employees pulling off an inside job, they know how to subvert the time-honored tenets of research to fit personal ideologies or ulterior motives. Here are a few common tactics:

- Using the media to exploit the bread-and-butter practice of presenting opposing viewpoints, which feeds the perception that scientists are equally divided. (As one example: lost in a two-person debate is the fact that 98 percent of climate scientists attribute global warming to human activity, while only 2 percent do not.)
- Highlighting the absence of black-and-white findings to imply uncertainty and division among scientists. (In fact, the role of science is providing a way to navigate uncertainty by weighing all evidence and building consensus, which takes time.)
- Dismissing findings as bogus while never submitting contrary evidence or studies for peer review. (Such criticism often includes cooking up sinister motives for existing science.)
- Creating a scientific façade through official-sounding institutes, conferences, speakers, and even published proceedings. (On the surface are the trappings of scientific integrity. Below the surface are dubious funding sources and lack of peer review.)
- Impugning the reputation of scientists who disagree with their positions. (This often includes vicious personal character attacks, unsubstantiated allegations, and misrepresentation by taking facts out of context.)
- Targeting donations and sponsoring endowed chairs at public institutions. (The clear intent is to create an apparently independent, well-respected source of information to disseminate a particular message that is favorable to the donor.)
- Using popular media to distribute sensationalized but official-sounding stories. (This rewards people seeking to affirm their own biases.)
- Invoking seemingly scholarly articles published in open-access journals. (Pseudo-online journals are the latest way to earn quick money. To illustrate the point, *Science* magazine submitted 304 versions of a bogus wonder-drug study with hopelessly flawed results to online

journals. Despite its glaring errors, the study was accepted by more than half, including two of the largest in the industry.)

The final leg in the platform for science is turning respect for science into the tactical rejection of scientific findings. While working at IICA, I received a call from my regional plant-health specialist in Central America. A virus causing citrus leprosis disease had been detected in a previously uninfected country. Transmitted by spider mites, the virus causes infected trees to drop their fruit prematurely and yields to decline significantly. More than ten types of citrus are susceptible, including mandarins, oranges, lemons, limes, and grapefruits.

Because the virus had just emerged, a window for action existed. A meeting with the minister was arranged and two scientists were flown in from Brazil, where the disease is endemic. The experts shared Brazil's experience trying to hold the virus in check. They pointed out that as much as half the cost of a box of citrus went toward acaricides to control the mite populations. Based on extensive evidence and fieldwork, they emphasized how critical it was to act fast and quarantine all orchards within the infected areas.

After the scientists left, the minister discussed the major impediments with my regional plant-health specialist. The infected areas included orchards owned by people with political influence. The imposition of quarantines would put the minister's job in jeopardy. He decided to play to the interests of a few—including his own—and do nothing. Citrus leprosis is now endemic throughout the country.

The United States has its own less-than-commendable record. Starting in 1960, FDA began permitting the wide use of antibiotics in animal feeds, leading to a sixfold increase in ten years. The National Academy of Sciences, the World Health Organization, the Government Accountability Office, an FDA task force, and an FDA national advisory committee all advised against the use of antibiotics in feed. Great Britain had already banned their previously planned usage. Yet the concerns of vested interests and the potential upending of FDA's budget by politicians overrode the science-based evidence. Today, 80 percent of all antibiotics consumed in the United States are destined for animals and agriculture. At least partly as a result, antibiotic resistance has become one of the most imminent threats to human health.

In 2017, under the direction of its administrator, Scott Pruitt (who has subsequently resigned in disgrace), the Environmental Protection Agency (EPA) began purging scientists from its Scientific Board. In their place would be representatives from chemical and fossil fuel companies. The role of EPA's Science Board is to review the scientific merits of research findings in fulfilling the agency's mission. EPA's mission is to protect the health of people and the environment. For food and agriculture, EPA regulates pollutants flowing into waterways, pesticides applied to crops, and contaminants released into the atmosphere. Retaining the appearance of a Scientific Board—while introducing conflicts of interest—is a blatant repudiation of the platform for science.

A beautiful afternoon overlooking the shores of Lake Michigan was the perfect backdrop for a summer barbecue and a chance to meet new friends. One was a physician, the other an automotive designer. The conversation flowed naturally, meandering through life experiences before turning to questions of what kinds of footprints we were leaving behind.

Readily acknowledging that our generation had irrevocably changed the world, we pondered what awaited our children and future generations to follow. Two of us were particularly concerned with issues like global warming, the availability of fresh water, our reliance on liquid fossil energy, and growing resistance of pathogens. In our minds, these issues represented weighty, complex problems that defied easy solutions. Perhaps hoping to jump-start our thinking, the third person declared his optimism, saying, "Science has always solved problems in the past. If future problems are important enough, science will find solutions."

Indeed, living in a world transformed by science, we are seduced into believing that science will save us from whatever perils are lurking on the horizon. By wishing it were so, we rest easier, assured that science is far ahead of us, pioneering new opportunities, neatly arranging everything to our liking, and cleaning up after us. Like a dessert tray the waiter wheels up to our table at the end of a delectable meal, we can choose *à la carte* the science that serves us best while ignoring the rest.

"We live in a society exquisitely dependent on science and technology, in which hardly anyone knows anything about science and technology," observed Carl Sagan. At one time the platform for science was firmly grounded in developing knowledge that advanced societal understanding. But as we began to think of science as simply another tool for enriching personal lifestyles, corporate profits, and political power, the platform for science was being sold off and dismantled.

What is happening is not new. As Thomas Hobbes noted centuries ago, men will argue about the rules of geometry if they find it in their interest to do so. But as our lives become ever more intertwined with science, there are increasing incentives and rewards for altering the platform for science for personal and corporate gain. The methods are often subtle and avoid directly attacking the science itself. In the course of my career, I have yet to meet another person conversant in science who did not endorse science as vital to our lives. Yet while each affirmed its importance, I've witnessed numerous efforts to weaken the platform for science by trying to cut funding, undermine the collection of data, or misconstrue the results and scientific methods whenever the science-based evidence threatened profits, market share, standards of living, or livelihoods.

The adage that "knowledge is power" comes from the Latin expression *scientia potentia est*, a reminder that science—objective evidence-based knowledge of the world around us and inside us—is the power that has transformed human civilization. That power transformed America's western deserts into fields of leafy green produce, and stopped worldwide hunger through the Green Revolution. Yet the same power is also evident in nuclear warheads and chemicals of mass destruction created to annihilate life. Or in the destruction of the Aral Sea, once the fourth-largest lake in the world and now one of the planet's worst environmental disasters.

The power of science is supported by a platform for science. Erode the platform by selling access, neglecting basic research, undermining the scientific method, or accepting science only conditionally, and the integrity of science is compromised. When any of this happens, science becomes an exercise in GIGO—garbage in, garbage out.

A belief that science should serve us subverts an understanding of how it actually works. The role of science is not to make our lives better. The role of science is to provide knowledge. What we do with that knowledge is what determines how our lives will change. Ultimately, the role of science is to inform, while the role of society is to decide.

The more we know about the role of science, the greater our appreciation of food and our surroundings. As we'll explore in the next chapter, this knowledge is important if we are to recognize that not everything of value comes with a price tag.

Chapter 7

Becoming a Market Society

Today, the logic of buying and selling no longer applies to material goods alone but increasingly governs the whole of life.

— Michael J. Sandel

With his mind set on defeating the Red Army and his pledge to "erase St. Petersburg [Leningrad] from the face of the Earth," in June 1941 Adolf Hitler ordered his forces to cross Poland and invade the Soviet Union. By early September, with the city all but surrounded by German and Finnish troops, he launched a calculated plan to bomb and starve its residents into submission.

For more than three years, the battle for the city dragged on at a cost of 1.6–2 million Soviet lives. While tens of thousands of civilians died from enemy fire, most of the 800,000 who perished succumbed to starvation and disease.[3] Among the civilian dead was a small group of scientists whose bodies were surrounded by bags of wheat, barley, beans, peas, and potatoes. They had chosen to preserve the seeds over saving their own lives.

For Hitler, conquering St. Petersburg, a city of immense wealth and strategic importance, would hasten the surrender of the Soviet Union and weaken the resolve of its allies. Among the most prized spoils of war would be the Hermitage Museum, home to one of the world's oldest and largest collections of history and culture.

Two days after German armies invaded the country, while Stalin was still grappling with how to respond, the museum's director launched a daring plan to safeguard over two million paintings, sculptures, jewelry, coins, and artifacts from the six hundred rooms of the Winter Palace. With the help of hundreds of volunteers and the support of the government, in six days more than a million and a half works of art were readied for secret storage in hidden vaults, a nearby cathedral, and the hinterlands of Russia. Seven weeks later, another 700,000 masterpieces, enough to fill fifty-three Pullman cars, were dispatched to Sverdlovsk, some 1,500 miles away.

A few blocks from the Hermitage, barely a hundred feet away from where Hitler had planned to make his victory speech on the balcony of the Hotel Astoria, stood a nondescript building housing the Research Institute of Plant Industry. Unbeknownst to St. Petersburg's residents, but not lost on Adolf Hitler, the institute's walls held another treasure—since 1894, more than 380,000 samples of seeds, roots, and fruits representing some 2,500 species of food crops had been collected from around the world.

To Nazi strategists, the institute's contents were more valuable than the museum's art and artifacts. In planning the invasion, Hitler had designated a special S.S. tactical unit—the *Russland-Sammelcommando*—to seize the seed collection for the Third Reich's future use. The conquest of fertile lands beyond Germany's borders would be incomplete without a rich reserve of plant varieties to produce more food.

Hitler and the Russian institute director, Nikolai Vavilov, may have had little in common, but both appreciated the fact that seeds alter human life. The institute's collection was a repository of genetic traits representing tens of thousands of years of natural selection and crossbreeding. For Hitler, such a genetic record would be invaluable in fighting crop diseases and pests, adapting to drought or cold, or protecting soil—just a few of the collection's many benefits. Learning from seeds had long unleashed human advancement. The seed bank contained not only a record of the past, but a map for the future of food.

Vavilov was a scientist with incredible vision and boundless energy. In the course of a quarter century, he had organized 115 research expeditions through sixty-four countries on five continents. Having gained the early support of Stalin, he directed all plant genetic research for the Soviet Union. But his methodical and scientific approach to collecting, testing, and selecting different varieties of seeds was slow. He could demonstrate consistent improvements, but he could not compete with the pseudoscience of another researcher, Trofim Lysenko. Playing to Stalin's demand for instant gratification, Lysenko had convinced the Soviet leader that simply cold-treating seeds would alter their development, hasten their maturity, and increase yields.

In the summer of 1940, Vavilov was arrested and held as a political prisoner. The official press release stated that he was helping Stalin craft a new strategy to feed the people. In reality, and unbeknown to his family as well as the institute's staff, he was dying from hunger. Intent on extracting a confession of squandering the state's resources to foolishly establish a seed bank instead of feeding the masses, the KGB was torturing Vavilov's emaciated body and mind. He died in prison— no confession was rendered.

Meanwhile, with virtually no support from the government, and no word from their director, the institute's staff carried on their work. Under extraordinary risk from both Russian and German armies, they collected, divided, and relocated seeds to different sites for safekeeping. At some point, "the scientists and curators locked themselves into the dank, unheated building, guarding the other set of seeds as well as all of their potatoes in the dark, damp conditions of the near-freezing basement. Numb with cold and stricken with hunger, the staff took shifts caretaking the seeds around the clock. Nine of Vavilov's most dedicated coworkers slowly starved to death or died of disease rather than eat the seeds that were under their care."

Each time I revisit their story, I am touched by their prescient understanding, which eluded their own government. They must have realized the hostility that awaited them should word of their actions— hoarding seeds that could keep fellow countrymen from starving—leak to the public. Yet they also understood the value of seeds to produce living tissues that could ensure the lives of generations yet born.

Knowing what they did, they devised a plan to preserve this treasure, then backed it up with a commitment greater than their commitment to their own lives. They were protecting not just a mere collection of seeds, but human sustenance itself. That knowledge sealed their fate, compelling them to withstand the relentless agony of emaciation and ultimately starvation.

Their sacrifice cries out with lessons worth heeding. What we dismiss as worthless may be infinitely valuable. What we measure may be woefully incomplete. What we cannot see may be critically relevant. And what we ignore may ultimately prescribe our future.

Part of my reverence for seeds came from wondering how colonial farmers got by before seed companies came along. What happened when crops planted in the current year succumbed to extreme events like drought, wiping out next year's seed supply? How did they protect seeds against inevitable damage from humidity and heat, not to mention invasions of insects and rodents whose voracious appetites could quickly devour precious seed reserves?

The other part came from observing my father at planting time. When I was old enough to help, I asked why corn seed was colored pink while wheat seed was turquoise. With a grin he said the colors kept mice—and me—from eating them before they were planted. In fact, the coating protected against fungi, bacteria, and moisture until the conditions were right for germination.

We planted winter wheat in the fall. Most everything else waited until spring. Preparing the land while the weather cooperated could be intense. But when the moment came to start planting, my father's next steps were cautiously executed. It began with a top-to-bottom inspection of the planter. Chains and gear drives were lubed, hoppers and tubes were examined, the depth and spacing of each planting arm was set, checked, then rechecked. When filling the hoppers, we handled the seed as if it were precious glass.

When planting began, he followed a precise plan without rushing. A few yards into the first pass, he shut down the tractor and checked each row for proper seed depth and spacing. At periodic intervals he repeated the process, while verifying each hopper was drawing down seed at similar rates. He insisted that the rows for each pass be straight; and I learned through experience that he had little tolerance for deviations.

Of the seeds we planted, the most intriguing for me was alfalfa. From a speck the diameter of a pinhead emerged a perennial plant whose taproot could penetrate fifteen feet or more belowground. Its deep roots improved soil structure and hosted bacteria that supplied it with nitrogen. Its flowers supported bees that produced honey. Its foliage provided habitat for wildlife, including cover for pheasants. Cut when it reached nearly three feet in height, alfalfa consistently produced three crops of hay each year, which we fed to cattle and occasionally sold to others.

More than any other crop, alfalfa drove the viability of our farm. Its added value was a fraction of the price paid. Even today, a pound of seed (some 200,000 seeds) sells for around three to five dollars in bulk. An acre (three-quarters of a football field) uses four million seeds. Back then, the cost of alfalfa seed was minor compared with the annual fuel bill or property taxes. We likely paid more for the baling wire that bound cut alfalfa together than for the seed that produced it.

Typical of farmers at the time, my father sometimes stored excess seed, shared it with other farmers, or experimented. Seed was to farmers what knives were to chefs or wrenches to mechanics. Not only did seeds and farmers go together, they defined what farming was all about.

It is not surprising to me that when Congress enacted the first Patent Act in 1790, seeds were not included. While its leaders sought to encourage innovations that were "sufficiently useful and important," they excluded products of nature. This was not because seeds were unimportant. It was Thomas Jefferson, the first patent office administrator, who said that "the greatest service which can be rendered to any country is to add a useful plant to its culture." And when John Adams assumed the presidency from George Washington, he directed overseas consuls to collect rare seeds, which were then shipped by the navy and distributed by the Treasury.

Awarding patent protection to seeds would have bestowed temporary monopoly power, as it were, to set price and limit access. While the country was all in on "useful art, manufacture, engine, machine, or device, or any improvement thereon not before known or used," letting private interests meddle with the nation's food supply through the control of seeds was out of bounds.

Though patent protection was not offered, the government played an active role in other ways. By the end of the nineteenth century, USDA had mailed some one billion packages of seed to farmers who planted, saved, and shared them, as well as carrying out their own experiments. Meanwhile, USDA and university researchers were conducting their own field trials, discovering, for example, how corn yields could jump significantly by tightly controlling pollination. From their research was born the "hybrid" seed, an offspring of two different varieties.

Small fledgling seed companies seized upon their research in order to grow their own varieties, which they marketed to farmers by promising higher and more predictable yields than if farmers saved their own seeds. The companies valued seeds by the profit they returned from each sale. Yet as they looked around and watched other agribusinesses growing larger, they saw only limited opportunities for themselves.

If, on the other hand, they could *patent* seeds, the companies could control prices, limit supply, and increase profits. After decades of lobbying Congress, they won a partial victory. The Plant Patent Act of 1930 granted patent protection for fruit and nut trees and plants reproduced asexually via budding, cutting, and grafting. But sexually propagated plants like wheat, soybeans, corn, and vegetables, and even tuber-propagated plants like potatoes, were still excluded.

Seed companies were undeterred, and the lobbying persisted. It took four additional decades, but in 1970, the Plant Variety Protection Act was passed. Up to twenty years of monopoly power was granted for seeds used to produce food. To appease opponents who saw patents as a threat to the food supply, the law allowed farmers to save, replant, and sell seeds, and researchers were given access to patented seeds for study.

When the bill was enacted, the seed industry was made up of some one thousand different-sized independent companies competing with one another to sell farmers seeds. A decade later, the smaller ones were gone; the bigger ones had been taken over by large pharmaceutical and petrochemical corporations. Three decades later, fewer than a hundred remained.

Prior to patent protection, seeds had been stewarded by society. Costs to develop new varieties had been underwritten through public research. Benefits had been shared widely. Except for hybrids, once seeds were in the hands of farmers they could be replicated cheaply without additional research. Now companies and their investors controlled seeds, jealously guarding their cash cows. When I joined Farmland Industries in 1985 in North Kansas City, Missouri, I never imagined that one day one of the largest chemical companies would become the world's largest seed company.

Years before, Monsanto, headquartered five hours away on the opposite end of the state, had purchased the rights to a molecule earlier synthesized by a Swiss pharmaceutical company and labeled glyphosate. Compared with other chemical herbicides used in agriculture, glyphosate had a shorter half-life or initial effectiveness. It was also less likely to contaminate the surrounding air or disperse into soil and groundwater. Some scientists had gone so far as to say that glyphosate "more closely approximates to a perfect herbicide than any other." With little evidence of natural resistance by plants, glyphosate (trade-branded as Roundup) quickly became a once-in-a-century blockbuster success.

But patents eventually expire, and this was true for the glyphosate patent, too. So well before its expiration, Monsanto went to companies like Farmland to discuss its post-patent options. At the meeting I attended, Monsanto presented examples of expired patents on pharmaceutical and chemical products. While each was different, all followed a similar script: the patent expired, generic production ramped up, supply expanded, prices fell, and the company's once-secure stream of profits vanished.

As I listened to Monsanto's representatives, one theme came through with absolute clarity—glyphosate was too lucrative to let go; the company was not about to relinquish control. Monsanto was already experimenting with altering the DNA of soybeans to resist glyphosate, enabling the entire field to be sprayed for weeds without harming the genetically altered crop.

Working in the company's favor, the Supreme Court had previously ruled that inserting foreign genetic material within a bacterium cell was patentable. That outcome led to the US Trade Patent Office ruling that farmers could no longer save and replant seeds that companies like Monsanto had patented; outside research was also forbidden. Later, the federal government decided that *genetically engineered* products were to be regulated no differently than traditional seeds, plants, foods, and chemicals.

Having grown up around farmers who prized their independence, I thought that a company telling farmers what they could and could not do with seeds was a bridge too far. Yet this was precisely what happened. Receiving patents for marrying glyphosate with seeds had granted Monsanto monopoly power to control access and price. The company had found a way to value seeds based solely on profits that they would earn.

But farmers went along. Convenience, lower fuel costs, and the ability to grow pristine fields of soybeans and corn with nary a weed in sight had convinced them to change how they farmed. No longer could they drop by local farm-supply stores and buy seeds. In fact, genetically modified seeds from Monsanto were not for sale. To "use" Monsanto's seeds, they had to sign a binding "technology use agreement" that obligated them to adhere to Monsanto's prescribed farming practices, which included granting the company access to their farm and all farm records. Should Monsanto determine that the farm was in violation of the agreement, the farmer agreed to pay all costs demanded by the company, including litigation expenses.

Restricted access did not end with farmers. Without Monsanto's prior authorization, any studies conducted by independent scientists also violated federal law. Even university field trials that compared seeds from multiple companies were now a punishable patent infringement. The tradition of unimpeded public research and sharing the results was over. Patent holders now determined what scientists could research and how results could be disclosed. Not until 2009, under pressure from EPA and a small group of scientists, did Monsanto acquiesce to partial access for research.

Continuing consolidation has produced a seed industry now dominated by three companies: Bayer-Monsanto, Dow-Dupont, and Syngenta-ChemChina (a Chinese state-owned chemical company). All follow the same strategy: bundle chemicals with patented seeds, pursue new patents, offer rebates to distributors and retailers, vigorously enforce use, and eliminate competition through acquisitions.

The value we place on seeds reveals how we value life. Seeds are the bedrock of life, an insight that helped sustain the scientists in St. Petersburg coping with severe food shortages and brutal cold that eventually claimed their lives. Similar insight was also evident in

America's founding fathers, whose wisdom transcended time. Seeds are part of nature. Nature determines survival. Whoever controls the seeds holds the power to control life. Such power is now concentrated in the hands of three corporations.

It is worth remembering that public resistance to patenting seeds for food lasted 180 years. The promise of new inventions was not enough. In order for market conditions to change and society to go along, the government had to enforce who could and could not have access to seeds.

Governments have been playing this role of access for a long, long time. In medieval Britain, for example, a hierarchy—from the king to lords, then to tenants and finally peasants—jointly shared the English countryside. While each had certain dominion over how land was used, none had absolute control over the entirety of land use. In the eighteenth and nineteenth centuries, when England's aristocrats colluded to seize outright control, their first step was to abolish the age-old hierarchical and communal arrangement. How? By erecting hedges to kept animals in and people out—and then requiring the government to enforce access.

From this precedent emerged modern property ownership. While the rich benefited, tenant farmers were locked out. No longer able to work the land that had sustained them for generations, farmers and their families starved and watched helplessly as sheep grazed or land was converted into houses and factories. The uprooting of millions of people became known as the enclosure movement, or "the revolution of the rich against the poor."

At about the same time, in the wake of its own revolution, the United States faced a related dilemma about land access. The newly independent country had plentiful land but little cash. President Washington's secretary of the treasury, Alexander Hamilton, valued land for the revenue it could provide. He proposed that large parcels be sold to wealthy individuals who could fill the Treasury's coffers.

However, the secretary of state, Thomas Jefferson, along with James Madison, "the Father of the Constitution," viewed Hamilton's plan as a return to aristocratic control. To avoid empowering a class of wealthy landholders who would rise up and control government, they argued that small parcels of land should be dispersed to individual farmers.

America's revolution had liberated the country from a web of loyalties and insider connections reminiscent of European rule. Just in time, Adam Smith's new book, *The Wealth of Nations*, set forward the formula for nationwide prosperity: ample numbers of buyers and sellers possessing the same information, all acting independently of each other without recrimination.

Jefferson's plan was summarily adopted. Aligned with market conditions laid out by Smith, and values espousing opportunity and independence, individuals initially received 160 acres of land. As some farmers became more productive and earned more profits, they bought more land. As mechanization and technology were integrated into farming, the cycle accelerated. Slowly but surely, the competitive conditions by which markets operated were changing.

In 1919, Thomas Campbell trumpeted that "the farm is a factory." Producing more food came down to "mass production, cost accounting, specialized machinery, and skilled labor." Wanting a larger factory, he bought the biggest tractors available and planted some 200,000 acres (312 square miles) in wheat in Montana and Wyoming. The farm thrived, a harbinger of things to come. In 1935, the total number of farms peaked near seven million nationwide before declining. The bulk of food production was gradually shifting toward the largest farms.

Though farms were consolidating, the businesses supporting farming were consolidating even faster. Farmers were having to deal with powerful banks and railroads. Ninety-five percent of farm implements were controlled by a single company. Meat processors had pooled their stocks into trusts and acted as a single business. Known as the "Beef Trust," their immense size and control made it easy to exploit both farmers and consumers.

From the public outrage that ensued, the government enacted antitrust legislation. A wave of "trustbusting" swept over the nation. Large businesses were broken up. Executives who colluded to fix prices were sent to prison. Ironically, breaking up the trusts had set the stage for their replacement—large corporations. As growth and consolidation continued, Jefferson's idyllic vision of competition, independence, and opportunity all but vanished.

My fascination with the way markets can change society started with learning about lantern oil made from sperm whales prior to the 1850s. As my professor in college explained, the light thrown off by candles was rather dim and easily snuffed out by a whiff of air. Whale oil, on the other hand, burned more steadily and made lamps simpler to transport, thus helping people to extend their mobility and the number of waking hours available each day. As people switched from candles to whale oil, demand shot up and the whaling fleet doubled in size in just thirteen years.

As whaling intensified to meet demand, the number of whales killed climbed rapidly, peaking near fifteen thousand per year before precipitously falling. Whales were poised for extinction until the appearance of a new product called kerosene, made from refining recently discovered crude oil. Its superior attributes all but snuffed out demand for whale oil, and the whaling fleets disbanded. By understanding how a market economy works, the professor told our class, it was easy to see how households benefited and sperm whales were saved.

As I studied more, I learned how market economics could be combined with mathematics to show all sorts of interesting numerical outcomes, including validation of Adam Smith's competitive conditions for optimal prosperity. As such derivations commanded more attention within the social sciences, scholarly agricultural-economics journals filled their pages with mathematical formulas and Greek symbols.

Then one day, I read an open letter from a journal editor whose tenure was over but who wanted to leave behind a few parting thoughts. There were certain problems, he reflected, that agricultural economists were unlikely to solve: what to pay for farmland, when to cut down a tree, how much fertilizer to put on crops. The reason why, he concluded, was that such problems lent themselves to elegant mathematics and few paid attention to the results. His second thought was more succinct—the more one runs over a dead cat, the flatter it gets.

I took his point. It was easy to get caught up in the mathematical trees and miss how the forests—or market conditions—were quickly changing. At the time, University of Chicago–trained economists were advancing the idea that breaking up big trusts and corporations was wrong. Big was better. Mergers and acquisitions benefited consumers through more efficiency, lower prices, and greater supply. Enforcing antitrust legislation was crippling companies who needed monopoly power to compete in a global economy. When Ronald Reagan assumed the presidency in 1981, his administration stopped enforcing antitrust laws. When Bill Clinton took over in 1993, he carried on the same practice "with even greater abandon."

As business journalist Barry Lynn summarized it, "If antitrust law exists to serve the consumer, and if consumers are best served by getting more for less, and if the best way to get more for less is to encourage business to be 'efficient,' and if the best way to be efficient is to build up scale and scope, then ergo, monopoly is the best friend of the consumer."

In the four decades since 1980, antitrust and competitive conditions have been largely swept away before most Americans realized what happened. A market economy still exists. But national prosperity is no longer tethered to independence and opportunity from having many buyers and sellers. Believing that lower prices make them better off, consumers have gone along. Once-important values, not always reflected in the prices and quantities recorded by markets, have fallen by the wayside.

Today, consolidation and control of markets dominate food production. Agribusinesses have grown larger by buying companies in the same line of production *and* buying companies that had previously provided them with raw materials or sold finished products. At Iowa State University, lawyer and economist Neil Harl warned that such two-way mergers and acquisitions were a "deadly combination." The ability to dominate markets across several sectors of food production made it easier to squeeze concessions, off-load risk, manipulate market transactions, and curry government favor. To believe that companies didn't take advantage of their newfound power was to pretend that sports cars were never driven above the speed limit.

I watched these trends unfold while at Farmland. Formed on the eve of the Great Depression, when farmers were legally sanctioned to "act together" in order to offset the control of large businesses, Farmland provided most of what farmers needed to produce and sell their products. With its trademark phrase "Proud to be Farmer-Owned," it was the largest agricultural cooperative in North America.

Revenues the first year I joined were five billion dollars, but losses were over $100 million. Given the company's long history, many saw the shortfall as a rough patch in the road. I was less sanguine. Farmland was competing with ever-larger businesses, who had deeper financial pockets and were marching along acquiring other companies, sometimes on the steps of bankruptcy courts.

As the consolidation trend intensified, to stay competitive Farmland made their own acquisitions by taking on more debt. When a combination of volatile markets and management missteps almost put the cooperative under, a new president was brought in from another company to turn things around. Though he was making progress, he was under intense scrutiny by Farmland's creditors. Everywhere he went, even the men's room, he once quipped, at least two bankers went with him.

In the midst of almost palpable uncertainty, when entire departments were disbanded and people who had worked for Farmland their entire careers were let go, he commissioned a public relations firm to create a new company logo. On a backdrop of green (the field) and blue (the sky) was a billowy white cloud and the name Farmland emblazoned across the front. When I learned how much it cost this company teetering at the brink of insolvency, I contemplated leaving while the lights were still on. In the end I stayed, intrigued by the value our president saw in Farmland that lay beyond what the markets were saying.

My decision to stay was a good one. Farmland regained its financial footing. When I later did choose to leave, its future looked promising. As the years went by, consolidation across food and agriculture continued and a new president at Farmland took over. When the economy took a sharp downturn, the advantage fell to those companies that had seized market control. Farmland was not among them.

In the story of Farmland, the pork industry perfectly exemplifies the trend in consolidation. In one generation, the number of farms producing hogs fell by almost three-quarters—while the median number of hogs per farm climbed from 1,200 to 40,000. Four companies would eventually control nearly two-thirds of all hogs processed. Its largest meat processor was also the largest retailer—Smithfield Foods. Upon Farmland's liquidation in 2002, Smithfield Foods snapped up Farmland's pork-processing assets—including its logo.

With four companies in control, individual contracts with farmers now cover some 95 percent of all hogs marketed. Traditional competitive markets are relics of the past. While contracts vary by company, the essentials are the same. The corporation owns the pigs and provides the feed and other supplies. The farmer puts up the land and finances the construction of the confinement building per the company's detailed specifications. The corporation prescribes the exact rearing practices. The farmer provides the labor.

At first glance, the dollar figures shown to potential farmers appear attractive. The corporation is providing the opportunity. Owning a business suggests independence. In a rural economy with limited options, the opportunity before them represents the new American dream, one that can be passed along to future generations. But the competitive markets of the past that ensured opportunity through many buyers and sellers, with no one firm having undue influence over market price, no longer exists. Instead, farmers are dealing with a multinational corporation whose sheer size allows the company to dictate the formulas by which farmers will compete and prices are set.

Looking even closer raises an obvious question. Why would well-financed, multibillion-dollar companies offer lucrative propositions instead of keeping all the profits for themselves? The short answer is that these contracts pass the lion's share of financial risk on to farmers.

Contracts adapted to pork production were first pioneered by Tyson, which was, decades ago, searching for ways to expand and integrate its poultry business and saw an abundant supply of rural labor with few opportunities for income. People signed up to be contract farmers. Years later, when the sole source of income was raising chickens under contract, 71 percent of the farmers studied were living below the poverty line. Tyson, coincidently or not, is number one in poultry and number two in pork.

The contracts reward performance—even though most of the performance variables are outside the farmer's control. The health of incoming pigs (or chicks), animal genetics, feed quality, inherent disease susceptibility, extreme weather, and climate are just some examples. Contracts may also require farmers to install and pay for company-mandated technology upgrades, disallow lawsuits by using forced-arbitration clauses, or omit transparency safeguards pertaining to standards and weights. Compensation is typically tied to a "tournament system"—a scheme whereby farmers compete against each other over a fixed amount of compensation.

Then there are the working conditions. Long hours are spent in a closed environment with thousands of animals living on slatted floors, beneath which is a waste pit of liquids and gases—ammonia, carbon dioxide, carbon monoxide, methane, and hydrogen sulfide—so toxic it can kill humans and the pigs should the ventilation system fail.

Contracts also contain nonperformance clauses. Should the company decide to revoke the contract, farmers have few options, especially since traditional markets are no longer viable. But contract or not, farmers are still on the hook to pay off land and buildings mortgaged in their name, even if unoccupied.

None of what I describe is breaking news. But it illustrates that modern farming can be the antithesis of independence and opportunity. In 2009, USDA used its legal authority to address anti-competitive behavior. When it did, members of Congress on both sides called hearings, wrote USDA letters, and withheld funding. In December 2016, a watered-down set of rules was released.

In 2017, the incoming Trump administration withdrew the rules. When they did, the National Cattlemen's Beef Association said, "This is a victory for America's cattle and beef producers—and it's a victory for America's consumers." The National Pork Producers Council added that the rules "would have had a devastating impact on America's pork producers. The regulations would have restricted the buying and selling of livestock, led to consolidation of the livestock industry—putting farmers out of business—and increased consumer prices for meat."

It's hard to read such statements without thinking of the "double-speak" of George Orwell's *1984* or perhaps his other dystopia, *Animal Farm*. The Justice Department and USDA had followed a methodical process, investing tens of thousands of hours and untold expenditures in nationwide hearings, interviews, investigations, and fact-finding missions. A long, drawn-out rule-making process followed afterward.

Yet none of that compared to the power of agribusiness and political spin.

At one time, Americans could distinguish between competitive markets and monopoly power—the former bolsters independence and opportunity, the later rewards control and avarice. Yet today, the lines have blurred and the values that once guided markets are on life support. What remains are contracts written by companies and enforced, if need be, by the government.

Dominance of the food system is not limited to meat and seeds. In seventeen of nineteen categories such as processing milk, milling flour, or refining sugar, the top four companies control from 46 to 95 percent of the market. In nine of the seventeen categories, market dominance exceeds 70 percent. At the global level, the top four companies in crop seeds, agricultural chemicals, animal health, animal breeding, and farm machinery control more than half of each market.

On the supermarket retail side of the food system, more than half (54 percent) is dominated by four companies, with Walmart controlling one-third of the entire market. Consolidation across retail product categories continues. As examples, Tyson Foods owns thirty-eight brands, while Smithfield Foods has at least fourteen core brands.

Each time I come across the Farmland logo, my mind takes me back to the moment the company president rolled it out. Those were desperate times—whether a farmer-owned company could withstand growing market control was an open question. The new logo embodied the hope of surviving an onslaught of monopoly power. But it was not to be.

Counting Smithfield Foods' purchase of Farmland's pork division, Smithfield now controls 27 percent of the retail pork market. The consolidation has continued. In 2013, in what was the largest-ever acquisition of a United States company by a Chinese business, Smithfield Foods was purchased by Shuanghui International Holdings. The United States government registered no opposition.

One American firm that supported the Chinese buyout was Goldman Sachs, an investment bank that held shares in Smithfield Foods and stood to make tens of millions of dollars in advising the company—until its shares in Shuanghui were revealed. For Goldman Sachs's president, potential conflicts in the securities business were a fact of life, one he believed the firm managed effectively. To the bank, food was just another sector in which to rake in profits.

For investors of the past, producing food had been fraught with uncertainty and low returns. This alone explained why the government's role has been crucial in providing or insuring financing on the front end for operating loans, buying farm machinery, and land. On the back end, farmers depended on the government for shoring up farm income through price supports and insurance. And throughout the food-production process, governmental support has been critical for funding research to advance knowledge and spur innovation.

But as farming cut back on labor, bought more-sophisticated machinery, and incurred more debt, private banks provided more loans. As larger agribusinesses and food companies began to dominate the modern food system, a host of financial institutions and markets, private equity consortia, asset-management firms, pension, and hedge funds climbed onboard.

Over time, putting financial capital toward food production became another category in a diversified portfolio that investors and bankers tweaked to balance short-term profits with long-term growth. Positive trends—from population growth, increasing trade, rising land values, and people eating more-expensive meat-based diets—suggested greater returns, which could go even higher by exploiting the agricultural commodities "futures markets."

Established in London in the 1700s and the United States in the 1850s, agricultural futures markets initially attracted little interest from mainstream investors and banks. Futures markets trade in contracts—binding agreements to sell or buy commodities like wheat at an agreed-to price and future date. For a farmer growing wheat, a futures contract is protection against low prices at the time of harvest, should a nationwide bumper crop cause wheat prices to fall. For a baker, worried about having sufficient wheat, a futures contract assures availability should a drought cause wheat harvests to plummet and prices to skyrocket. Farmers and bakers are called hedgers; they are physically tied to wheat and want a practical way to hedge risk.

Other traders are called speculators—they buy and sell contracts based on variations in current market prices versus future prices. They are after short-term profits, and their actions provide liquidity by making sure large distortions in price do not happen. To ensure that futures markets operate smoothly, hedgers and speculators follow different rules.

For a century and a half, futures markets chugged along with hedgers and speculators staying within their respective lanes of conduct. Then came the deregulation of the 1980s, which relaxed the rules and blurred the roles. Financial institutions like Goldman Sachs and other bankers began crafting and selling to investors speculative index funds that included prices of basic food commodities like wheat. To minimize financial risk from their *own* index funds, bankers hedged their actions by buying futures markets contracts—in effect, preventing futures markets from reconciling physical supply and demand. As one trader testified before Congress, such companies were engaged in "virtual hoarding via the commodities futures markets," in anticipation of earning higher returns.

All speculative bubbles inevitably crash. When it happened in mid-2008 for wheat, an additional 130 to 155 million people in developing countries reliant on wheat imports for sufficient food were pushed into poverty and malnutrition. Goldman Sachs and others claim they are not responsible for what happened. Yet no evidence has ever shown that deregulation and changing the rules improved performance—the futures market was not broken and it did not need to be fixed. As Bill Clinton, whose administration helped encourage deregulation, later said, "We all blew it, including me when I was president. We were wrong to believe that food was like some other product in international trade."

Futures markets for agricultural commodities had been a tool to manage the uncertainty of providing food. Its rules of order provided stability to smooth over unpredictable events like weather on wheat harvests. For countries that needed wheat, futures markets helped ensure sufficient food to feed their people. Many of these countries were home to some of the most vulnerable populations in the world.

But deregulation relaxed the rules and conditions by which markets operated. For investors, futures markets for food represented financial gains and losses. Depending on the wealth strategy they chose, higher food prices translated into higher profits. Whether or not those higher prices pushed people into poverty was not part of the investors' financial objective or moral calculation.

As sophisticated financial strategies are grafted onto the modern food system, more mergers and acquisitions by ever-larger multinational companies follow. Food is no longer valued for its ability to sustain life, but only for its ability to generate profits. Whether higher returns come from squeezing farmers under contract to grow pigs or poultry, creating a monopoly on seeds that can by doused with chemicals, or selling food laden with cheap calories makes no difference.

"We all blew it" applies not only to futures markets but to a cavalier acceptance of markets. The phrase "free markets" is bandied about as if questioning free markets is on par with challenging gravity. The plain fact is, though, that free markets are more illusion than reality. As Dwayne Andreas, the former CEO of ADM (one of four largest grain traders in the world) unabashedly put it, "There isn't one grain of anything in the world that is sold in a free market. Not one! The only place you see a free market is in the speeches of politicians." The closest America has come to free markets were the competitive conditions outlined by Adam Smith, which, at least in the modern food system, no longer exist.

This is not to say that markets have no role. A market economy can help organize productive activity. In a food system, a market economy helps assemble the biological drive for food, the resources to produce it, the governance to regulate shared interests, and the science to spur advancement. A market economy can span geography, national boundaries, languages, and cultures.

But when the utilitarian mindset of a market economy takes over and absorbs peoples' outlook on life, the whole of society is in trouble. When market-oriented thinking becomes so ingrained in peoples' psyches that they rationalize away once-important values, then a market economy has become a market society.

In a market society, everything is for sale (if you have the money to buy it) and anything without a price tag is deemed unimportant. No market, no price, no value—which includes the contributions of nature. With no market for wild honeybees, for example, their value is unimportant and wild bees are forgotten. In their place have come monoculture crops, whose market value comes from plowing up habitat that wild bee populations need to survive.

A market society does not question how intensive food production has changed rural America, whose local businesses have crumbled and whose educational opportunities have dried up. A market society goes along with a seed industry controlled by three multinationals, whose obligation is to their shareholders, not to present and future generations. In a market society, farmers, ranchers, and farm laborers (along with fishermen and foresters) have a higher rate of suicide than do other occupational groups in America.

Our Achilles heel from becoming a market society is how its financial rewards ruthlessly reinforce what people want to value—all the while ignoring irrevocable laws of nature. No matter who controls the market or holds the most money, food is and will always be a product of the environment. The evidence is all around us. For good reasons, corn is never grown in Death Valley and banana plantations are not found in Alaska. This seems like an obvious point, yet it is one we ignore every day. As we will cover in the next three chapters of the book, this oversight comes at a cost. The consequences of our grand food bargain never stop, no matter how much Americans pretend otherwise.

PART III

UNEXPECTED CONSEQUENCES

Chapter 8

The World's Safest Food

The US enjoys one of the world's safest food supplies.
— FDA, USDA, NOAA Joint Statement on Food Safety

He was a soldier's soldier. A career military man who embodied toughness and grit. So when President Polk feared that war might erupt with Mexico over America's annexation of Texas, he knew just who to send to defend the border—General Zachary Taylor. Known by his men as "Old Rough and Ready," Taylor had no hesitation leading his army against forces more than three times larger. Not satisfied with driving Mexican troops out of Texas, he defied orders and marched his troops well south of the border, leveling a crushing blow that ended Mexico's claims over what is now the American Southwest.

Overnight, Taylor had become an American hero. As his popularity soared, citizens pushed him to run for president. Although Taylor had no interest in pursuing political office, let alone the presidency, he was eventually persuaded otherwise. On March 4, 1849, General Zachary Taylor became President Zachary Taylor. Sixteen months later, he found himself in another war, this one waged from within by an adversary too small to see, yet too powerful to be defeated.

The battle began on Independence Day, 1850, with heat so stifling, it was said, that only flies and insects were out in force, taking advantage of the capital's primitive water and sewage infrastructure. Taylor's packed schedule began with a Sunday school recital. At the future site of the Washington Monument, he spent much of the afternoon under the hot sun while speechifying politicians rambled on to commemorate the occasion.

Upon returning to the White House, he purportedly ate cherries in iced milk. A few hours later, he fell ill with nausea and cramps. Believing he could tough it out, Taylor initially refused the medicine offered by his physician. Five days later, Old Rough and Ready was dead. The cause of death was listed as *cholera morbus*, which we know today as viral gastroenteritis or stomach flu—the result of ingesting unsafe food or liquid.

Another half century would go by before public consciousness that microscopic organisms might be lurking about in food would catalyze action. Behaviors did not change overnight. Old beliefs that disease could emanate spontaneously (arise from anything, even out of thin air) persisted. Understanding of disease transmission in food lagged. And the risk of illness (and possibly death) needed to outweigh purported claims that food would become unaffordable. Until then, people accepted his death as a tragic event, then carried on preparing food following familial, religious, and cultural traditions practiced over hundreds of generations.

My mother inherited some of those traditions from her mother. My mother's command of the kitchen had no equal. She seldom looked at a recipe or opened a cookbook. Multiple measuring spoons and cups got in her way. She knew the ingredient proportions and when to add them. Dialing up the correct temperature on the oven or stovetop was second nature, as was her keen sense of when bread, a casserole, or a pot roast was ready. Her ease in preparing food allowed our family to take her skills for granted. Later in her life, I tried to coax out details on how to prepare some of my favorite dishes. My questions flummoxed her—why couldn't I see what to her was so obvious?

Yet when canning season began toward the end of summer, she pulled out a well-worn set of index cards with specific directions. For the next several weeks, she filled a pantry about half the size of the kitchen with everything from dill pickles to apricot jam. Unlike the rest of the year, when her mastery of the kitchen seemed effortless, now her movements were fastidious, her measurements exacting, her attention toward two well-used pressure cookers unwavering.

Between the daily tasks of rewashing last year's bottles, snapping green beans, and peeling peaches, she constantly referenced her notes and kept an eagle eye on temperature and time. As she removed the lid of the hot cooker and lifted out each bottle using tongs, she carefully wiped away the water, then placed each one upside down as an added measure. After the bottles had cooled, she re-inspected each for air bubbles. The occasional one that failed to meet her standards never made it to the pantry.

Those dog-eared index cards that my mother checked and rechecked contained specific safe-canning protocols, her safeguards against real threats such as botulism, a bacterium whose spores produce one of the deadliest toxins ever linked with food. She understood what was at stake. Her vigilance was our protection that the food we ate was safe.

Long hours of toiling in the kitchen were part of the daily rhythm. Farm life also meant that, each spring, freshly turned soil was prepared and furrows were marked off for planting tomato and strawberry seedlings. Rows of vegetables like cucumbers, sweet corn, varieties of squash, and beans were also sown. A few short months later, the harvesting began and continued until ground covers placed at night no longer protected the last remaining vegetables from autumn's frost.

Our farm was reminiscent of an earlier era. Step back in time to a fledgling nation when most people produced and prepared the food they ate and farm life dominated an entire economy. As the harvests rolled in, attention turned toward preservation and preparation. From past traditions and their own experiences, they learned how inadequate cooking or ill-conceived shortcuts sometimes had real consequences—including death. Passing along fundamental safe-food-handling skills to counter often unknown microscopic organisms, toxins, and physical impurities was a matter of survival.

Yet as the modern food system gradually took over American life, generationally transmitted lessons, culinary practices, and cultural expectations changed. Consumers turned their attention toward ready availability and affordability. Food providers, at least some of them, saw an opening to make more money by adulterating the food they were selling.

Cottonseed oil was added to butter and lard. Sawdust, coconut shells, rice bran, and other foreign substances were mixed into spices. Metallic additives and poisonous colorings were blended into candies. Cane syrup and glucose were put into honey. Brick, sand, copper, and gypsum dust showed up in tea. And poisonous preservatives were added to meats and meat products, including "embalmed meat" sent to soldiers during the Spanish–American War.

In the 1870s, a "pure-food" movement of consumers and scientists petitioned Congress to pass laws requiring that all ingredients be disclosed. When well-connected food manufacturers convinced Congress to ignore the outcry, the movement organized an exhibition of over two thousand adulterated products collected from every state, each with a label listing their contents as verified by independent chemists. Unfazed, food manufacturers argued that the questionable additives were actually preservatives and should remain outside the government's purview.

Ridding the modern food system of adulterants was not the only challenge. The "Beef Trust" (the cartel of meat processors that pooled their stocks into trusts and acted as a single business) had built an empire that extended well beyond meat packinghouses to include thousands of refrigerated railcars, warehouses, and fruit and vegetable canneries. If growers wanted to ship fresh produce from California to the East Coast, they needed to do business with the Beef Trust. Meanwhile, just as food prices were going up, industrial magnates were raising the prices of other essentials like energy and steel. Taken together, such business practices stoked social unrest and provoked calls for reform.

At the same time, knowledge of "germ theory"—microscopic organisms too small to see but capable of invading humans and causing disease—was itself spreading across America. Articles in the press seized on germ theory to suggest that unprincipled practices by large companies were fomenting illness and death. Attention zeroed in on the unsanitary conditions inside Chicago's meatpacking plants. But two government-sponsored investigations and articles in *The Lancet*, the respected British medical journal, went nowhere. Not until Upton Sinclair's novel *The*

Jungle and President Theodore Roosevelt's own probe and his forceful use of the "bully pulpit" was Congress cajoled into action.

In 1906, Congress passed two laws to address food safety from different perspectives. In one, manufacturers were to be held responsible for ensuring that adulterants were not added to food. To make sure they complied, products were pulled from store shelves, tested, and verified. Violations could result in fines and possible imprisonment. The agency in charge was the predecessor to today's US Food and Drug Administration (FDA).

The other new law took a different tack. Instead of putting the meatpacking plants in charge of compliance, government inspectors were responsible for rooting out contaminants. Their criteria: "meat and meat food products which are unsound, unhealthful, unwholesome, or otherwise unfit for human food." Their leverage: if the government refused to inspect meat, the plant could no longer operate. Already displeased with the government's approach, meatpacking companies secured a provision requiring taxpayers to pay for inspection.

Having public officials inspect and approve meat for sale took companies off the hook. But the outcome set up an unending battle to limit government oversight in determining what is safe—a battle that continues to this day. The agency in charge became the USDA Food Safety Inspection Service (FSIS).

My immersion into public food safety practices began at USDA with a novel bovine disease that scientists called *bovine spongiform encephalopathy*, which had appeared in 1996 in Great Britain. Because it's not a name that easily rolls off the tongue, journalists had promptly dubbed it "mad cow disease," setting up endless satire but also heightened fear.

As the epidemic spread across Britain, anxiety was building on this side of the pond as well. I was asked to lead a study addressing whether the disease would land on American shores and, if so, where it would first show up. To better assess the full impact and to interact with scientists on the front line, a few of us traveled to England.

Observing the outbreak firsthand, I saw the public's raw reactions to perceived threats outside their control. Demand for beef had plummeted despite expert belief at the time that beef could be eaten safely. To buoy public trust, the minister of agriculture invited camera crews to record him and his four-year-old daughter eating hamburgers. Only later was it discovered that beef muscle containing small bits of central nervous system tissues posed a risk to health—231 individuals in twelve countries were eventually infected and later died.

For me, a widespread foodborne threat that lacked a straightforward explanation and resolution was cause for serious concern. It was fundamentally different from the stories I'd heard while growing up of individuals falling ill at a church supper or neighborhood gathering. There, it was easier to pinpoint the offender—foods like deviled eggs or potato salad that were not properly refrigerated, allowing harmful bacteria to multiply. These were isolated incidents that affected a small number of people and never made the national evening news.

Several months after the mad cow disease risk assessment was completed, I was handed another assignment for our small center in Colorado— *Escherichia coli* O157:H7 (*E. coli*) in cattle. This time we were asking where the contaminated ground beef was coming from and being distributed.

The assignment was prompted by a foodborne outbreak particularly devastating to children. The problem first appeared in Washington State, where parents had fed their children hamburgers from Jack in the Box restaurants. Some of those children had ended up in hospitals. Unlike foodborne outbreaks confined to a unique local source, this one had spread across the Pacific Northwest. More than seven hundred people were affected, four children died, and at least 178 others suffered permanent kidney or brain damage.

The pathogen was identified as *E. coli*, a bacteria benign to cattle. Somewhere between the slaughter of cows and the preparation of hamburgers, *E. coli* had found safe passage from the guts of cattle to those of people. When not repelled by the stomach's acid, it quickly multiplied. Otherwise healthy individuals experienced nausea, vomiting, cramping, and severe pain, but generally recovered within a few days.

For young children, older adults, or anyone whose immune system was less than robust, the invasion could turn deadly. The bacteria tore apart cells in the intestine, streamed into the circulatory system, blocked kidneys from functioning, attacked other major organs, induced stroke, and sometimes resulted in death. Hospital staff could only manage the symptoms. If the patient survived, the pathogen sometimes left behind permanent brain damage, paralysis, epilepsy, or kidney damage requiring dialysis.

Yet what happened was preventable. A year before the outbreak, Washington State had issued new regulations requiring that meat patties be cooked to 155 degrees—fifteen degrees higher than federal rules called for. A few months afterward, a restaurant shift leader faxed a suggestion form to corporate headquarters stating, "I think regular patties should cook longer. They don't get done and we have customer complaints." The company headquarters acknowledged receipt of the fax, but longer cooking time meant longer preparation time per burger. The suggestion was ignored, as was the state's cooking-temperature regulation. Profit was a function of volume, which went up with the number of burgers sold per grill.

As news of the outbreak unfolded nationwide, an angry public clamored for an investigation. Those responsible had to be punished. The discovery of multiple violations by Jack in the Box substantiated their negligence. Congressional hearings, trials, and lawsuits followed. Ironically, many of those infected had eaten the deeply discounted "Monster Burger" special, sold with the slogan "So good, it's scary!"

In their defense, Jack in the Box pointed out that *E. coli* came from cattle on farms whose meat and bacteria passed through multiple slaughter and processing plants. What had happened was a modern food system failure. But shifting attention to systematic causes was too great a reach. The public had fingered Jack in the Box—whose own admissions left them holding the smoking gun.

For some of us, the outbreak underscored a new reality: as large agribusinesses and food companies expanded geographically, widespread outbreaks were sure to follow. While consumers were eating individual hamburgers, the meat it was made from could have included culled dairy cows in Wisconsin, feedlot steers in Colorado, coarse meat grind from Texas, and imported meat scraps from Australia, Canada, or Latin America. Based on price and buyers' specifications, different combinations of trimmings and coarse grind were being moved around the country in two-thousand-pound "combo bins" before being fabricated into patties. The efficiency of the ground-beef system was offset by the reality that the meat and fat in any one hamburger could not be tracked.

While the Jack in the Box outbreak had captured the public's attention, it was not the first widespread occurrence tied to *E. coli*. A decade earlier, the *New England Journal of Medicine* reported a rare serotype of *E. coli* identified in two outbreaks in two different states. This time the restaurant chain was McDonald's, and the states were Oregon and Michigan. The rare serotype was O157:H7. Its implication for future widespread outbreaks garnered little attention.

As we prepared our report, the question I mulled over was what that future would look like. The number of beef cattle on large feedlots had increased by over 50 percent in one decade. The dairy industry was likewise consolidating. The odds of finding *E. coli* on any livestock operation increased with herd size and samples taken. Beef scraps were arriving from overseas. Bins of fat and protein were crisscrossing the country. Ground beef profitability came through volume. And consumers were eating more food prepared outside the home. All these trends were sure to continue. Then the realization set in: the system that made products like ground beef so readily available also served double duty as a superhighway disseminating pathogens farther and faster.

Well into my adult years, I was pretty much impregnable to microscopic threats—or so I thought. I had a strong constitution from good genetics and hard work on the farm. Very seldom was I ever under the weather. For several years I had been living in Costa Rica and traveling throughout the Americas, as well as many parts of Africa, Asia, and Europe, without any memorable bouts of foodborne illness.

At one point, I traveled to Colorado with plans to rendezvous with my daughter Tamara, who was now on her own, working near Denver. We were to meet that evening at a friend's home outside Fort Collins. Arriving in the afternoon, I met my friends and another couple at a restaurant in Fort Collins. When we finished dinner, Monty tossed me the keys to their home and said they would be along later.

As I drove along country roads, I began to feel an uncomfortable pain in my gut, accompanied by slight nausea. Instead of subsiding, the pain intensified, as if I were being stabbed. Gritting my teeth, I willed myself the last few miles and pulled into their driveway. As I struggled to the porch, my cellphone rang. While trying to answer the phone, fumble with keys, and open the front door, I lost consciousness.

What happened next still seems surreal. I remembered staring across the concrete porch with its brick edging. Nearby were my crumpled eyeglasses. One side of my face stung from hitting the concrete. I had no strength to move. I heard a faint voice calling my name, but several moments passed before I recognized it was Tamara imploring me to pick up the phone. I mumbled a response but could not locate the phone, which had fallen beyond my line of sight.

She kept talking, trying to keep me awake to ask my location and call for help. As she spoke, the cloudiness slowly lifted. I remembered where I was and noticed I was bleeding. After a couple of minutes, I managed to lift my head. Before falling, I had unlocked the door. Mustering what strength I could, I staggered to the bathroom for an experience I hope to never repeat or even describe. When Monty and Jeanice arrived, the worst was over. They found me lying on the floor, too exhausted to move. Never before had I felt so helpless and vulnerable. Still weak, I handed the phone to Monty and drifted into sleep.

A week went by before all my strength had returned. When I reported the event to the county's public health office, they jotted down my information and said they would call, but they never did. No one else in our group fell ill. As is the case with most foodborne illness events with no medical follow-up, an etiologic agent was never identified. Wanting to put the whole incident behind me, I let it go. After no recallable foodborne illnesses until then, I experienced two additional bouts in the next three years—all in the United States.

Nowadays, we know more about food-related threats than ever before. As human populations have increased, microscopic organisms that see us as food (or vacation destinations) have also proliferated. As the modern food system became part of our surroundings, pathogens did likewise. With millions if not billions of years of adaptation, they were not about to roll over and go extinct.

Starting long before people appeared on Earth, the sole objective of microbes (and other living organisms) has always been to conquer any obstacles that threaten their survival. In the pathogens' world, time is meaningless, natural selection is eternal, and the modern food system has become an ally to help them invade and reproduce. Even though their actions can take us out, thereby depriving themselves of a suitable host, they continue to march on. What we call "advances in science to thwart microbes" are nothing more than temporary detours.

In the aptly titled *Bad Bug Book*, FDA describes the most common and dangerous foodborne pathogens. Start with *E. coli* (O157:H7), which became an ominous threat for humans by picking up the genes to produce the deadly Shiga toxin. As few as ten to one hundred organisms can induce infection (ten thousand are needed to fill the head of pin). Over time, the spores of the extremely potent neurotoxin known as botulism (*Clostridium botulinum*) adapted to be heat-resistant and to thrive in low-oxygen environments like canned foods. *Listeria* evolved to be tolerant of cold temperatures and salty environments. Some natural toxins found in fish, shellfish, and mushrooms can linger in food despite washing, cooking, and freezing.

Among major pathogens in America, the most lethal bacteria is *Listeria*. The one most likely to send you to the hospital is *Salmonella*. As bacteria and parasites go, the number of *Salmonella* cases exceed all others combined.

Another pathogen likely to invite itself inside your body is the norovirus. Vomiting, diarrhea, fever, and stomach cramps announce that you are its latest residence and food source. Over a lifetime, expect it to drop in about five times, each episode accompanied with varying severity. Norovirus travels through food, water, contaminated surfaces, and contact with infected individuals. Exceedingly opportunistic and hard to eliminate, norovirus hangs out in places serving food—restaurants, hospitals, and cruise ships. It is the leading foodborne cause of illness, and outbreaks in the United States infecting some nineteen to twenty-one million people each year.

Overall, between twenty-nine to seventy-one million foodborne illnesses occur annually, which works out to be about three-quarters of the population of California on the low end, or the population of the thirteen Western states plus one-fifth of Texas on the high end. Of those infected, 63,000 to 216,000 require hospitalization. Between 1,500 and 5,000 ultimately die.

For a country like the United States, rich in technology and fortitude, such imprecise estimates of illness, hospitalization, and death are one indicator of the priority accorded food safety. Another is disparate, century-old laws that still serve as the main tools of national action. As the country's population increased, the modern food system went global. Food imports shot upward and widespread outbreaks became common. Congress responded not by rethinking its approach in light of underlying trends, but by tacking on ad hoc, makeshift additional laws and calling for new regulations on top of what already existed. What Congress has never done is set out to design a food safety system that matches the complexity and scope of the globally expanding modern food system. Their approach has always been a patchwork.

It's no surprise that this mess of laws and rules is, as Marion Nestle describes, "breathtaking in its irrationality." Formally, it is cobbled together using twelve to fifteen different agencies, thirty to thirty-five separate laws, and more than fifty interagency agreements. Informally, it requires extraordinary efforts of time, communication, and coordination. Food safety in America is held together using the policy equivalent of baling wire and duct tape.

The food-safety legal system's inequities begin with its two main agencies, FSIS and FDA. FSIS is responsible for 10–20 percent of the food supply, but has traditionally received 60 percent of the two agencies' combined food-safety budget. FDA is responsible for 80–90 percent of the food supply, but has operated with one-third the staff.

Disparities are also found at the state level—often the front line in responding to foodborne outbreaks. Over a ten-year period, Minnesota investigated and resolved 267 separate state-level foodborne outbreaks. During the same time frame, Texas, with five times the population, resolved eighteen cases.

Over the last three decades, demands on FDA have shot up, staff levels have declined, and funding has remained erratic. In 2007, the agency oversaw imports of fifteen million lines of products. A decade later, the number had increased to forty million. In addition to a greater number of outbreaks, the outbreaks were more widespread. Included in these trends were nationwide cases found to involve egregious criminal fraud leading to a half-billion eggs needing to be recalled, and pathogen-tainted peanuts knowingly shipped to forty-six states. By 2010, public confidence was sufficiently shaken that Congress was finally forced to act.

As had happened before, the National Academies and the Government Accountability Office pushed for a single agency. "The time had come to modernize the nation's food safety system," said a National Academies report, recommending that "the federal government move toward the establishment of a single food safety agency." Instead, in 2011 Congress tacked on another law, the Food Safety Modernization Act (FSMA), by which FDA's newest mandate was to stop reacting to problems by preventing them from ever occurring in the first place.

The act was touted as "a sea change for food safety in America" that would bring about "sweeping improvements to the security and safety of our nation's food supply." Others said it was historic, the first time in "more than seventy years since our nation's food safety regime was overhauled top to bottom." The senator authoring the bill remarked that "the FDA finally has all the tools it needs to ensure the food on dinner tables and store shelves is safe."

Well, not quite. Congress's own budget office said that the FDA needed an additional $1.4 billion for implementation over the next five years. Instead, the bill was enacted as an unfunded mandate. FDA still needed to convince Congress that more money was needed.

At FSMA's core was an expectation that growers, processors, manufacturers, importers, transporters, retailers, etc. would voluntarily implement what FDA mandated. Meanwhile, as FDA was preparing new comprehensive standards, the agency was still expected to provide oversight and technical support, ensure compliance, strengthen the global food-safety system, enhance protection of public health, deliver training, serve as a repository of science and expertise, provide leadership for innovation and action, ensure that firms are consistently implementing effective prevention systems, enhance partnerships with states and other government counterparts, build robust data integration and analysis systems along with information-sharing mechanisms, significantly expand its inspection and surveillance tools to include a wider range of inspection including sampling, testing, and other data-collection activities, and—as always—respond when food-related problems and outbreaks emerged.

Openly acknowledging that it had neither the funding nor staffing "to provide the elevated assurances of food safety envisioned by FSMA," FDA reaffirmed that it would rely on voluntary compliance, and on technology to identify possible violations, and on third parties for inspection. Consumers had demanded a robust governmental response to food-safety concerns; what they got instead was FDA deputizing foreign governments and private businesses to act on their behalf.

The USDA Food Safety Inspection Service, on the other hand, was beset with its own challenges. FSIS had been created over a century ago, before society fully understood how meat could harbor pathogens, but after the meat industry had already locked itself into a high-volume, assembly-line way of conducting business. Inserting government inspectors into the processing line, with the job of evaluating each carcass through sight, smell, and touch, immediately caused friction if companies were unable to increase line speed, or worse yet, had to slow the line down.

A century later, while working on *E. coli*, I would see how line speed was still sacrosanct. While I had been inside abattoirs before, I had never witnessed one that slaughtered up to five thousand cattle each day. Arriving well before dawn with two other colleagues, we entered a massive, windowless concrete building and walked long cement corridors alongside workers coming on shift. In the changing room we were outfitted with ear plugs, hairnets, hard hats, safety glasses, white smocks, and knee-high rubber boots, then escorted to where the line began. As expected, blood was being splattered about, and the noise from motors, chains, and saws made it difficult to be heard.

The rear legs of warm, freshly killed cattle were shackled to the overhead line that serpentined through the plant before exiting near the cold-storage lockers. Workers standing next to each other were draped in eight pounds of chain mail as protection against an errant knife or hook. Underneath the layers of safeguards were people who repeated the same repetitive task thousands of times for at least eight hours each day. Behind them were supervisors who walked back and forth, making sure their section of the line kept pace. Profitability was measured in volume, volume was measured in efficiency, and efficiency was measured by ensuring no worker slowed down the line. High rates of injury made meat-packing one of the most dangerous jobs. Whenever a worker was injured, a "floater" was quickly brought in as a replacement.

As we moved along, I watched workers synchronize their movements with a machine that peeled the hide from each carcass. Afterward, another person reached deep into the cavity and eviscerated the animal by cutting away the connective tissues without puncturing the viscera and spilling out its contents, which would contaminate the carcass. Other workers cut off the heads, split each carcass into halves and washed each with antimicrobials to neutralize fecal matter that may have landed on the meat.

A bit farther along, we watched as a different line wound around us carrying the suspended skulls. Then, without any warning, the power went out, engulfing us in darkness. We stood motionless in the sudden silence and stillness. Moments later, flashlights darted about and emergency exit lights blinked on in the distance. The light cast a long shadow across the line of cattle skulls, highlighting their red skeletal tissues, and illuminating their still-fibrillating eyeballs—twitching about, as if to remind us they were still alive.

As I stared into the darkness while maintenance workers were scrambling about, I realized why line speed meant everything. Once workers were at their duty stations, any line stoppage instantly cut into profits. But the opposite was also true: increasing line speed beyond the break-even threshold was pure profit. For a plant turning out millions of pounds of finished beef each day, the connection between pushing workers to do more and higher returns was obvious. I understood why volume was idolized, why line speed had continually been ratcheted up over time, and why who determines whether or not meat is safe had always been problematic.

FSIS's mandate includes "assuring that meat and meat food products are wholesome, *not adulterated*, and properly marked, labeled, and packaged" [italics added]. For nine decades, meatpacking plants were inspected for hygiene and visible signs of disease. Even if meat was suspected of harboring pathogens, no one ever declared it was *adulterated*—until *E. coli* came along.

In 1994, a new FSIS administrator, Michael Taylor, announced at a meat industry convention that the agency was not meeting the public's expectations. Henceforward, *E. coli* in ground beef would be considered an adulterant—making its sale illegal. With some eight billion pounds of ground beef produced annually, the industry sued. But FSIS was prepared, and the courts upheld the new standard; a new benchmark for food safety had been established.

Two-plus decades later, *E. coli* (O157:H7 and six closely related serotypes) remain the only pathogenic microbes still considered adulterants in food—and only if they are found in ground beef. Companies have increased processing line speeds to as much as 10,500 poultry birds, 1,300 hogs, and 390 cattle per hour. Determining what is safe has shifted toward controlling potential hazards. Instead of the government, FSIS has adopted programs where companies themselves now assume more inspection and testing responsibilities for pathogens.

One such FSIS program for hogs promised to demonstrate that increasing line speed did not compromise food safety. Then, in 2013, USDA's Office of Inspector General took a closer look. The report pointed out that since the program's inception fifteen years earlier, no study had ever been conducted to determine whether food safety had measurably improved. Its auditors had inspected thirty plants, including one processing up to nineteen thousand hogs per day. The report found that "enforcement policies do not deter swine slaughter plants from becoming repeat violators of food safety regulations."

Each year, FSIS is responsible for safeguarding "the processing of more than 150.7 million livestock carcasses and 9.26 billion poultry carcasses." Printed on packages of meat products in supermarkets are the words "inspected for wholesomeness." What the label does not disclose, and consumers may not know, is that "wholesomeness" does not mean free of pathogens.

In a perfect world, meat ready for purchase would be free of pathogens. Some strains of *Salmonella*, for example, are highly antibiotic-resistant. But because we do not live in a perfect world, and the risk of foodborne illness is always present, what is permissible within products sold to consumers is important.

Several years ago, the European Union identified *Salmonella* as a systemic threat across their food system. Reducing its prevalence became a priority. In 2016, *Salmonella* was found in 6.4 percent of some 25,000 samples taken from processing plants or retail outlets. In America, what is permissible is set by FSIS. For packaged poultry parts, 15.4 percent of packages can contain *Salmonella*. For ground poultry, the cutoff is 25 percent. With good reason, FSIS advises consumers to *not* rinse raw chicken, as the bacteria splashing about can contaminate other foods and kitchen surfaces.

This is a good moment to check in on who benefits from our grand food bargain. Yes, consumers are getting more food for less effort, as is clear from our growing waistlines and the money we spend on prepared food. But food providers are benefiting as well, not just by producing and delivering more food on a larger scale but also through global consolidation. As they become larger, their influence over countries, their regulations, and how markets operate has grown.

This makes comprehensive food-safety oversight across the entire food system even more important. In the European Union with its twenty-eight countries and differences in culture, language, and levels of economic development, food-safety oversight is led through one agency. In the United States, oversight is a fragmented combination of laws and regulations spread across multiple agencies with different underlying missions. Calls for a single food-safety agency, by the government's own accountability office, continue to be ignored by Congress.

Why? What might appear to be broken to some, works perfectly well for others. Establishing a unified agency could jeopardize the leverage food providers have over how laws and regulations are passed (or not passed) and enforced (or not enforced).

The existing approach, which muddles who decides whether food is safe, provides room to cut costs and increase profits. At one time, the meatpacking industry afforded a respectable blue-collar middle-class lifestyle, paying more than most other manufacturing jobs. Meat packers were a proud and highly visible segment of the American food-production system. The National Football League's Green Bay Packers, for example, took their name from the Acme [Meat] Packing Company. In the 1980s, the meat industry successfully broke the union hold on meat workers. Shifting to immigrant laborers, who went along with approved higher line speeds with few complaints about working conditions, allowed companies to cut hourly compensation by almost one-half.

Food providers have also profited by steering toward more imports. Benefits of trade are commonly sold to the public in terms of reciprocal benefits—for instance, Central America ships bananas while the United States sends walnuts. The 1970s and '80s was an era of global expansion through trade and promised prosperity. So-called free-trade agreements encouraged the outsourcing of entire food product lines because off-shore labor costs were lower.

In recent decades, much of America's food imports are "value-added products," owing to additional processing or related services. Food imports are growing faster than are exports because value-added products take advantage of cheaper offshore labor, ingredients, and other production factors. Over 90 percent of the seafood consumed in the United States is now imported, though most is caught by American fisherman, exported to Asia for processing, then shipped back to the United States.

For domestic meat slaughter and processing, the largest operating expense is labor. Though it was cut by half through mostly immigrant labor, by 2016 average meatpacking wages had crept up to $13 per hour. By comparison, hourly compensation in China in 2016 was $3.60, a difference of $9.40 per worker per hour.

In 2013, FSIS representatives traveled to China to determine whether food-safety practices in four Chinese plants were equivalent to United States standards. A positive finding would mean that chickens raised in the United States could be eviscerated, frozen, shipped to China, processed into parts, and reshipped as cooked product to the United States. (Because China is not recognized as free of two poultry diseases, shipping uncooked poultry to the United States is not allowed.)

When questioned about using Chinese labor to increase profits, a spokesperson for the National Chicken Council scoffed at the idea, saying, "Economically, it doesn't make much sense. . . . I don't know how anyone could make a profit doing that." In 2016, FSIS ruled that China's poultry processing was equivalent to that of the United States. The new approach could begin. A year later, Qingdao Nine-Alliance Group of China, one of the largest privately owned chicken companies in China, claimed to be the first. No country of origin label was required.

So what does trade have to do with food safety? Much of the trade among 164 countries is governed through some thirty separate agreements that countries have negotiated. The World Trade Organization (WTO) facilitates the execution of these agreements, though countries themselves are the ones providing the WTO's leadership, decisions, and resolutions.

One agreement ties international trade to health. The Agreement on the Application of Sanitary and Phytosanitary Measures (SPS) affirms that countries have the right to take "measures necessary for the protection of human, animal, or plant life or health." To avoid the influence of politics, measures should be scientifically justified.

For many years, I have worked with expert professionals within the WTO and officials from developing countries on the implementation of this one agreement, which specifically affirms the priority of science and the rights of each country. When it comes to animal, plant, and human health and trade, the role of science is crucial.

Throughout this chapter, I have repeatedly referred to who determines whether food is safe. This was intentional, typical of how we think— but also a bit misleading. Every time we take food in, we are accepting a risk. The risks vary depending on the food, but they never disappear altogether.

A more appropriate question may be, Who decides what those risks will be? The common response is letting scientists tell us. But that answer takes us down the wrong track. What science does well is informing us about what pathogens, chemicals, or other impurities may be present in food, based on our expectations for precision.

Thus, the answers science provides are relative, not absolute. Living with absolute answers would rule out eating many foods, and many other foods would be made unaffordable. In other words, while science is good at informing, deciding what is safe is our job as a society. Food safety really comes down to what consumers demand of their government. When those demands are unspoken or unheeded, others insert themselves, with their own criteria, to decide for us.

The results are unnecessary acute illness and sometimes death. In 2013, an outbreak of *Salmonella* started on the West Coast and spread to twenty-nine states and Puerto Rico. All the government's epidemiologic evidence pointed to a Foster Farms poultry processing plant in California. But because *Salmonella* has never been declared an adulterant, and before FSIS would take regulatory action, the agency wanted a perfect genetic match linking the specific plant to *Salmonella* in an infected consumer who ate poultry coming from that plant.

So public funding for scientists and investigators were poured into finding a consumer sick enough to report their illness, but who had kept uneaten product and its label. Eighteen months and an estimated 18,400 illnesses after the outbreak began, a genetic match was found, confirming the earlier evidence.

In June 2017, FSIS proposed that China be allowed to export chickens, ducks, and turkeys *it* raises. Inspection of products after arriving in the United States would be at the discretion of FSIS. What is decided in one meat sector can guide what happens in another. Smithfield Foods, you will recall, is a Chinese company that controls one of every four pork products retailed in the United States. Their influence with the pork industry's trade association, the National Pork Producers' Council, cannot be overstated. To no one's surprise, the president of the NPPC wrote in favor of the rule.

In 2018, FSIS proposed a voluntary inspection system for pork. Under the arrangement, slaughter plants would determine which foodborne pathogens to monitor. Per the USDA acting deputy undersecretary, "We would be removing the generic *E. coli* (testing) requirement and really allowing establishments to choose what they want to sample for." Also, she went on, in an effort to "remove unnecessary regulatory obstacles to innovation," plants could operate at whatever line speed they wanted.

The presence of pathogens in meat belies a larger issue: what is sitting in supermarket display cases—as well as home and restaurant refrigerators—is not always safe to eat without consumers taking added precautions. Industry-friendly regulations put the onus on consumers to mop up risks while companies reap the profits.

Industry-friendly regulations also apply to FDA. The food industry overwhelmingly pushed for passage of the Food Safety Modernization Act, which gave the agency more responsibility to make sure that preventative practices were working. The new mandates, however, required additional funding and staffing. When little was provided, the food industry went silent. Adding responsibilities only exacerbated chronic funding and staffing shortages.

Meanwhile, the mandates have not gone away. In the agency's own words: "Hundreds of thousands of growers and processors worldwide are producing food for the US market . . . and making millions of decisions every day that affect food safety." Imports arrive from some two hundred different countries, mostly less economically advanced countries. Around 70 percent are processed food products. Only about 1 percent of imported food is examined, which can range from a closer inspection of the manifest to a quick visual check of the product to dispatching samples for laboratory analysis.

More recently, the agency's inability to execute effective food recalls has come under harsh criticism from the Office of the Inspector General. Sampling thirty recalls from 1,557 cases over thirty-two months revealed systemic deficiencies in evaluating health hazards, carrying out audits, ensuring compliance where recalls were initiated, tracking, and maintaining accurate recall data.

FDA's challenge is to prove that the 2011 FSMA law isn't compromising public health. So far, they can't. My experience with scientists and regulators is that they take their responsibilities seriously. But when working in a fragmented system that is dogged by funding and staffing limits even while being handed more mandates, they resort to practicing triage.

Outbreaks serious enough to show up on the national public radar receive high priority. Resources are found and investigations follow. But overreliance on back-end responses presumes that foodborne risks are accidental and transitory, akin to being in the wrong place at the wrong time. In reality, other outbreaks are also occurring—we just don't know about them.

Ideally, no triage should be necessary. Providers and consumers should have the same understanding of whether food is safe. The national food safety system would be as agile and advanced as the underlying food production system. Standards of food safety would not be contested trade-offs between individual health and corporate profitability. Foodborne outbreaks would become less and less frequent.

As is, when an outbreak is severe enough to grab the national spotlight, a government official often assures the public that "The US food supply remains one of the safest in the world." My first reaction is always: Compared to what? Burkina Faso in Africa? Probably so. Similar countries in Western Europe? I have my doubts, unless some substantiated data somewhere exists. Notwithstanding different opinions, saying America's food supply is safe implies there is little to improve on—as if to say this latest outbreak was an aberration, a circuit breaker that momentarily tripped, but remain calm as power will be restored shortly.

One of the biggest threats to food safety is surrendering to the fact of widespread foodborne outbreaks as an everyday part of life. In 2002, there were eight multi-state outbreaks. In 2016, the number had jumped to thirty-eight—more than three per month. Foodborne outbreaks are less and less front-page news. Were the Jack in the Box outbreak to occur today, would the public be sufficiently enraged to redefine what was safe?

Whether we as consumers will accept the charge to establish what is safe remains an open question. It's worth asking ourselves: What are we willing to pay for? The lion's share of food safety expenditures are channeled to FDA and FSIS. In 2016, their combined food-safety appropriations, including user fees, were just over two billion dollars—almost three hundred times less than what was spent on national defense. Or, looking at it another way, for every hundred dollars in food expenditures, taxpayers anted up around fifteen cents for food safety.

Over a century ago, outraged Americans demanded that their government intercede to ensure that the food they purchased was safe to eat. But wealthy, politically influential food manufacturers resisted. In the end, consumer indignation and an emboldened president prevailed. Today, multinational food companies are larger and more consolidated than those of the antitrust era. They are well financed, technologically sophisticated, globally connected, business-savvy, and politically astute.

They do not turn a blind eye to food safety. Within their immense scale of operations, they can deploy sensors, conduct testing, and implement food-safety practices. Having to deal with foodborne outbreaks is not good for business—but neither is not meeting growth and profitability expectations.

For many, chasing biological, chemical, and physical hazards can resemble fighting an imaginary foe. As one food-safety veteran of nearly forty years with the same company told me, the priority that management assigned to food safety cycled up and down. When the issues were unavoidable, investments were made in technology, processes, and people. As time went on, their importance was forgotten and food-safety expenditures were cut in the name of profitability, which eventually triggered a new cycle. When risks seem low, he said, it's easy to forget the need for sustained vigilance.

Ultimately, it's up to consumers to decide whether or not food safety is important. Walking away by leaving our oversight to what others decide is a sure way to lock us into more of the same.

Chapter 9

The Perfect Formula

People in this country eat what is set before them, asking no questions for economy's sake provided it suits their taste. We are a generation of sugar and fat eaters. The one-sidedness of our dietary is a result of the one-sidedness of our agricultural production.

— W. O. Atwater, 1891

I was twelve years old the first time I stepped inside a restaurant. The waitress asked if I wanted "soup or salad," but I heard "super salad" and said yes. She repeated the question twice more; each time I responded affirmatively. Once he stopped laughing, my neighbor, who had invited me there, translated.

Five years later, the first all-you-can-eat buffet restaurant opened two towns away. For a set price, one could chow down on deep-fried battered chicken, cuts of roast beef, heavy creamed soups, and decadent deserts. From eating out, I was learning that proper nutrition was something people preached but not necessarily practiced.

Two decades later, while working for USDA, I was invited to Washington, DC, to learn more about the origin and execution of food and agriculture policies. Joining me were two dozen other professionals whose backgrounds spanned industry, government, and academia. One was Laura Sims, at that time dean at the University of Maryland and former administrator of the Human Nutrition Information Service (HNIS) in USDA.

Laura's career in nutrition policy and mine in food production were at the opposite ends of the modern food system. One evening, we tried to identify a single program, task force, or individual that linked our two worlds together through USDA. She thought that the mission statement of USDA might do it, but it did not. The best we could come up with was the role played by the USDA secretary himself. Not surprisingly, what little I knew about nutrition policy was contained in USDA's Food Guide Pyramid.

Laura, on the other hand, had a bird's-eye view of the growing divide between nutrition and food production. Her small staff of mostly nutritionists had the Herculean task of preparing and promoting dietary guidance for American consumers, as required by law. Coming up with guidelines supported by science was the easy part. Navigating them through political landmines was quite another, especially if they hinted at reducing consumption of certain foods.

Aside from the politics, dietary guidelines needed to appeal to consumers, while also conveying the importance of variety and moderation. It was Laura's office that had researched and pilot-tested formats before settling on a food pyramid as the most effective way to reach consumers. Final layout and supporting text had been cleared internally within USDA. But on the eve of the food pyramid's release, a new secretary of agriculture yielded to the meat and dairy industry, which feared that demand for their products could decline. A last-minute decision to withhold release of the food pyramid made headline news.

Though Laura had returned to academia before the rollout, the secretary's decision did not surprise her. This was just the latest step in delegitimizing a nutrition policy that actually focused on health. The food pyramid message of moderation and variety was already outgunned by a well-funded modern food system bent on producing and selling more. Muted phrases like "use sparingly," "avoid too much sugar," or "eat a variety of foods" were already muzzled messages. Absent were candid calls to eat fewer foods high in fats, sugars, and salt.

The secretary's equivocating quickly became fodder for major newspapers. A year-long protracted David-versus-Goliath debate ensued—a small band of nutritionists adhering to science versus food producers with the political muscle to lean heavily on USDA. In the end, after purportedly spending a million dollars to improve the original pyramid design and description, a more politically palatable version was released.

At the time, I interpreted the outcome as typical Washington politics. Yet in my dismissiveness, I had overlooked the most crucial element—an ongoing pattern to block or at least water down nutrition policy whenever it threatened the grand food bargain. Without realizing it, most Americans were ceding their long-term health to a culture of more.

In the decades since, little has changed. When compared with sixteen peer countries, the United States is near the top in terms of wealth but near the bottom in terms of health. Per person, we spend more on health care and less on food. We also consume more calories per person than any other country. And we are dead last in chronic maladies like obesity, diabetes, and heart disease, the leading cause of death.

In the United States, almost seven out of ten adults are overweight, with more than half obese. One in three adults suffers from hypertension; 30 percent maintain high-risk cholesterol levels. An estimated one of three cancer deaths is linked to excess body weight, poor nutrition, or physical inactivity. Even those most likely attuned to nutrition—Caucasian, college-educated, upper-income, insured—are in worse health than their peers in other countries. The disconnect between nutrition and food production has not served America well.

Today's food system did not start out at odds with nutrition. Though the initial 1894 dietary recommendations never mentioned vitamins or minerals, the public already knew that citrus could prevent scurvy without knowing how. Nutrition science would later record the presence of vitamin C in citrus, the importance of minerals like iron to stem anemia, and the value of iodine to avert developmental disabilities like thyroid enlargement.

When vitamins like B1 (thiamine), B3 (niacin), C, and D were documented in specific foods, boosting consumption of foods containing these nutrients became a public health priority. Dietary recommendations included basic food groupings such as fruits and vegetables, cereals and grains. Diets consisting solely of corn or potatoes were deemed insufficient.

Meanwhile, the ability to produce more food than necessary was fast becoming food providers' biggest challenge. To boost consumption, producers touted the micronutrients in their foods as essential for optimal health and longevity. For a brief period of time, food providers and nutritionists were in alignment—eat more food of greater variety.

This alignment unraveled as additional research showed that all foods were not created nutritionally equal. As American diets fell below targets for key foods, new dietary recommendations specified the number of servings and serving sizes for each food group.

In the 1960s, amid the continuing struggle to rein in overproduction, many learned about hunger and malnutrition among low-income Americans. Public demand to tackle undernutrition in the Southeast and Appalachia provided an opening for simultaneously addressing diseases from overconsumption. But dietary advice that favored more whole grains, fruits, vegetables, and fish while reducing meat, eggs, and whole milk meant picking winners and losers.

Staunch opposition from farmers and food manufacturers quickly followed. The subsequent maneuvering marked a turning point— nutrition policy had become a political hotbed. To reduce backlash to forthcoming dietary guidelines, phrases such as "decrease consumption of meats" were scrubbed in favor of sterile reminders to "avoid too much fat, saturated fat, and cholesterol."

The fight over nutrition was a surrogate battle over the direction of the modern food system. Foods loaded with sugars and fats were no longer rare treats, but standard fare. Any recommendations to limit their intake was akin to throwing a wrench into a well-oiled gearbox designed to pump out more and more food.

The result has been malnutrition in all its forms—undernutrition, insufficient micronutrients, and obesity. In a paradox particular to the grand food bargain, overconsumption and malnutrition live side by side in America. It's all too common for fatty, sugary food to have almost zero nutrient value.

How did it come to this? One answer is that we broadened our definition of *food* to include anything edible, so long as it did not make us immediately sick. At one time, before the grand food bargain, nutrition and calories were two sides of the same coin. Today, we are awash in empty calories, and eating more no longer means eating better.

When I was a kid, each summer brought Strawberry Days, the celebration of what was once a viable farming enterprise in the valley. Residents from nearby towns gathered for the annual parade of floats, horses, fire trucks, and the Strawberry Days queen and her court. Afterward, farmers sold produce, especially large, juicy strawberries. Homemakers displayed crafts along with delectable home-baked pies and breads. The traveling carnival opened its amusement park rides and concession stands. But the feature attraction was always the rodeo.

For three nights, a professional rodeo circuit with bucking broncos, calf roping, bull riding, and clowns played to full bleachers of spectators. In the background, volunteers served up a steady stream of soda, hamburgers, hot dogs, french fries, ice cream, and candy bars.

For some reason, my father was always in charge of the two refreshment stands situated at opposite ends of the arena. Each night, while spectators filed out, I helped move unsold food and drink, grills, and ice chests to be kept in the larger of the two stands until the following evening. Because the stand was a simple wooden structure with minimum security, someone always needed to stay on the premises each night. As compensation, any food or drink consumed was on the house.

I desperately wanted to be that overnight person and experience the culinary euphoria of eating my fill of rodeo fare. Such food was not served at home, and its allure was too tempting. Notwithstanding my best lobbying efforts, the overnight vigil always fell to an older brother. I was "too young" became the patent answer. Undeterred, I bided my time and, while doing farm work, schemed about what I would do when my turn came.

Then one year, as we pulled onto the arena grounds to set up for the evening, I saw it—a newly built refreshment stand with brick walls, lockable metal doors, serving windows, and shutters. An overnight sentry was no longer needed. I slumped back in the seat saying nothing. When the rodeo ended, I went about moving food and supplies just as before. When finished, my father turned to me and asked if I would be willing to stay overnight—"just to make sure," he remarked. As long as the same benefits applied, I responded, count me in.

His parting instructions were to not burn the place down, and then he left. I waited a few minutes, half-expecting he would return, then fired up the grill. On tap for the evening was a full night of high-octane eating, one that did not include squash, green beans, tomatoes, corn, peaches, or cherries—foods I ate plenty of at home. My sights were on juicy cheeseburgers, hotdogs, candy bars, and ice cream. I would start by eating one of everything, including every kind of ice cream bar and every brand of candy bar. The second round would be similar. My father would be back in a matter of hours. Time was wasting.

My best-laid plan was a bust. The fatal flaw in my scheme was feeling satiated too quickly. I never made it through the first round. After a cheeseburger, hotdog, ice cream bar, and two candy bars, I felt stuffed. My body was not up to the task. So I cleaned the grill, stored everything away, and settled in for the night. When my father returned the following morning and asked how I fared, I recounted what happened. He wryly responded that I needed more practice.

The food I ate that night cost more than food I ate at home. In the future, rodeo fare would become cheaper per calorie than the fresh fruits and vegetables I took for granted. Fast-food restaurants would dominate the food landscape. Little did my father know how easy it would be to get more practice consuming unneeded calories.

As the modern food system was becoming more proficient in producing food and convincing people to eat more, medical science was busy reducing the incidence of infectious diseases and making procedures like open-heart bypass surgery common practice. With the spotlight on medical breakthroughs, it was easy to ignore how food and diet contributed to chronic ill-health and diminished life expectancy.

Not until 2001 did the surgeon general officially acknowledge America's national obesity epidemic. By then, chronic diseases were becoming a new cultural norm, though most people were reluctant to acknowledge it. Behind growing waistlines, vital organs like the heart and liver were being encased in morbid layers of fat.

Human genetics evolved when food was scarce and lots of energy from food was needed for daily physical activity. Getting enough calories was key to survival. But American culture wanted convenient food, with little physical effort to get it. Food manufacturers were all too happy to oblige, turning out rich processed foods with captivating tastes, textures, aromas, appearance, and even sound. Perfecting this formula was money in the bank. For consumers, meanwhile, learning not to succumb to overeating was becoming a daily struggle.

Not until living overseas did I fully appreciate how culture can dominate genetics at the expense of health. As soon as I walked out of the airport in Brasilia, Brazil, and greeted my colleague José, he announced that I was to dine with him and his wife that evening. During my last business trip, I had teased José that Argentine grass-fed beef and *asado* (barbecue) was the best South America had to offer. Not to be outdone by rivals to the south, José had planned ahead. Brazilian pride demanded that we eat at one of Brasilia's finest *churrasqueira* restaurants.

Restaurants like these existed for a singular purpose—to serve as much meat as patrons could consume. After we arrived and were seated, José gave me a personal tour. Along an entire wall was a long open grill. Sizzling on top were large skewers made up of appetizing cuts of beef, pork, lamb, and assorted wild game. To titillate the senses, the choicest cuts were being grilled with a thick layer of fat still intact.

While returning to our table, José pointed to the small salad bar tucked off to one side. It was there just in case. For most of the patrons filing through the front doors, lettuce and garnishes could wait another day. They were there to sate their primal want for calorie-dense meat. Leaving satisfied meant arriving early and staying late, while eating lots of animal protein and fat in between.

As we settled in for the evening, servers circled our table presenting hot skewers of meat and slicing portions onto our plates until we said stop. The quality of the meat mirrored Brazil's growing prosperity and advancing food system. Brazilians had tamed vast land holdings to produce food animals tailored to local conditions. The abundance supported a vibrant restaurant sector and an enthusiastic meat-eating culture.

Early on, sensory overload prodded me to try different cuts and varieties. But as the evening wore on, I was no match for José, who was more skilled at pacing and packing food away. At some point I blurted out "*Não mais,*" as if hoisting a white flag in surrender. On the way to the hotel, when he asked me if I was ready to retract my statement about Argentine beef, I mumbled that I was too full to talk. Bursting into laughter, he knew that he had his answer but said he would join me for breakfast in the morning. The thought of more food in a few hours made an already upset stomach ache even more.

I passed the night more awake than asleep. A full evening of gluttony brought on fitful dreams of servers slicing more meat on already full plates. Between the tossing and turning, I realized that eating with impunity was over, even though readily available calories and not enough physical activity were growing trends that were spreading worldwide.

While America has never been known for *churrasqueira* restaurants, it is the land of all-you-can-eat buffets, fast-food restaurants, fine dining, food courts, gas station convenience stores, supermarkets, specialty food stores, and vending machines. Culture has made convenience and sensory pleasures available at every turn.

These calorie-rich, nutrient-poor foods prompt the production of chemicals like endorphins and dopamine that regulate the brain's reward center and overpower hormonal signals to stop eating, notwithstanding our understanding of the health consequences. More than 90 percent of Americans eat multiple times throughout the day. Close to half say they cannot get through the day without a snack.

In *The Road to Wigan Pier,* George Orwell wrote: "A man dies and is buried, and all his words and actions are forgotten, but the food he has eaten lives after him in the sound or rotten bones of his children." Our legacy is fast becoming one of sugar, fat, and salt (though salt contains no calories). At the time of the American Revolution, individuals consumed about four pounds of sugar per year. By 1850, the amount had increased to twenty pounds. By 1994, it stood at 120 pounds. Today, the number-one food group consumed is added fats and oils, followed by processed flour and cereals, meat and eggs, and added sugars. In 2018, Americans are on track to set a new record for meat and poultry consumption at 222.2 pounds per person—almost double the recommended amount.

Orwell also wrote that "the human being is primarily a bag for putting food into." Crass as it sounds, finding ways to stuff more food into the human bag is just another day at the office. Behind the 21,000 new or updated food products rolled out each year, there are techniques like mapping the "bliss point"—that is, finding the precise amounts of sugars, fats, and salt that keep consumers coming back for more. Or tinkering with fat globules to alter rates of absorption, enhancing sugars to amplify sweetness, and physically altering salt, even pulverizing it, to trigger a boost in flavor.

All of this is part of the perfect formula that helps explain why so much fat is used. Why three-quarters of products in the food supply contain some form of sweeteners. And why three-quarters of dietary salt comes from processed foods.

The perfect formula also explains why eating a variety of foods today means something quite different than it once did. Historically, scarcity of calories in food encouraged greater diversity of diet. Variety could come from up to 300,000 edible species of plants that existed throughout the world. In the modern food system, most calories come from four crops (corn, wheat, soybeans, and rice) and three animals (cattle, pigs, and chicken). Variety now comes from combining sugars, fats, salts, chemical flavors, and other additives in endless ways.

Two years before the surgeon general's report on America's obesity epidemic, CEOs and presidents from eleven of the largest food manufacturers and suppliers met in Minneapolis at a rare and secretive meeting. As Pulitzer Prize–winning author Michael Moss chronicled in his book *Salt, Sugar, Fat*, the agenda had one item: how to respond to the emerging obesity epidemic. Two companies led the discussion, citing parallels with the tobacco industry's efforts to obfuscate the dangers of smoking. They urged the other companies to join together and proactively find ways to improve public health. One CEO strenuously objected. The others remained silent. In the end, they each went their separate ways.

Reform efforts by individual companies have wilted under stockholder scrutiny. Kraft, which ironically was owned by tobacco giant Phillip Morris, tweaked product formulations to improve nutrition and sought permission from the US Food and Drug Administration (FDA) to amend product labels with more nutrition information. When sales of its new products faltered and other reliable brands underperformed, the share price tumbled and the CEO was replaced.

Campbell Soup tried improving the nutrition profile of select soups by reducing salt content and adding fresh herbs and spices. Salt is cheap. Adding more herbs and spices is not. When costs rose, product competitiveness fell, and market share suffered, Wall Street downgraded the company. A new CEO was brought in, whose turnaround plan included adding salt back into soup.

For several years, major cereal manufacturers like General Mills, Post, and Kellogg offered breakfast cereals with reduced levels of sugar; some sugary brands were even discontinued. But having watched cereal sales decline by 11 percent in five years, in 2018 they brought back the sugar and reintroduced old brands. Those with sugar are outselling some of the healthier versions. As one executive put it, "Taste is king."

Companies also plot to guide consumers on nutrition and health. When PepsiCo rolled out its new food categories, comprising half of the company's sixty-six billion dollars in sales, the CEO said, "We have never seen food consumers as confused as they are today." With that introduction she announced three categories—"good for you," "better for you," and "fun for you." Quaker oats were in the "good for you" category. Fritos corn chips were assigned to the "fun for you" category. Of course, a "bad for you" category was never announced. The strategy was less about resolving consumer confusion and more about promoting sales.

When food is manufactured according to the perfect formula, messaging matters. Advertisements and food labels are integral to driving up sales. Yet more than a century after food manufacturers were legally compelled to be transparent about what was in their products, what can be said or withheld is as contested as ever.

In the 1980s, as awareness grew about food's role in chronic disease, a more health-conscious public called for additional transparency, particularly for processed foods. A renewed interest in labels emerged. Claims that foods were "low fat," for example, had no standardized baseline for comparison.

In a marketing ploy to sell more All Bran cereal, Kellogg's had featured on their boxes the National Cancer Institute's recommendation to "eat high-fiber foods"—not-so-subtly implying that All Bran cereal helped prevent cancer. Similar actions by other companies followed. Multiple states initiated lawsuits. At the federal level, divisions were widening across regulatory agencies over permissible information on labels, advertising, and enforcement. To find a solution, consumer advocates, food manufacturers, and oversight agencies agreed to uniform labeling.

While agreeing to uniform labels seemed logical, its execution was not. Health and nutrition professionals wanted more disclosure, while food manufacturers maneuvered for less. Both claimed that their positions were in the best interests of consumers. Battles were fought over which foods, ingredients, and nutrients would be included or excluded. What constituted serving size, percent of daily value, total daily calories, label format, and contents were hotly debated—not only among industry and scientists but also FDA and USDA.

As the process dragged on, testing different label formats and designs on consumers provided more opportunities for political posturing and further delays in implementation. Each side angled for policy provisions that supported their interests. Restaurants and small food manufacturers fought for exemptions, citing high costs of compliance. Knowing that adding health descriptors like "light," "lean," "extra lean," "enriched," "low fat," or "fortified" sold more products, food manufacturers fought for more lenient baselines; advertising food as "low fat" based on 20 percent less fat versus 50 percent sold more products. Food manufacturers also lobbied hard to include broad claims such as "improves health." In the absence of an established scientific link between their products and particular health advantages, a vague association would suffice to grow profits.

Despite the setbacks, uniform labeling was finally implemented, arguably the high-water mark in nutrition awareness. More than three decades and several revisions later, consumers *should* be able to walk into a grocery store feeling confident in their ability to interpret what manufacturers have printed on the labels. But can we? Or does obfuscation still reign in the name of transparency?

Food and ingredient manufacturers love to use *natural*, a word so phonetically close to *nature* that whatever they are selling just has to be healthier and more wholesome. But words can mislead, and *natural* is near the front of the pack. In the context of food, FDA is mostly hands-off but considers *natural* to imply an absence of artificial or synthetic additives. So when Cargill used the word *natural* to describe Stevia, an artificially manufactured sweetener from the stevia plant, it wasn't FDA but private parties that filed lawsuits. Though a settlement was reached, the company admitted no wrongdoing and retained all rights to using the word in the future.

Real, as in "real fruit juice," makes busy shoppers think they're buying actual fruit, just in more convenient liquid form. What the label does not reveal, is how much actual fruit has been added, whether its fiber content has been stripped and replaced with artificial fiber, or what percentage of the fruit's juice has been substituted in favor of cheaper sugary alternatives.

When food labels describe nutrient contents, more-specific rules apply; for example, only approved, recognizable nutrients like vitamin B12 or selenium are permitted. Creative labels sprinkled with a dash of truth like "super-mega vitamin C complex" are out of bounds. Qualifier terms like *free, low, high, good source*, etc. must follow prescribed usages.

Free is another opaque word. "Calorie-free" means less than five calories per serving, not zero calories. "Sodium-free" stands for less than five milligrams per serving. Similarly, *no* does not equal zero. "No trans fat" is no more than 0.5 grams per serving. Though partially hydrogenated vegetable oil is being phased out, check to see if it appears on the ingredient list just to make sure.

Passive consumers create opportunity for producers. Plastering a "no cholesterol" label on vegetable oil is factually true—*all* vegetable oil is cholesterol free. Manufacturers are constantly jiggering package sizes and quantity, or offering lower prices on higher quantities, on the safe bet that people will buy more. Labels on soups, chips, and cookies show nutrition information for one serving when the package actually contains more. Manufacturers know that people will read the label but still eat the entire contents of the package (a practice the newest labeling requirements try to address).

When processed food is dressed up to appear nutritious, labeling gets even more nuanced. For manufacturers, attaching any sort of health claims sells more products. But for consumers, parsing through such claims is not easy. In descending order of scientific rigor and evidence, there are health claims, qualified health claims, and structure/function claims.

Health claims must be backed by "significant scientific agreement." The use of such claims is limited to products proven to reduce disease risk. Health claims that imply a diagnosis, cure, mitigation, or treatment are out of bounds. Also, wording must be precise, such as: "Three grams of soluble fiber from oatmeal daily in a diet low in saturated fat and cholesterol may reduce the risk of heart disease. This cereal has two grams per serving."

Qualified health claims require less scientific evidence and usually include an asterisk and footnote. Wording such as "supportive but not conclusive research" is a tip-off. Finally, structure/function claims describe in broad strokes how ingredients can affect the normal structure or function of the body. Think of yogurt with probiotics added to promote digestive health. Or how "calcium builds strong bodies."

Even revered organizations like the American Heart Association are wading into the food-labeling morass, lured by the promise of revenue. Akin to the Marine Stewardship Council's stamp of approval for seafood sustainability (discussed in chapter 2), AHA now offers its own endorsement—the AHA Heart-Check Food Certification checkmark. Its use comes with a licensing fee, of course, and not just *processed*-food manufacturers are paying up. The AHA believes consumers need their guidance in deciding whether whole fruits and vegetables like pears and sweet potatoes are good for health.

So are Americans more informed? Is their health getting better? Do people understand that labels *associating* processed foods with better health do not mean they actually *deliver* better health? Is the proliferation of health claims degrading the value of science? Or is marketing hype making it harder to arrive at sound decisions?

The labeling morass points to a broader problem with food regulation. Consumers assume that the government has their backs, ensuring that food is safe. We like to think that all those unpronounceable additive names on the ingredient list have been properly vetted. But have they?

Concerns about additives dates back to 1958, when Congress prohibited adding substances "which had not been adequately tested to establish their safety." At that moment, some eight hundred ingredients, including pepper, vinegar, salt, vegetable oil, and preservatives like sorbic acid, already had a long history of use. Congress exempted these from further review, since they were widely recognized as safe. All others were to undergo a rigorous FDA evaluation using scientific data.

Today, more than ten thousand substances are allowed. Why so many? When the growth in new additives surpassed FDA's capacity to assess safety, the agency came up with a new approach—let the companies decide if they were safe. In essence, the original exemption in the law became the new rule. Companies would self-determine whether their additives were GRAS—"generally recognized as safe." If the companies said they were safe, FDA could not overturn their decision without first substantiating the harm to consumers. When the Government Accountability Office evaluated FDA's rule, they looked for similar approaches in other countries. None was found.

Several years ago, the Pew Charitable Trusts wanted to know whether the GRAS provision was working. Among their findings: food companies had no obligation to even notify FDA of their determinations. An estimated one thousand substances were introduced into food without FDA being informed. It was unclear how the agency could investigate such substances with no direct knowledge of their existence.

Pushing their investigation further, and knowing that many food companies rely on third parties in making their determinations, Pew looked at 451 findings where FDA did receive voluntary notifications. To evaluate whether third parties were free of conflicts of interests that could bias the results, Pew used criteria developed by the National Academies' Institutes of Medicine. Their conclusion: none of the third parties met the criteria.

In practice, even when a substance is identified as harmful, removing it from the food supply can take decades. Artificial trans fat, or partially hydrogenated oil, is made by adding hydrogen to solidify liquid vegetable oils. It was covered by the original 1958 exemption. Because trans fat is inexpensive, tasty, keeps food from spoiling, and can be used multiple times in deep fryers, food providers love it. But for consumers, trans fat raises bad cholesterol (LDL) and lowers good cholesterol (HDL), a one-two punch against good health. Despite decades of research consistently pointing out its dangers, FDA did nothing until a petition and lawsuit were filed in 2009.

Instead, the leadership came from New York City, which boosted public awareness by creating its own ban, thereby prompting some food retailers to voluntarily withdraw trans fat from their products. Not until June 2015 did FDA rule that trans fat be phased out over three years. Their ruling, however, was not a prohibition but a statement that trans fat was not safe for consumption. Companies could still seek permission for specific uses. Also, usage and enforcement in non-interstate commerce like local restaurants was left to each state.

America's once localized food system is now global. Food arrives from at least two hundred different cultures and food systems around the world. My first brush with unexpected foreign practices was decades ago while living in Argentina. Tree-ripened, brightly colored navel oranges are at the top of my favorite-fruits list. While I was growing up, they were only available for a few short weeks around Christmas. That recollection accompanied me to Argentina, where one day, while walking past a roadside produce cart, I spotted that round familiar orange glow on display. The oranges felt overly firm, but their color and my memories won me over. While expensive for my tight budget, I splurged for a few and happily strolled away.

It only took a few minutes of tossing the fruit back and forth from one hand to the other before I noticed that my hands had turned orange. It had never occurred to me that someone would paint unripe oranges in order to sell them as ready-to-eat fresh fruit. I had been duped. Welcome to the world of fraudulent foods and products.

Years later, while at USDA and researching bovine spongiform encephalopathy (BSE), I was drawn into a world most Americans never think about. Beyond the meat, milk, and leather coming from cows are other bovine by-products. Historically, they have included gelatin from bones and skins, used to make ice cream, salad dressings, and calcium supplements; pericardial tissue harvested for heart surgery; purified blood processed into coagulants; fibrin used to repair internal organs; glands and organs manufactured into hormones, enzymes, or medicines such as epinephrine, estrogen, testosterone, and antigens; and many more.

One prized product is fetal bovine serum, a growth medium used in medicine and biopharmaceuticals to culture cells outside the body. The polio vaccine, for example, came from research using cell cultures grown in fetal bovine serum. Harvested from the fetuses of pregnant cows during slaughter, it is the gold standard.

Its limited supply made the serum expensive. Countries free of specific diseases like BSE, foot-and-mouth, and scrapie in sheep commanded a premium price. From a country's cattle population, I could estimate potential supply. Yet when I looked at serum being traded internationally, significant discrepancies emerged. Serum exported by select countries free of the aforementioned diseases far exceeded my estimates of the available supply. After talking with experts and rechecking the data, the most plausible explanation was that serum was being shipped and relabeled as originating from disease-free countries. It was my first introduction into potential fraud on a global scale.

International trade can benefit both commerce and consumers. But it also creates opportunities for unethical behavior—behavior that governments are poorly equipped to detect, let alone deter. While most trade is legitimate, fraud does happen and can often persist with few, if any, consequences for the perpetrators. Imported honey is one example.

Beekeepers who maintain their own hives are my preferred source for honey. Typically offered in small local stores or at farmers' markets, it is commonly sold in mason jars, along with a free story or two. For more than three decades, honeybees have battled a host of new viruses, fungi, parasites, and pesticides. What scientists call Colony Collapse Disorder still defies answers. Prime bee habitat is dwindling as more land is developed or planted in monoculture crops. Over the last two decades, honey production per colony has trended downward by more than a pound per year.

Meanwhile, honey imports are skyrocketing—a thirty-four-fold increase over four decades. Typically arriving in fifty-five-gallon steel drums, imports now supply two-thirds of all honey consumed, of which 70 percent goes directly into manufactured foods. (Honey is just one of at least sixty different ways that sugars are added to foods without drawing attention to any one ingredient.)

In 2002, so much honey was arriving from China at bargain prices that the United States levied antidumping tariffs, effectively tripling its cost. No matter, Chinese production continued to increase, and honey imports from a host of other countries, particularly countries with little previous honey exports, more than doubled in a twelve-year period. Pollen in honey provides a geographic footprint as to its origin. But pollen can be removed and water or cheap sweeteners such as sugar or corn syrup can be added. When honey is adulterated and "laundered" by relabeling the country of origin, that sticky substance may still taste sweet—but it is not honey.

In 2010, the largest case of food fraud to date was brought against a German food conglomerate trying to evade eighty million dollars in honey import duties. Three years later, charges were brought against two domestic honey processors for likewise trying to evade $180 million in duties. In 2015, another illegal shipment of Chinese honey was seized in Houston.

These investigations were triggered because customs agents were looking for importers trying to skip out on fees. When US Customs and Border Protection (CBP) keyed in on "blue" steel drums, typical of honey shipped from China, honey showed up in drums painted other colors. When officials questioned why so much honey was coming from countries with little history of exports, more honey started arriving through other countries.

Ultimately, FDA was drawn in and discovered that some honey contained chloramphenicol, an antibiotic given to bees but not approved in the United States because it can cause cancer and damage to DNA in children. When chloramphenicol became a marker for illegal Chinese honey, other residues of prohibited drugs, including fluoroquinolone and nitrofurans, showed up instead. FDA has now issued six import alerts, the latest in 2018 covering fourteen countries and forty-two importing companies, meaning that shipments can be detained without physical examination.

This is a start, but except for high-profile cases, sleuthing out criminal commerce is a thankless job. Stopping fraudulent food becomes another underfunded mandate for an already overburdened agency. As is, FDA relies on published rules with the threat of legal action as its primary deterrent—a strategy akin to posting speed limits on highways and threatening enforcement, leaving street-smart motorists to figure out that few cops are on the beat.

In fairness, organized food fraud is not confined to the United States. In January 2013, Irish food inspectors found horsemeat in frozen beef burgers. Millions of processed foods like lasagna, packaged ground beef, and hamburgers were pulled from supermarket shelves and fast-food restaurants across the European Union.

Europeans were outraged, particularly that they may have consumed contaminants like anti-inflammatory drugs used in horses but banned for humans. In Great Britain, the fraud touched a societal nerve. As details emerged, public outcry prompted an outside review.

Leaks from the interim report were so hard-hitting that the final release was purportedly delayed for months to tone down its findings. Sanitized as it might have been, the report still underscored that food fraud was not a random, isolated, or victimless act. The evidence pointed to substantial organized crime.

Yet what had happened was self-inflicted. Agency budgets had been cut, boundaries between government departments were blurred, political interference was tolerated, and enforcement authority had been stripped away. Regulators lacked the experience and expertise to combat organized crime. Apathy from suppliers, politicians, and consumers had fostered a culture in which food fraud could flourish.

Less than two years after the initial outbreak, authorities announced another horsemeat trafficking crackdown. This time, it involved seven European Union countries, and once again Great Britain. The main tool used to inject illegal meat into the human food supply—simple falsification of official health documents.

Whether in Europe, the United States or beyond, there are no limits to ingenuity in defrauding consumers. Fraudulent ketchup packaged in premium Heinz ketchup bottles was only detected after counterfeit bottles began exploding. Poultry meat covered in feces and slime was cleaned up with chemicals and then relabeled and sold to consumers. Olive oil extracted from the fat of olive skins and pits using heat and chemical solvents like hexane was marketed as "100% pure olive oil." Meat made from rats, minks, and foxes was marketed as beef and mutton. Melamine (an industrial toxin) was added to milk (and pet food) to spike tests for protein content and higher prices. Pork meat was contaminated with clenbuterol (an illegal feed additive). Shrimp were injected with gelatin. Cabbage was treated with formaldehyde. And cooking oil sold for human consumption began as "gutter oil"—sewage oil collected, heated, and treated with chemicals.

Even leaving aside blatant fraud, food is not as innocent as it once was. With the grand food bargain, we got the cheap, easy, addictive products we wanted, but not without their consequences. Initially, more food came from conscripting more energy. But before long, a staid diet of whole grains, vegetables, fruits, and limited animal protein was supplanted by foods engineered to evoke pleasure and stimulate taste. Today, diets are dominated by refined carbohydrates, processed flour, loads of saturated fat, plenty of added salt, and minimal amounts of fiber. Consuming more than what our bodies require is tied to at least thirty different medical conditions and diseases.

Yet food companies are not slowing down. Instead, they are consolidating, gaining power and leverage over government. Even in the early days of regulation, government agencies hardly amassed a stellar track record of protecting public health. If the past is any clue, governments will continue to be reactive—responding to scandals that grab headlines. Only consistent political pressure will force politicians to initiate real reform.

For consumers, the laws of nature still apply—the more calories we eat, the more weight we gain. Our economic model doesn't help: on a per-calorie basis, it's cheaper to fill up on unhealthy foods than nutritious fare. And while physical activity has never been more important for overall health, it's hard to exercise your way to weight loss when food is so caloric. Few of us will work out for an hour just to burn off a slice of pizza.

Moreover, our metabolisms are not cooperating. The average American dieter attempts to lose weight four times a year. Most who try will eventually put the weight back on, plus some. A study of contestants on television's *The Biggest Loser* revealed some disappointing news: to maintain their weight loss, they needed to eat significantly fewer calories than most people their size. Their metabolisms had slowed down, allowing their bodies to put the weight back on more easily.

Perhaps the best dietary advice was given by W. O. Atwater, a bona fide pioneer in nutrition science. His counsel: avoid a diet that is "one-sided or badly balanced—that is, one in which either protein or fuel ingredients (carbohydrate and fat) are provided in excess."

As I look back, I can see that I was the beneficiary of advice such as Atwater's. Yet my favorable edge had nothing to do with choices I made personally when starting out life. My good fortune was not having access to foods I wanted because of their cost. As it turned out, consuming wholesome foods like plenty of fruits and vegetables in my formative years was akin to winning the nutritional lottery—even if I failed to see it when I was yearning for rodeo fare.

The challenge that today's parents face is creating a similarly nutritious diet when the economic incentives are just the reverse. Families need a healthy food system that takes advantage of the depth and breadth of good food that is now available, rather than loading up on empty calories.

Such a system would begin with the principle that people are not bags for putting food into and getting money out of. Paradoxically, the danger of ever more food was already known shortly after the grand food bargain took hold. As W. O. Atwater put it, "The evils of overeating may not be felt at once, but sooner or later they are sure to appear perhaps in an excessive amount of fatty tissue, perhaps in general debility, perhaps in actual disease." Atwater wrote that in the year 1902.

Chapter 10

Controlling Nature

Whether we and our politicians know it or not, Nature is party to all our deals and decisions, and she has more votes, a longer memory, and a sterner sense of justice than we do.

— Wendell Berry

In a restaurant on the outskirts of Toledo, I met up with a long-time friend. He and his wife had once lived in Ohio and traveled throughout its four corners. Now they were back to visit and see what had changed. One of their pleasant memories from this state, Roy told me, was seeing the immaculately kept farms and fields of crops with nary a weed in sight.

I could relate. Having traveled many of Michigan's rural roads on two wheels, with the wind in my face and the smell of fresh crops in the air, I was often drawn in by picturesque country landscapes: well-kept white farmhouses, gambrel roofs on red barns, and gently rolling green hills in the background.

Occasionally, I would chance across a farmhouse that looked as if it were drawn by Norman Rockwell, with its wraparound porch, stately trees, colorful flower beds, and white picket fences. The mailbox would be perched on an old wagon wheel or moldboard plow, the lawn neatly manicured, the driveway wide and inviting. The homestead would be encircled by green crops uniform in height, glistening in the sunshine. It was easy to imagine the family who lived inside, sitting on the porch swing at night after finishing the chores and listening to the crickets chirp, watching the moon gliding through the clouds as the wind gently stroked the leaves on the trees.

For those who love the countryside, these scenes inspire dreams of a utopian existence: the ultimate harmony between civilization and Earth. In this world, roofs of barns are not collapsing inward, broken farm equipment is not rusting away on cement blocks, and weeds are not cluttering ditch banks or crowding out crops.

"How do they do it?" Roy asked. For decades he had routinely planted the same half-dozen vegetables in his backyard garden plot, only to see weeds and ravenous insects overrun it if he happened to be away for a few days. "How do farmers grow hundreds of acres of crops free of weeds?"

The answer was many farmers are planting seeds engineered to resist pesticides. By genetically altering the seeds' DNA to withstand compounds and chemicals like glyphosate, dicamba, or 2,4-D, farmers can blanket spray their fields, killing everything but the crops. Following a long line of precedents, GMO crops are one of our latest—and most controversial—attempts to control nature.

Some of my earliest memories are of people's attempts to *take on* the environment. On cool fall days while walking home from school, I still remember dark streaks of black smoke wafting skyward against a backdrop of blue sky. Discarded tires had been lit on fire, then dragged by chains across canals and ditch banks. The sound of dried brush crackling into flames and the hiss of burning tires filled the air. Yet once the fire died out, the smoke soon dissipated and the blue skies returned. Charred, blackened banks were the only lingering evidence. By spring, order had been restored as plants reclaimed the land. The environment had reaffirmed its resilience, and new life had once again regained its impunity against those who confronted it.

Signs of the environment's robustness were everywhere. On nights before I went fishing, I could walk into a field and sink a shovel head into the soft soil, parting the earth to reveal night crawlers under the glow of my flashlight. No less amazing was how wheat planted in the fall came back to life no matter how cold the winter or deep the snow. In the garden, ladybugs always landed on my forearms and crawled along tomato vines. All were symbols of the resilience of the natural world.

So too were pheasants. Our alfalfa fields not only grew hay, they provided habitat. With their long feathered tails and the males' vibrant colors, pheasants were wily birds that, when threatened, preferred to run rather than fly. When they did breech their cover, they launched without warning; their flapping wings nearby never failed to startle me.

One summer day, I was riding along with my father when he suddenly stopped the tractor and powered down the mower. A male pheasant had been decapitated. He put the bird into a box and had me carry it to the house with instructions to ask my grandmother (his mother-in-law, who was visiting) if she would prepare it for dinner. I did as he asked, but my mother made sure the request was never repeated!

When I was old enough to take over the mowing, I kept one eye on the mower's cutting bar and the other on steering the tractor. Sometimes, a pheasant would fly up in front of me. Other times, I saw alfalfa leaves stirring about as they scurried for safety. Some birds waited until the last possible moment to run, barely escaping the knives on the cutting bar's far end.

When the mower kept breaking down, my father purchased a swather. The new machine, with its nearly ten-foot cutting bar, metal paddle reel, and dual pinching rollers, dwarfed the old mower. The swather not only cut alfalfa, it compressed and pushed the cut hay out the back, forming neat windrows ready for baling in a couple of days. With the swather, the time required to cut and prepare hay for baling dropped by half.

It was only after I picked up a bale of hay, smelled the pungent remnants of a pheasant carcass, and saw bits of buried feathers that I realized what was happening—the swather was too wide for some pheasants to outrun. It was an early lesson that I could damage nature, even without meaning to.

Regrettably for the pheasants, they held little value to anyone but bird hunters and a few farmers. As time passed, pheasants all but disappeared, unable to escape modern farming equipment or find habitat in the midst of urban development. As party to their disappearance, I witnessed how the environment did not always bounce back in the way I wanted.

Dating back some ten thousand years, Mesopotamia is often called the "cradle of civilization," a precursor to modern cities supported by rural farming. Its semiarid climate and abundance of fertile soil and sunshine were similar to conditions in California's Central Valley, the primary source of America's produce and tree nuts. And just like the Central Valley, Mesopotamia relied on an extensive network of aqueducts and canals to deliver water to its fields.

For thousands of years, as water flowed from rivers through canals, farmers grew barley, emmer (wheat), nuts, herbs, beans, lentils, green vegetables like lettuce and garlic, and fruits such as apples, melons, grapes, pomegranates, and figs. Sheep, goats, pigs, and, later, cattle, donkeys, and oxen were also used for food and for labor. With ingenuity, people tamed the environment and society flourished.

The area that was once Mesopotamia still exists today. Nestled between the Tigris and Euphrates rivers, it encompasses what is Iraq, portions of Turkey, Syria, and Iran. But the water that once flowed through its canals and aqueducts, along with its periodic floods, changed the land long ago. Silt particles too small to see were deposited on the top layers of soil, making them impermeable. As the water evaporated, the salt left behind accumulated, preventing seeds from germinating. Where the land was sandy, water passed through the soils too quickly for plants to hold on to moisture and nutrients. The environment was forever changed. The flourishing Mesopotamian era was over.

Today, a different environment now characterizes the region. Large expanses of irrigated fields that once produced a cornucopia of fruits and vegetables have disappeared. Pastures of animals that provided a bounty of meat and milk are also gone. What remains is severe desertification, with intense dust storms that loosen and then sweep up layers of dirt to be scattered about by strong winds. Similar phenomena are happening in California and other states. The only difference is the severity and rate of change.

History teaches that we can alter the environment, but we cannot control what happens afterward. When potatoes were introduced in Europe, people enjoyed a new abundance of food. While one acre of wheat or barley had yielded around 1,400 pounds, the same acre planted in potatoes provided some 25,000 pounds. Potato production took off in countries like Ireland. Within two centuries, its population had grown from 1.5 million to 8.5 million people subsisting on a diet of mostly milk and potatoes.

Meanwhile, on islands off the shores of Peru, vast reserves of guano had been discovered. Guano (excrement deposited by seabirds) was brought to Europe as fertilizer to put on crops like potatoes. But along with the guano came a pathogen that, during an unusually damp spell, spread throughout Ireland and destroyed most of the potato crop. Before it was over, the resulting famine claimed one million lives and chased two million people from their homeland.

Explorers, conquerors, and settlers crisscrossing oceans were doing more than claiming new land and expropriating the riches they found. They were also bringing along microscopic organisms, introducing exotic bacteria, viruses, fungi, pathogens, and pests that redefined the environment and decimated native populations.

New microbes were not the only unwelcome change. Back in America's Great Plains, in the half century leading up to the 1930s, homesteaders plowed under drought-resistant grasses and planted non-drought-resistant wheat. Ranchers co-opted and overgrazed millions of acres of unattended public lands. "Suitcase farmers," who were attracted by seemingly plentiful rains but who had no intention to stay and homestead, showed up just long enough to plant then return to harvest their crops. Total land cultivated increased from 12 million to 103 million acres.

But then the rains ceased and the moisture in the soil evaporated. Without the native grasses to hold topsoil in place, sand and dirt were lifted by prevailing winds to form dust storms. Suitcase farmers stopped coming around. The Dust Bowl was under way and the widespread erosion that followed persisted for a decade. "Funnel storms" carried dust four miles into the atmosphere and transported it to cities like New York and Washington, DC. Chicago was blanketed with up to four feet of dust from a single storm. In the Southern Plains, black storms turned day to night and paralyzed travel.

Six years into what is now known as the Dust Bowl era or the "Dirty Thirties," an estimated four out of every five acres across the Great Plains were in some stage of erosion. Farmers placed the blame on drought and seasonal winds, refusing to believe that "one man cannot stop the dust from blowing but one man can start it." Ultimately, the government ended up paying farmers to conserve their land through strip cropping, terracing, and planting trees as windbreaks.

The environmental disaster subsided. The taxpayer bailout had rewarded farmers for changing course without having to change their minds. Many remained unconvinced that they were complicit in creating the Dust Bowl. When your livelihood was at stake, it was easier to blame the weather than yourself; as a landowner, you had the right to do as you pleased. The government had reinforced this belief through financial incentives, creating a dangerous precedent that there would be no penalty for environmental destruction, even when it directly damages others.

Once in a while, we do learn when things are going wrong. On our farm, no one wanted to see a cow get sick and die. Yet periodically, one would become lethargic and lie down. When attempts to coax the animal to stand, eat, or drink failed, my father sterilized a glass syringe and a stainless steel needle in boiling water. Then taking from the refrigerator a bottle of Combiotic, a veterinary drug comprised of two antibiotics, he drew down the needed dosage. Back at the barn, I restrained the animal while he plunged the needle through the dense hide and into the muscle, emptying the contents. Giving an injection was infrequent enough that I never paid attention to details like dosage per animal weight.

One summer while my parents were away, my brother pointed to a recumbent calf in the pasture. In the days prior, we had noticed its energy level was falling. The calf refused to stand or take nourishment. Fearing it could die on our watch, I prepared a syringe of Combiotic, just as I had seen my father do. Unsure of the dosage, I scanned the label for directions, but I was also hurrying, scared of what would happen if I waited too long. While my brother held the calf, I took the syringe in hand and gave the injection.

As I pulled the needle out, a new fear swept over me—had I just overdosed the calf? Rereading the instructions, I realized I had injected a full adult dosage. In my teenage mind, I had just administered a lethal injection like those given to prisoners on death row. I expected the calf to die shortly. The possibility of implicating my brother crossed my mind. But as the older son, I would be the one who would be held to account.

For the rest of the day, I rehearsed my explanation. When I checked on the calf later that evening, to my surprise he was marginally better. Over the next several days, the calf received more attention from me than any other before or since. When my parents came home (and long before the military started using it) my strategy changed to one of "don't ask, don't tell."

I lucked out. I had known just enough to be dangerous. Antibiotics interact with microscopic organisms to alter nature and you can never be certain what will follow. The calf had taught me that antibiotics are not to be trifled with.

The rollout of penicillin to the general population in 1943 marked a new era in treating bacterial illness. Before then, it was all too common to survive battlefield wounds or surgery, only to be felled by infection. Almost overnight, antibiotics proved to be an astounding medical breakthrough, earning the label of the "crown jewels of medicine." Two decades later, the surgeon general declared, "The time has come to close the book on infectious disease. We have basically wiped out infection in the United States." Few at the time realized that immunity to penicillin had already started three years prior to its rollout.

Antibiotics were initially confined to treating infection, in both humans and animals. Then in 1950, and quite by accident, scientists discovered that adding antibiotics to livestock feed accelerated their growth; their use in animal production exploded. Exactly how they promote growth is a mystery, even today. What proved less mysterious was mounting evidence of bacteria thwarting the drugs intended to kill them. As scientific concern increased that people would "find themselves back in the pre-antibiotic Middle Ages," the FDA tried to rein in usage. But a Congress heavily influenced by agricultural interests would have none of it.

Today, 80 percent of all antibiotics consumed in the United States are destined for animals and agriculture. While farm animals consume the majority, antibiotics are also used in aquaculture, honeybees, and companion animals, and they are even sprayed on fruit trees like apples, pears, and peaches. Antibiotics paved the way to raise large numbers of animals in confined spaces. From an average of 355 chickens per farm in 1950, large operations now produce over 500,000 birds annually; and a handful of corporations control thousands of operations. Similar trends have redefined pork production, and beef is not far behind. Using antibiotics, nutrition, and genetics, farmers raise animals to put on more weight more quickly. In 1925, it took 112 days to raise a 2.5 pound chicken. Today, a five-pound bird takes less than fifty days.

Proponents of agricultural drugs argue that they made food more affordable. But this success overshadows an inconvenient truth that not all bacteria are being killed. An antibiotic that is 99.9999 percent effective still leaves one in one million organisms alive. A single resistant bacterium capable of dividing every thirty minutes, like *E. coli*, can become a population of over 2.5 trillion in one day. Antibiotics are not killing off *entire* pathogen populations. Rather, antibiotics are creating hardier bacteria, genetically resistant to drugs that once eliminated them.

So long as new classes of antibiotics were rolling off pharmaceutical manufacturing lines, resistance was easily ignored. A generation after penicillin was brought to market, thirteen new classes of antibiotics had been introduced. Confidence in newer, better drugs ran high. If one class of antibiotics did not work, another one would. But pharmaceutical companies were moving on. Developing drugs for treating chronic, lifelong illnesses like cholesterol, diabetes, or high blood pressure was more lucrative; after all, antibiotics are taken for a couple of weeks, then stopped. In the last half century, only two new classes of antibiotics have come to market.

With fewer choices available, say hello to "superbugs"—bacteria resistant to multiple antibiotics. Superbugs, found in foods, hospitals, and playgrounds, are now a permanent addition to the environment. They are to be feared. One called MRSA (pronounced "mirsa") invades from a scratch, small cut, or scraped knee, then floods the bloodstream or lungs with deadly toxins. Potent yet highly toxic antibiotics have become the treatment option of last resort, where the goal is to kill the bacteria before the antibiotics kill the patient. Each year, MRSA accounts for an estimated eighty thousand invasive infections and eleven thousand related deaths.

Another ominous threat is called CRE, a group of some seventy bacteria, including toxic strains of *E. coli*, that can reside in the digestive systems of meat animals. With mortality rates of up to 50 percent, they are resistant to nearly all antibiotics. Called "nightmare bacteria," they *pass along* their resistance to other bacteria.

Overall, at least two million people per year become infected with bacteria resistant to antibiotics; some 23,000 die as a result. Neither statistic accounts for those who die from other conditions complicated by antibiotic-resistant infections. Bacteria have developed resistance to *every* antibiotic ever created. Still, sales of antibiotics worldwide continue to shoot up. In the next two decades, annual usage is forecast to grow from 63,000 tons to 106,000 tons.

Four decades after FDA failed to regulate antibiotic use in agriculture, the agency was back with a new tack—a voluntary approach with nonbinding recommendations. Part of their pitch to the animal industry was to emphasize principles like only using drugs "considered necessary for assuring animal health." The initial good news is year-over-year sales in 2016 were down 10 percent for the first time since 2009. The not-so-good news: antibiotic consumption rates in the United States are five times higher than in the United Kingdom.

Antibiotics are not the only human invention spawning resistance. We face a similar problem with synthetic chemicals, introduced into the modern food system a century ago. Before then, farmers used substances like nicotine sulfate (from tobacco plants) and lead arsenates (poisonous salt compounds) to kill off weeds and insects. They also rotated crops, pulled weeds, and resigned themselves to losing a portion of each year's harvest. After all, competing with other species over food is part of nature.

But synthetic pesticides promised to be a virtual fence that would kept out unwanted riffraff. Exterminating competitors meant higher yields and less need to rotate crops. Pesticides allowed farmers to do less and keep more.

Most pesticides are the by-product of research into chemical warfare. After World War II ended, Congress passed legislation governing their sale and intended use—but not their long-term effects. In just five years, ten thousand new pesticides were registered. Over the next forty years, fifty thousand different pesticides came into use across America's farms.

The most infamous was dichlorodiphenyltrichloroethane—DDT. Originally used to kill mosquitoes carrying malaria and lice-spreading typhus, the pesticide won its inventor a Nobel Prize. Newsreels in the 1940s showed children in swimsuits playing under a shower of DDT while mosquito-control trucks sprayed neighborhoods. Believed to be safe, DDT soon found other uses like eliminating pests plaguing farms.

Yet DDT was never benign. Though highly effective, it failed to kill *all* mosquitoes (or other insects). Just as antibiotics bred resistant bacteria, populations of DDT-resistant mosquitoes flourished as susceptible ones were killed. Meanwhile, research by the United States Fisheries and Wildlife reported that DDT was killing fish, mammals, beneficial insects, and, indirectly, agricultural crops. The National Institutes of Health branded DDT a carcinogen and FDA said it posed serious health risks. Farmers were warned in 1947 not to use DDT on food plants, but many continued to do so, letting profits override public health concerns.

Not until scientist and author Rachel Carson published *Silent Spring* in 1962 did public sentiment turn against DDT. Carson described how spraying DDT to kill Dutch elm disease was decimating bird populations, leading to an eventual "silent spring" devoid of birdsong. The book became a best seller.

When DDT was banned, other pesticides filled the void. Though each carried varying levels of toxicity, all were touted as safe with few environmental downsides. But the messaging did not stop there. Chemical manufacturers crafted narratives that stressed higher yields and greater profits for farmers, and more-affordable and more-wholesome food for consumers. Without pesticides, food production would plummet, prices would soar, exports would drop, global markets would go elsewhere, tens of thousands of jobs would disappear, and the poor would suffer. Nothing less than economic prosperity, feeding families, growing the economy, protecting America, and creating a better future was at stake.

Leading the charge was Monsanto, a manufacturer of DDT and Agent Orange, a defoliant used in Vietnam. Embroiled in lawsuits over dioxin, a known carcinogen and highly toxic by-product from manufacturing Agent Orange, the company banked heavily on its new pesticide, Roundup. Roundup and its active ingredient glyphosate were touted by some as safe enough to drink and fast became farmers' go-to pesticide. But the clock was ticking on Roundup's profitability. As glyphosate patents neared expiration, Monsanto sought USDA approval to market Roundup-tolerant soybeans, the first of many genetically modified seeds in the pipeline to be coupled with chemicals. With millions of dollars sunk into development, and desperately needing approval, the company wrote in its application, "It is highly unlikely that weed resistance to glyphosate will become a problem."

Before Roundup, there had never been a pesticide that didn't provoke resistance. But Monsanto believed its products were different. Besides Roundup, other seeds were genetically altered using a naturally occurring species of bacteria called *Bt*, which was toxic for despised insects. Company scientists, some in academia, government regulators, financial investors, and many farmers had convinced themselves that genetically modified seeds were new miracle elixirs capable of permanently subverting nature.

With Roundup taking care of weeds, planting the same crops in the same fields year after year promised to earn farmers higher returns. Previously, as a measure of defense against damaging insects like European corn borer and corn rootworm, farmers rotated soybean and corn fields. Because *Bt*-engineered seeds would not kill every insect pest, EPA proposed that one of every two acres be planted in a non–genetically modified crop (known as a "refuge" crop). Planting the two crops alongside each other was designed to ensure that *Bt*-resistant insects did not come to dominate the population.

But with so much money on the line, Monsanto fought back, and eventually EPA relented, settling on one of every five acres. Though some farmers still rotated their crops and planted refuge crops, others sought higher returns by planting the same crop each year, and reducing or ignoring refuge-crops requirements.

So along with superbugs, say hello to "superpests" and "superweeds." Two decades went by before weed resistance from glyphosate was finally acknowledged. Since then, thirty-five glyphosate-resistant weed species worldwide have been documented, sixteen in North America. In thirty-eight states and four Canadian provinces, common weeds like pigweed, horseweed, and ragweed are back with a vengeance.

As superweeds were taking over the environment, chemical-seed companies like Monsanto and DowDuPont adopted a different strategy—new seeds engineered to withstand older, more-toxic legacy chemicals. Because of known environmental and health risks, EPA classifies such chemicals as "restricted use." On their list: dicamba.

No sooner was dicamba rolled out than the complaints began. Recall that federal approval for genetically modified seeds and treatments is based on company-provided data, not independent studies. When dicamba-resistant seeds came on the market, most, if not all, university extension scientists had played no role in their evaluation.

Farmers who had never used dicamba-resistant seeds suffered crop damage from neighbors who applied dicamba. When sprayed, the product was drifting. One university scientist estimated over three million acres were affected. Missouri's largest peach farm, in the heart of soybean country, suffered extensive damage and filed a lawsuit. Monsanto countered that farmers were to blame for not following directions.

In a greenhouse in Arkansas, a university scientist demonstrated how pigweed could develop full-blown resistance to dicamba in just three generations. Other scientists, having looked at patterns in damaged fields, suspected it was more than drift. Trays of dirt from a sprayed soybean field were placed between rows of an unsprayed soybean field. Dicamba was not staying in the soil but was turning to gas and dispersing. As it evaporated, surrounding soybeans were damaged—the product was volatile. Arkansas passed a law limiting its usage. Monsanto filed suit. As of this writing, restrictions are being considered in other states, and the legal battles continue.

EPA's response has been to tweak its rules while continuing to green-light dicamba usage. At stake for Monsanto, DowDuPont, and BASF is billions of dollars in revenues. Paradoxically, farmers who had no plans to use dicamba may be forced to buy dicamba-resistant seeds at premium prices just for protection. Farmers who crafted markets around non-GMO crops may suffer the greatest losses.

Strip away the drama, lawsuits, and counterclaims, and what remains are profound differences in how people perceive the environment. At one end are university extension scientists who understand that resistance is inevitable, and that humans do not control nature's response. At the other end are companies with deep financial pockets who believe that technology can conquer all, including the environment.

The EPA has approved some seven hundred restricted-use pesticides. But such designation does not limit how much can be sold and applied, nor does it address the cumulative effects over time on health and the environment. As more land and crops are sprayed, more people are exposed. Organophosphates such as chlorpyrifos, diazinon, and malathion were originally developed by Nazi Germany as chemical weapons of war. Extremely toxic, they operate like nerve gas.

Chlorpyrifos-based products are widely applied to produce foods like soybeans, nuts, citrus, and fruit trees, as well as specialty crops like brussels sprouts, cranberries, broccoli, and cauliflower. Except for pest control, they are not sold for home use. Professionals who apply chlorpyrifos pesticide must don protective clothing and respirators. Fields should not be entered for up to five days after spraying.

Research from animal models and young children show that even low exposure levels are associated with irreversible brain development and impaired cognitive functioning. Studies of juvenile salmon documented that brain damage and death far exceed predictions when mixtures of organophosphates are used.

Government scientists compiled an official record more than ten thousand pages in length, outlining threats to nearly every endangered species. EPA's own biological evaluation concluded that some 1,800 animals and plants were likely adversely affected. In 2015, the agency proposed zero tolerance for chlorpyrifos in food residues, effectively banning their use in food production. In 2016, EPA's revised human health risk assessment affirmed that expected residues on food crops and drinking water would exceed allowable standards. By all accounts, using chlorpyrifos to produce food was on the ropes.

But in 2017, a more business-friendly administration under Donald Trump prompted letters to the EPA from the chief executives of three chemical manufacturers. They contended the studies were flawed— offering up their own scientific studies as unbiased proof. Chlorpyrifos manufacturer Dow Agrosciences led the effort, saying it was "committed to the production and marketing of products that will help American farmers feed the world, and do so with full respect for human health and the environment." Against a backdrop of White House friendships and allegations of influence-buying, the EPA reversed course, rejecting its own science and suspending further action. Sales of chlorpyrifos would not have missed a beat, and EPA's next review would not have occurred until 2021. The suspension was appealed to the Ninth Circuit Court, which in August 2018 gave the agency sixty days to "revoke all tolerances" and "cancel all registrations." Whether or not vested interests will once again triumph over the body of science-based evidence is still being contested.

You might think that Dow's "respect for human health and the environment" would compel the company to take a precautionary approach to pesticides, particularly in light of peer-reviewed scientific studies about irreversible brain damage. Instead, like most manufacturers, Dow continues to tout its products' safety notwithstanding mounting evidence otherwise. It can do so because studies showing definitive long-term health effects are much more difficult to carry out than those showing the absence of acute, immediate harm.

In an environment where thousands of synthetic chemicals abound, teasing out the long-term confounding effects is complex, time consuming, and expensive. Such are the challenges of regulating pesticides in the United States. Though DDT was banned in 1972, almost two generations ago, its residues live on in the environment and in human blood samples. While levels are lower, the long-term effects remain unknown.

In 1966, the richest man in the world launched a scheme that most people have never heard about. Daniel Ludwig set his mind to turning four million acres of the Amazon rain forest into food and wood products. This self-made billionaire abhorred publicity, as it stole from his mercenary drive to make more money, however and wherever possible. His business empire, operating in twenty-three countries scattered around the world, included mining, dredging, ship building, oil and cargo transportation, banking and financial services, land development, housing, hotels and casinos, office towers, refining, petroleum and gas exploration, and agriculture.

Well connected politically, Ludwig paid three million dollars for a tract of Brazilian land equivalent to the size of Connecticut plus half of Rhode Island. Located along the banks of the Jari River deep within Brazil's rain forest, Ludwig's proposed "Jari project" would be five hundred miles downriver from Fordlandia, an earlier and likewise ambitious project undertaken to produce latex for making tires. Launched by another Michigander, Henry Ford, "Fordlandia" was eventually sold for a fraction of its cost and was then abandoned twenty years later.

Ludwig showed no interest in Ford's failure, including how blight and parasites had plagued its rubber trees. His brilliance was extracting immense wealth, be it from governments, war, natural resources, labor, or the environment. His engineer's mind, market acuity, and supreme confidence in his own judgments had made him wealthy. Subordinates who disagreed with his decisions were easily replaced.

Enthusiasm for the Jari project soared when one of Ludwig's chemical engineers identified in Africa a fast-growing tropical tree, *Gmelina arborea* (known simply as gmelina). Ludwig instantly foresaw domination of the global market for hardwood and pulp products. The potential for riches had parallels with America's earlier petroleum barons. Saying that he "always wanted to plant trees like rows of corn," Ludwig set about reordering the environment by importing massive tractors dubbed "jungle crushers" to clear 250,000 acres of rain forest.

Once the land had been cleared, and workers began planting gmelina seedlings in neat, straight rows, his first of many missteps soon became evident. In removing the native trees and undergrowth, the jungle crushers had stripped away the thin layer of top soil, exposing the subsoil to bake in the hot sun, and then harden. The land became so compacted that the seedlings' roots could not penetrate the soil.

Over the next decade and a half, the mistakes compounded. Plantations of rice were doused so heavily with pesticides that insect populations grew immune. More recurrent and heavier applications killed off bird and fish populations. As had happened with Fordlandia, planting the same species of trees so close together had removed natural barriers against pests, requiring trees to be sprayed more frequently.

Ludwig was learning that soil types varied widely across his land. To compensate, ammonium sulfate was imported to bolster the lack of nutrients. Gmelina trees were yanked out in some places and replaced with Caribbean pines. Land stripped of native vegetation and turned into pasture to raise cattle now required the addition of synthetic fertilizers.

The Jari project was to have been Ludwig's swan song at the close of a lucrative career. Instead, as he sank more money into the effort, the criticisms intensified and the setbacks continued. With nothing but red ink and a damaged environment, a tired Ludwig gave up, ceded ownership back to the Brazilian government, and walked away.

After fifteen years of intense effort and more than a billion dollars expended, the environment Ludwig set out to conscript remained beyond his control. The Jari project had met the same fate as Fordlandia. Both Ford and Ludwig had come with vision, ingenuity, money, and the latest technology. They possessed immense wealth, power, and drive to impose their will. They did indeed change the environment, but not in the way either imagined.

I first learned of the Jari project in my early twenties, just before Ludwig gave up. He had gone all in. Though I admired his determination, I also wondered what might have been, had he himself not become the biggest obstacle. Others knew that the soil beneath the Amazon canopy was nothing like Midwestern farmland. Likewise, others knew that transplanting the same species of trees so close together, especially in a tropical environment thick with insects, would set off a domino response as living organisms competed for habitat and food to survive, thrive, and reproduce. Others knew that trying to sow, cultivate, and harvest tens of thousands of acres of foreign crops in atypical farming conditions was bound to trigger some nasty surprises.

But what if Ludwig had taken the environment into consideration? What might the outcome have looked like? After all, nature abounds with examples of innumerable species and diverse phenomena that somehow foster harmony. Bees pollinating flowers leads to more honey and more flowers. Birds picking ticks off cattle benefit both cattle and the birds themselves. Cottonwood trees utilize wind currents for propagation. Prairie grass depends on fire in order to rejuvenate and come back stronger.

Countless such phenomena are well known, and yet, more often than not, wisdom about the planet seems to be limited to hindsight. From Mesopotamia, the Dust Bowl, glyphosate, antibiotics, dicamba, DDT, the Amazon, and more, one overarching lesson never changes—attempting to control the environment and its inevitable response eventually fails.

A decade ago, while traveling the dry, open plains of Burkina Faso in Africa, I watched gusts of wind blow plastic bags across the road as though they were tumbleweeds. The Burkinabé professor hosting me commented that plastic had become a threat to ruminant animals like cattle, sheep, and goats. The bags were gumming up their digestion, causing a host of problems including bloating, weight loss, and reduced milk production. Similarly, plastic in soil was preventing water from percolating and seeds from sprouting.

From plastic bags, the conversation turned to the more general problem of refuse piling up in countries around the world. In one such country, though it could have been many, I recounted climbing a riverbank covered in garbage to reach a small city originally built to overlook the river. The seeming acceptance of trash with its insidious environmental consequence and diminished quality of life perplexed me. To my question about why this was being tolerated, my colleague responded: "If one chooses not to see the problem, is it still a problem?"

Nowhere is his question more illuminating than with global warming, the most existential problem facing the Earth's inhabitants—starting with ourselves, the human race. How carbon dioxide can retain heat in the atmosphere was known more than 150 years ago. In the early 1900s, scientists were already concerned with gases and other residues from burned fossil energy trapped in the atmosphere and possibly altering the Earth's climate. In the 1960s, President Johnson brought the matter before Congress. Only when crop failures, drought, and famine drew attention to changes in climate in the 1970s did the threat of a warming planet even appear on the global radar.

Scientists have provided volumes of peer-reviewed analyses on rising temperatures and sea levels, glacial melting, thermal expansion, and elevated levels of carbon dioxide in our oceans and atmosphere. Among

1,372 scientists who conduct research on climate change, nearly 98 percent concur that humans are most responsible for a warming planet. Yet a substantial portion of Americans choose not to see the problem or to accept the evidence.

Unfortunately, ignoring what is happening does not immunize us from the results. As unpleasant consequences go, the modern food system's contribution to global warming is enormous. Energy from fossil fuels is to powering food production what the money supply is to promoting the market economy. It powers the engines that plant and harvest food. It produces synthetic fertilizers and pesticides. It is the backbone of food manufacturing and packaging. It distributes food to where consumers live. And it exposes the reality that society is overwhelmingly vulnerable in its absence, yet we stroll along as if on a Sunday walk on the beach with no backup plan or imminent concern.

A major reason why is our fixation on short-term benefits. Be it food safety, chronic food-related diseases, or adverse environmental impacts, our actions have favored what is known in the present, not what we learn over time. Not acknowledging that the absence of evidence is not the same as the evidence of absence, we have set up our health and the environment as a high-stakes gamble with long-term consequences.

These contradictions and their results are on display seventy miles north of where I live. On the west edge of Midland, Michigan, a garden more than a century in the making beckons visitors to come and enjoy year-round. Alongside its paved walkways are some twenty thousand annual varieties of flowers and plants. Species like milkweed and butterfly bush illustrate the symbiotic existence between plants and pollinators. Others such as basil, lavender, sage, lilac, and boxwood offer up pleasing sights and scents. So also does the vast selection of tulips and roses chosen for their delicate allure.

The garden's orchards produce cherries, plums, pears, pawpaws, and over seventy varieties of apples. Quiet groves containing blue spruce, elm, balsam, hemlock, and birch trees invite reflection. In the glass-walled conservatory, wintertime is active with nonnative banana plants, orchids, and poinsettia. Springtime features thousands of brightly colored butterflies from around the world in their tropical environment. All around are well-manicured lawns and meandering streams. Everything on display is a moving reminder of the diversity and beauty of the Earth's environment. The garden, begun in 1899, was the creative outlet for Herbert Dow, founder of the Dow Chemical Company.

Leaving the gardens, I travel south feeling the delight of the wind against my face. Off to my left is Herbert Dow's other legacy, the second-largest chemical-production company in the world. The overcast skies silhouette the chemical-storage towers, metal buildings, and endless miles of pipes of this 1,900-acre manufacturing facility abutting the Tittabawassee River. Chemical operations started here two years before Dow began his garden.

This is the site where over a thousand organic and inorganic chemicals and by-products have been produced, including napalm and Agent Orange, the latter leaving behind dioxins—highly toxic compounds that can lead to cancer, reproductive and developmental problems, immune system damage, and disrupted hormones. Dioxins were discharged directly into the river and then built up in its banks and surrounding floodplains. The contamination extended over fifty miles downstream and into the Saginaw River that empties into Saginaw Bay and Lake Huron, one of the five Great Lakes.

It may have been the contrast between the dull shades of industrial gray and the rainbow of colors from the garden. Or the miles of tall wire fencing encompassing small lakes and once-open wildlife areas no longer habitable. Perhaps it was the risks to human and animal health that will persist for centuries. But in any case, the juxtapositions of beauty and ugliness I experienced that day in north-central Michigan removed any lingering doubts of how we often compartmentalize the environment to avert our eyes from life-threatening problems.

Just as we can believe in infinite amounts of finite resources, we can also choose to believe that the environment will never fail us. We can enjoy the beauty and diversity of a Dow Gardens without acknowledging the purpose of a DowDuPont chemical plant just down the street. We can ignore that neonicotinoids (nicotine-like insecticides) are threatening bee populations; or the reasons behind a dead zone the size of New Jersey where the Mississippi River empties into the Gulf of Mexico. Or how industrial farming is primarily responsible for toxic algal blooms in Lake Erie. Or that the ocean is becoming acidic, coral reefs are dying, methane and nitrous oxide are trapping heat in the atmosphere, pests and weeds are increasingly resistant to pesticides.

So long as there are luscious gardens, picturesque farms, manicured green lawns, photo-perfect orchards, and plenty of food, we can console ourselves that all is well. Alas, we are the one species on this Earth with the cognitive capacity to reject the environment—or the one species on this Earth that can pause and reflect on what really matters.

On special days, when we tune out distractions and tune in the splendors of nature, we can see glimpses of the world around us as a living organism. We have the ability to value the delicate balancing role the environment provides. How in the atmosphere, carbon dioxide is exchanged with oxygen. How a layer of ozone protects us from ultraviolet radiation from the Sun that would otherwise sterilize the Earth's surface. How clouds form and rains fall to regulate temperature, not just everywhere else but where we individually live. How varied habitats protect us against storms, control floods, and provide recovery from drought. How watersheds create snowpack, natural lakes, and aquifers. How flowing rivers provide water for growing food as well as transportation for commerce and pleasure.

If we are tuned in to what surrounds us, blowing winds are reminders that rock is being weathered, organic matter is accumulating, and soil is being formed and renewed. Above and beneath the surfaces we live on, microscopic organisms are supporting ongoing cycles of life, bringing nutrients and other elements. Naturally occurring geological and biological processes are treating waste, detoxifying compounds, recovering nutrients, and abating pollution. Predators are keeping prey in check. Different landscapes and climates are providing meat and wild game, habitat for migration and protection for resident populations. At least 200,000 species are serving as pollinators, leading to edible plants, nuts, and fruit.

Forests are providing wood and timber, binding soils and moisture, preventing erosion, creating microclimates, and maintaining habitat for wildlife. Oceans are absorbing carbon dioxide, creating habitat for marine life, moisture for precipitation, and energy for transportation. Through Earth's immeasurable diversity of living species, comes the genetic resources and biological matter we use every day in medicine, science, and food.

From what surrounds us, food and sustenance become common realities. Recreation, eco-tourism, sport fishing, long bike rides, and scenic hikes become everyday options. Being the one species that can meaningfully appreciate the environment affords us the inspiration we crave for embodying the aesthetic, artistic, educational, and spiritual values that imbue life with meaning.

Beyond what we see outwardly, we can also look inward at how our lives cling to a niche existence. We are limited to about 4 percent of the Earth's surface that must be above sea level and below fifteen thousand feet in altitude. Even though we are surrounded by water, almost all of it is undrinkable or locked up in ice. We rely on an invisible layer of gases to retain sufficient heat and keep temperature extremes within physiologically tolerable limits.

We know that all species must adapt to the environment in order to survive, yet we purposely try to reorder our habitat rather than strive for greater harmony. The more we succeed in exerting our will, the more control we presume to have—and the less respect we accord in return.

Perhaps if we can pause long enough, we might see that the environment is a marvel of completeness we can never match. We might realize that decades of divisive debate about trade-offs and need to protect the environment have not served us well. The environment never negotiates, nor does it need protection. It's not at risk—we are. We are the ones locked into a niche existence. We are the ones with our heads on the chopping block.

Lack of a niche habitat for us means no food or human life. All the money and technology in the world cannot change this reality. When it comes to survival, not to mention well-being, our best shot is forgoing presumptions of control and embracing harmony and respect with the one and only partner available to us.

Part IV

Decisions You'll Make

Chapter 11

Live *and* Learn

*If they can get you asking the wrong questions, they don't have
to worry about answers.*

— Thomas Pynchon, *Gravity's Rainbow*

When life expectancy hovers around eighty years, it is hard to grasp geologic time—the eons of subtle shifts in the land, air, and water. As the Central American isthmus was forming, the open waters between North and South America were closing, permanently changing the planet's ocean currents, weather, and temperatures. This land would become home to countries like Costa Rica, Honduras, and Nicaragua, some of our newest neighbors on the American-continent block. For me, taking up residence eons later in Costa Rica, and then being awakened and shaken by earthquakes, watching red lava spit from the bowels of an active volcano, and being drenched by storms and blown by trailing hurricanes as they lashed this lush paradise, were continual reminders that what began five million years ago still carries on to this day.

One fall afternoon in 1998, in the safety of my home outside San José, I stared outside and saw dark clouds open up and torrents of heavy rains pour down. As rainwater surged off rooftops, streets were flooded and embankments were washed away. I was witnessing the fringe of the deadliest Atlantic hurricane since 1780. At its worst, rain fell at up to four inches per hour while winds approached 180 miles per hour. Homes, roads, and bridges were torn apart. Water and mud washed out entire communities. By the time Hurricane Mitch made landfall in South Florida as a tropical storm and eventually faded into the Atlantic, an estimated 22,000 people had been killed, almost all in Central America.

Costa Rica was lucky. Despite the seven deaths and tens of millions of dollars in property damage reported, the country had gotten off easy. Mitch had saved its worst for two of the continent's poorest nations, further north—Nicaragua and Honduras.

One of every five Hondurans was left homeless. Seventy percent of the country's crops were lost. Up to 80 percent of its transportation infrastructure was destroyed. Among the two million people affected in Nicaragua, as many as 40 percent lost their homes. Thousands were buried under mudslides extending up to ten miles long and five miles wide. At least a thousand bodies were found floating in rivers or washed up onshore. Staple crops like beans, rice, sugar, bananas, and coffee were wiped out.

The aftermath defied description and comprehension. Not only were homes gone, but the flooding and erosion had wreaked havoc on the land. Though humanitarian aid was flowing in, picking up the pieces would be long and hellish. When the news coverage trailed off, the rest of the world moved on; the plight of the hurricane's victims was soon forgotten. Entire communities were starting over, but had little to start with.

The heavy damage inflicted included large farming operations. The hurricane had laid bare their dependence on modern systems like banking to offer loans, agribusinesses to provide machinery, fertilizers and pesticides to boost yields, and public infrastructure to maintain roads, bridges, and ports. With no products to harvest, their customers were lost to other countries. Convincing businesses, bankers, and buyers they could rebuild, take on more debt, and withstand another catastrophe, were it to happen, would be an uphill battle.

These pre-hurricane farms had followed the blueprints of their counterparts in Western countries like the United States. To compete internationally, they had turned to capital and technology to dial up as much food production as possible. But the trade-off for high-yield harvests was relinquishing self-reliance and forgoing resilience in the face of unforeseen events.

Post-hurricane, the only option, they concluded, was to rebuild. Their recovery would rely on support from their own governments, who in turn would rely on international loans and monetary relief.

As much as it could, my organization, the Inter-American Institute for Cooperation on Agriculture (IICA), assisted in the response. But as time passed, life went on and my memory might have faded, had there not been an Ibero-American Conference held later in Havana, Cuba. The theme was food and agriculture. To ensure that all Spanish- and Portuguese-speaking nations could participate, IICA helped finance the travel of representatives from Central America. I was invited to accompany IICA's director general.

Once in Cuba, I set out to spend time with individuals whose countries Mitch had unceremoniously turned inside out. Their stories were raw; the challenges they faced remained daunting. Setbacks in securing aid had delayed rebuilding roads and infrastructure, reestablishing production, and reclaiming old markets. The daily grind of uncertainty had taken its toll. As they talked about what lay ahead, a cloud of quiet desperation hung low over our conversations.

Eight years earlier, Cubans had similarly been thrust into their own crisis. For decades, the country had supplied the Soviet Union with sugar, citrus, and nickel in exchange for wheat, petroleum, chemicals, and machinery. Then, apparently without any warning, the Soviets had nullified the arrangement. The region's largest importer of petroleum and agricultural chemicals suddenly had none. Modern farming practices no longer worked; tractors sat idle, rusting in fields. Making the crisis worse, poor weather had dried up ready supplies of fresh water. Government efforts to boost productivity on state-owned agricultural farms had failed. From 1990 to 1994, the average Cuban lost twenty pounds.

Yet by the time of my visit, despair had gradually given way to determination. State control of farmland had been partially relaxed.

Peasant farmers were granted more autonomy. At their behest, Cuban agronomists were helping to advance non-petroleum-based technologies to rejuvenate the soil, control weeds, fight pests, promote plant diversity, rotate vegetable crops, encourage natural predator and parasite control, and otherwise rework farming practices for local conditions.

Cuban pride and optimism were on display in the farms I visited and in the stories I heard. Yields on small plots of land had steadily climbed. Additional food was being produced and sold at local markets. The road back had not been easy, but farmers expressed a sense of having more control and being less reliant on others.

Cubans often referred to these initial years of struggle as "the special period," as if it were a proving ground they had successfully conquered. As one farmer said to me, "We knew that nobody was coming to help us, so we pulled ourselves up by our bootstraps and made it happen." Then, as if to make sure I understood his point, he reached down and tugged on the top of his boots for emphasis.

For me, the contrast between Central America and Cuba highlighted what it meant to live *and* learn. Both areas were broadsided by devastating events, yet they responded very differently. Large farming operations in Central America fell back on what they already knew, while Cubans took a new tack. After early government initiatives had fallen short, rather than hold out hope for petroleum imports and external aid they had channeled their energy into producing food differently. Outside assistance would come from nature. Restoring food production would hinge on greater harmony with the environment.

When food comes easily, living without learning becomes easier. Any concerns about scarcity are countered by simply ratcheting up additional food production. Having more food comes from increasing the size and scale of production—not rethinking the modern food system. True learning, on the other hand, requires us to question common assumptions.

A case in point is the frequent assertion that *to feed a growing population, food production will need to double by the year 2050.* For many, this claim is self-evident. The United Nations estimates that the global population will reach 9.8 billion people by 2050. Projections about how much additional food will be needed have varied, ranging from half to twice as much as existing levels.

For those wanting to turn out more food, these statistics provide the perfect justification: more people means that more food is needed, which calls for greater food production. To disagree is to line up on the wrong side of humanity. Researchers seeking grants, countries wanting loans from international banks, and nonprofit organizations seeking donations all fall back on this assumption.

In addition, agribusinesses use it to rationalize new fertilizer plants or to market more pesticides. Politicians leverage it to secure votes or defend taxpayer subsidies. Farmers use it to reinforce existing production practices. When it comes to propping up modern food systems around the world, the question is not so much who relies on such statements as fact, but who doesn't.

But the idea that more people require greater production presumes there is barely enough food in the world as is. The related presumption is that food is already efficiently produced, distributed, and consumed. Backers of this idea show us images of starving children, not the two billion plus who are overweight or obese where food is readily abundant and needlessly wasted.

Indeed, food waste is chronic. Across the world, from one-third to one-half of food grown is never consumed at all. In developing countries, more than 40 percent of loss happens near the farm in storage, transportation, and processing. In countries like the United States, less food is lost on the front end, while more is wasted in stores, restaurant tables, and home refrigerators, where up to 40 percent is never eaten.

The food system converts different kinds of energy into edible calories, but Western diets squander most of that energy. Two-thirds of the energy harvested from cropland goes to feed animals, not people. Energy within grains and forage are transformed by animals into fat and muscle, but not before most of it is lost in the conversion or used to fuel the animals' metabolism. After taking into account all the energy loses from feed to food, only a small percentage of edible calories remain: from chickens, about 12 percent; hogs, around 10 percent; cattle, in the neighborhood of 3 percent.

People choose to eat meat and fat because of their genetics and culture, not because meat and fat are efficient sources of delivering edible calories. The caloric (or energy) waste goes up as people overeat. In four decades, global obesity rates have tripled. In too many countries, rates are rising faster in children than in adults.

Our focus on endlessly ramping up food production also discounts the drawdown of finite resources. Land used to raise animals, either to provide pasture or to grow animal feed, comprises 75 percent of all agricultural land. Annually, agriculture is the world's largest consumer of water, with irrigation accounting for some 70 percent of global fresh water used.

Our belief in the continual need for greater production is reinforced by a similar belief that America must *feed the world*. While sharing food is laudable, it has also been a façade for self-interest. Unloading excess food on other countries is a longtime public policy strategy to raise farm prices domestically. More to the point, surplus food is not automatically destined for those populations most in need. Government donor programs such as "Food for Peace" must first satisfy America's domestic and foreign-policy objectives; addressing malnutrition is secondary.

Feeding the world from surplus is not the same as helping the world feed itself. Mozambique, neighbor to South Africa, offers one example. For decades, the country relied on local food sold in small stores and open-air markets. Then came supermarkets, and with them, food produced abroad. On a trip to the nation's capital, Maputo, I went with my hosts to a well-stocked modern supermarket. In the meat department's frozen-food section, a display case was loaded with broilers, imported from Brazil, whose original destination was the Middle East. When those countries refused the shipment, then—as always happens whenever food is rejected—it was shopped to other countries. Eventually landing in Mozambique, the meat was priced low enough to disrupt the country's fledgling broiler chicken sector.

More than seven in ten farms in the world are smaller than one hectare (about 2.5 acres). Unlike in the United States, few farmers count on an abundance of resources, massive transportation infrastructure, access to financial capital, or farm and export subsidies. What these farmers can offer is biological diversity and resilience built up over generations to cope with harsh environments. Out of necessity, they have made do with very little.

But when others undercut their only means of livelihood, many ultimately migrate to urban areas, only to find themselves dependent on their country's ability to navigate the world of high-stakes trade, diplomacy, and international finance. If they cannot find jobs and secure food, some inevitably join uprisings or emigrate to other countries.

Such was the case in one country that had little annual rainfall but whose leaders foresaw prosperity in modern crop production and international exports. They poured money into extracting underground water and diverting rivers to grow water-intensive crops. As the amount of available water grew, so did the mismanagement and corruption. Water usage soon exceeded historic levels. When a severe drought settled over the region, water supplies were severely depleted.

Four years of unrelenting drought, falling food production, and escalating uncertainty triggered rural migration to urban areas, already under stress from a million-plus refugees fleeing war-torn Iraq. The country was Syria. The history of its brutal war includes actions and consequences not covered on the evening news. Behind the uprising and killing is a story of food prices that spiked in international markets, exploitation of scarce resources, indifference to the world's subsistence farmers, and misguided confidence in intensive agriculture.

The need for more food that can only come from perpetuating the existing modern food system is more myth than reality, which like most myths, needs good iconography. Pictures plastered on semi-truck trailers, ads on television, and product placements in social media and retail outlets would have consumers believe that their food came from a small family farm just down the road. Why such an approach? Farmers sell food—a food system, not so much.

Crafting a narrative around the family farm benefits the entire modern food system. On the outside of a paper bag that came from a quick-serve restaurant chain is a barn with a gambrel roof, typical of farms from an earlier era. In large bold letters the inscription declares, "Thank You, Farmers" and "Family Farm Fresh." The accompanying text applauds the customer, too, because their purchase will "help support hard-working farm families everywhere."

The subtle ploy is to bond consumers with small farmers, with the restaurant playing the neighborly role of bringing everyone together. The paper bag had held a chicken sandwich and ice cream sundae, with the cost totaling $6.95 plus tax. The farmer's portion, after others in the food system have taken their cut, works out to be a penny or so for the wheat made into a bun, maybe a nickel for the milk and sugar that became the ice cream, and a few cents for having raised the meat. (Few poultry farmers actually own the chickens or the feed, the two biggest expenses.) From the customer's decision to stop by and purchase ready-to-eat food, hard-working farm families earned a dime, maybe fifteen cents. The rest was gobbled up by expenses like transportation, processing, packaging, preparation, cleanup, wholesaling, retailing, labor, advertising, profit, etc.

All but the top 1 percent of farms are called family farms. One in ten farms account for more than three-quarters of value produced. Nine in ten farms account for less than one-quarter. Household income for the top 10 percent of family farms ranges from $186,000 to $1.7 million. Nine percent of farms receive two-thirds of all government subsidies. Seventy percent of farms receive nothing.

Subsidies began at a time when farms were more alike, facing similar challenges. Then as now, farmers made decisions months before harvest. So long as non-farmers were employed, there were buyers for what farmers produced. Then came the Great Depression. As the economy nosedived and savings dried up, volunteers and nonprofit relief agencies were overwhelmed. Some of the unemployed resorted to foraging through garbage cans, digging for roots in public parks, and sending their children begging door-to-door.

Farmers were also in dire straits. They had food to sell but not enough buyers able to pay for it. Unsold milk was dumped in ditches, piglets were slaughtered, fields were left fallow. Surplus farm products piled up. Farmers needed money to keep farming, but the unemployed had none to spare. Millions cried out for public assistance.

America had provided such assistance previously—to other countries. When World War I ended, the United States dispatched food to starving Europeans. But President Herbert Hoover viewed America's depression differently. In his mind, a sluggish economy did not merit national intervention. Overproduction and hunger were temporary anomalies that volunteers and nonprofit relief agencies could bridge until markets realigned themselves.

Notwithstanding his rationale, a moral question loomed—how could a country with so much food not share it with those in need? If the jobless had no income with which to buy farm products, and an oversupply of food dropped prices below what farmers needed to stay afloat, then channeling surplus food to unemployed urban workers would solve both problems. Hoover's defeat in the presidential election of 1932 cleared the way. As one official put it, "We got a picture of a gorge, with farm surpluses on one cliff and undernourished city folks with outstretched hands on the other. We set out to find a practical way to build a bridge across that chasm."

So in 1933, with the promise of more food and stable prices, taxpayers climbed aboard as Congress stepped in to rescue farmers by raising farm income. During the Great Depression, food comprised one-quarter of household expenditures, and unemployment peaked at 25 percent. Only government had the capacity to expediently reconcile excess production with the widespread need for food assistance.

Nonetheless, what followed became a missed opportunity to live *and* learn—a missed opportunity that continues to this day. At the time of the depression, people believed that farmers deserved help and that unemployment was temporary. Addressing questions of what should be the proper role of government post-depression fell by the wayside.

Before the decade was over, and despite steady growth in farm income, subsidies and protections became a permanent feature of ongoing farm legislation. Likewise, though the economy recovered and unemployment fell, leveraging hunger with public safety nets would become a tool for politicians to accumulate influence with the public to stay in office (political capital) and for businesses to sell more food and enrich profits. The opportunity to structurally address, rather than exploit, the connection between subsidies to produce food and food assistance to arrest hunger would be squandered.

Over the decades, other sectors of the economy also found ways to benefit or cash in. For the military, food-assistance programs became an issue of national security as malnutrition from lack of food had been the number-one reason military recruits had failed their physicals during World War II. The military's advocacy proved pivotal in launching the National School Lunch Program.

Wholesalers and retailers convinced Congress to funnel more business their way. The Food Stamp Act was the result, designed to tie surplus farm products to additional retail purchases. Eventually, electronic benefits (think: debit cards) replaced food stamps, and the program was rebranded as the Supplemental Nutrition Assistance Program (SNAP).

In recent decades, the moral questions asked earlier have not centered on why food production continues to be subsidized, or why excess food should be shared, but whether or not recipients of food assistance are *truly* in need. While there are fifteen separate food-assistance programs, SNAP receives the lion's share of funding, criticism, and zeal for reform—and both political parties have acted to limit eligibility.

For the record, SNAP enrollment climbs when the economy falters, and falls when the economy recovers. Ninety-two percent of SNAP benefits go to households below the poverty line. Nearly 90 percent of recipients are in households that include a child under age eighteen, an elderly person sixty years or older, or a member with disabilities. Children younger than eighteen make up 44 percent of all recipients. The benefit per meal—$1.40—is calculated from USDA's definition of a bare-bones, nutritionally adequate diet.

Traditionally, Americans' number-one volunteer activity is charitable food assistance. Americans help at soup kitchens, work in food banks, support food drives, and donate time, money, and effort to food relief causes. Whether it be a meal delivered to a home when a loved one passes away, or a welcome invitation to break bread with another, food reinforces a common bond with humanity, a reminder of vulnerability, a recognition of how we depend on other living beings for nourishment. The sharing of food is part of what defines America.

So why have food-aid programs like SNAP become so acrimonious? When help is abused, those doing the giving can feel burned and their resentment can be long-lasting. Any wrongdoing becomes fodder for agendas that oppose public aid. Reports of hucksters exploiting public assistance and living a life of slothfulness are perceived as the embodiment of a broken system financed on the backs of hard-working

Americans who get up every day, go to work, and do their part. The resentment lingers and trust erodes. Programs like SNAP are construed as rotten to the core, benefiting no one, including those most in need. Cutting funding and limiting benefits and eligibility become humane ways for moving forward. As the programs are starved into elimination, so the assumptions go, volunteers, churches, and nonprofit agencies will magnanimously take over.

Yet neither empathy, indignation, nor financial motives address the question once posed by food historian Janet Poppendieck: "If virtually nobody wants hunger in our affluent society, and nearly everybody supports some approach to its elimination, and there is plenty of food, why can't we get rid of it?"

Food aid has become too important a source for political capital and business profits. From 2010 through 2017, more than a half-*trillion* SNAP dollars were spent in some 260,000 retail outlets. Providing food assistance has become an essential revenue stream within the modern food system.

Walmart takes in close to one in five dollars of SNAP program benefits. Amazon, whose valuation by Wall Street is already greater than rivals Walmart, Costco, Target, Macy's, and Kohl's combined, is scheduled to accept SNAP grocery orders. Brushed aside is the fact that Amazon's median annual salary is only $28,466—well below the poverty line for a family of four. And the fact that one-third of its employees depend on SNAP for food. SNAP is the latest subsidy Amazon will receive on top of other tax breaks, infrastructure improvements, and financial incentives—all paid for by taxpayers. Expect food manufacturers and retailers to spend heavily lobbying Congress for food aid continuation.

And therein lies one of the most pernicious consequences of the grand food bargain—*availability* of food is not the same as *access* to food. The mindless drive for more food made food more abundant or readily available. No other country can turn out a greater volume of food at lower prices than can the United States. Yet those who go hungry are not beleaguered by whether or not food is available, but rather by whether they have access to it.

In America, access to food relies on a growing, vibrant economy whose benefits flow to *all* through viable jobs and livable wages. This idealized economy for all, however, no longer exists. The average worker's wages, adjusted for inflation, peaked more than forty years ago. While opportunities for those in the top income strata have continually improved, average workers' wages have barely budged, and those in the lowest income strata have fallen further behind. As household budgets have tightened, so also has access to food.

In the current environment, businesses and politicians are benefiting twice over. First, taxpayers are financing access to food for the most vulnerable, making it easy for politicians and businesses to avoid resetting public policies and business practices that undercut broad economic opportunity. Second, any calls to rein in oversupply by cutting subsidies to the food system are easily spun to the public as cruel measures that will cut off access to food by those most in need.

This willingness to blur access and availability, and unwillingness to address structural economic causes that limit opportunities for the most vulnerable, shows no signs of abating. Coming out of the post-2008 economic recovery, three of every five new jobs were mostly low-wage service positions. Such jobs remain the fastest-growing segment in the employment market. Keeping profits high and worker incomes low, American businesses outsource jobs overseas, deploy immigrant labor, and eliminate benefits through part-time positions (while often expecting workers to be available full-time). The service sector is also in the crosshairs of technology, with humans being replaced by artificial intelligence, automation, and self-service retail.

As more-desirable employment opportunities have withered, people have juggled multiple jobs, forgone health benefits, relied on extended families for day care, and applied for food assistance. As the number of service-sector jobs expands in proportion to total employment, low-income families make trade-offs—pay for utilities or purchase more food? Budget for maximum calories to dampen hunger or for better nutrition?

The vast majority on food assistance are working families, including military households. As incomes stagnate, their numbers will grow. Eighty percent of monthly SNAP benefits are typically spent by the end of the second week. These struggles serve as reminders that the ghosts of the Great Depression are still with us.

In a cruel twist of irony, those who rely most heavily on food aid are agricultural and food-service workers. These are the people who plant, harvest, process, prepare, deliver, and clean up after us. They serve in banquet halls for wedding receptions and conferences. They dutifully comply with requirements to throw away untouched plated food when guests fail to show up.

Admittedly, there are some who game the system, just as there are affluent people who cheat on their taxes, slough off at work, defraud friends and family, or renege on contracts. Overall, the most vulnerable in the country are no different from most Americans striving to fashion a better life. But as part of the lowest-income strata in society, they hold little sway with politicians.

Until we choose to live *and* learn, and demand better of our elected officials, it is worth remembering that more than one in five children now live below the poverty level (close to one in four in rural America). Those who receive SNAP benefits fare better as adults in health and education than eligible children who do not. These least fortunate live in the shadows, observing how those with easy access to food liberally waste food while determining their access to food.

Focusing attention on who deserves food assistance draws attention away from far greater subsidies. Subsidies, it is worth remembering, are benefits received without compensation. If nature were valued for the ongoing "public assistance" it provides, each of us would be guilty of receiving subsidies at levels that dwarf all other social and government programs.

In other words, all of us are freeloaders. Without nature and the environment there would be no fresh, filtered water transporting nutrients, petroleum for powering tractors, wood for cooking, or food and fiber from other living organisms. The evolution of genetics that enhances yields, the life-sustaining temperatures and climate that keep us alive, the ongoing cycling of carbon and nutrients, and the formation of new soil to grow plants are just a few of the countless subsidies we receive—for which we contribute nothing. Worth remembering is that these planetary forces can carry on just fine without any of us—while the reverse can never be said. When it comes to sustaining life on this planet, the environment holds all the cards.

The answer to freeloading was supposed to have been sustainability. In theory, sustainability embodies an appreciation that humans are one small part of a delicate environment and tenuous existence. The practice of sustainability was intended to give back instead of always taking.

But for all the honorable aspirations, sustainability is guided by few social norms; its importance is largely in the eye of the beholder. So while the word *sustainability* was being tacked on to scores of initiatives, its power to inspire societies was fading. Businesses set their own finish line, then declared themselves victorious. Questions about "greenwashing" mounted, then faded away.

Thus, when seafood in supermarkets was labeled as "certified sustainable," there was no guarantee that the fishery was indeed any more sustainable. Why? Third-party certifying organizations do not regulate, set catch limits, control marine biology and habitat, or ensure that illegal fishing is not happening.

When crop farmers enrolled in proprietary programs with names like SUSTAIN, they were offered promises that these programs would enable them to "keep nutrients and sediment where they belong— on farm fields." While such programs might help with placement and timing of fertilizer applications, there were never any assurances that less fertilizer would be used or water quality in streams and waterways would improve.

Petroleum-based "biodegradable" plastics were offered as a partial solution to plastic waste filling the oceans, ending up in fish and ultimately in the people who eat them. But when university researchers compared plastics containing the additives to make them biodegradable versus those without, no differences were detected.

In the corporate world, sustainability initiatives and reports were used to boost companies' public images. In 2014, Volkswagen Group, at the time the world's largest car manufacturer, declared that the company "has a long tradition of resolute commitment to environmental protection." Then it rigged eleven million vehicles to circumvent environmental rules before Volkswagen was caught. The year afterward, the company repeated the same pledge verbatim.

In 2006, to preserve the Amazon rain forest a moratorium on planting soybeans was enacted, to wide acclaim. Henceforth, beans grown by deforesting the Amazon would be rejected for purchase and export. Nonprofit agencies would use satellite imagery to carry out surveillance. Multinational grain-trading companies would enforce the rules. Sustainability of the Amazon was about to happen.

Before the agreement, soybean acreage had expanded by 30 percent in just two years. One year afterward, expansion was less than 1 percent. For retailers like McDonald's and Walmart, nonprofits like Greenpeace, and trading companies like Bunge and Cargill, a public relations nightmare had been filleted into a public relations triumph.

I was heartened when I read the press accounts, and I featured the moratorium in teaching materials and presentations as one example of forward-thinking agriculture. I also congratulated associates I knew in Cargill. But after eight years and two independent studies published in *Science*, a darker picture emerged. The moratorium, it became clear, only pertained to part of the Amazon, and the big decline in acreage planted was misleading. Land cleared prior to the moratorium was being used to accommodate further expansion. Pasture previously created from deforesting was also being planted in soybeans. Farmers had turned to clearing native vegetation and planting soybeans on land just outside the moratorium's boundaries. If need be, harvested beans were being "laundered" through other properties.

Indeed, as market opportunities for farmers beckoned and governments chose not to act, moratoriums provided cover for deforestation to continue. Beginning in the summer of 2015, in less than a year, more than two million acres were deforested in Brazil. In neighboring Bolivia, deforestation shot up by more than 80 percent in a decade.

My misstep was accepting the moratorium at face value. I wanted to believe the publicity that this was a promising new trend. I never bothered with confirming the results. In the midst of endless bad environmental news, it was natural to want progress. But living *and* learning requires vigilance in addition to hope.

The same applies to questioning the productivity of American agriculture. Over the last several decades, to turn out more food we have relied heavily on more fertilizer, chemicals, water, monoculture crops, and concentrated animal feeding operations. Using more to produce more without questioning what comes afterward is hardly a recipe for a sustainable food system.

Because what goes up invariably comes down, food productivity will eventually fall. A more technical term to describe this transition is *peak-rate*, which also serves as an indicator of sustainability. As the modern food system expands internationally, what happens at the global level takes on added importance. For crucial staple foods like wheat, for example, peak-rate indicates that wheat harvests will next plateau, and then decline. Recently, researchers looked at whether the peak-rates for major foods and related resources at the global level were in decline. For fifteen of the sixteen most common staples like dairy, eggs, seafood, meat, poultry, soybeans, wheat, and corn, the answer was yes. For related resources like land to grow crops, water to irrigate those crops, and nitrogen to provide nutrients, the answer was also yes.

While the environment's role in food availability is irreplaceable, such importance is seldom acknowledged. Over time, shifts in the environment have led to mass extinction of species. Five such extinctions have occurred, caused by meteor strikes, volcanoes, and natural climate. Today, we are experiencing the sixth mass extinction. But unlike the previous five, this one is due to heat-trapping molecules in the atmosphere from burning fossil fuels.

Extinction rates always vary by species and changes to habitat. As the planet warms, weeds, insects, and parasites are fanning out geographically. As they spread, entire ecologies of needed microbes, beneficial insects, food plants, and food animals are threatened. When habitats that once supported life begin to perish, genetic diversity falls and traits that gave us greater yields at harvest, resilience to weather, or resistance to pests and competitors are at risk of being lost. Nutrients like zinc and iron in grains and legumes decline. Food plants and animals, already weakened by higher stress as temperatures rise, succumb to the growth and attacks of bacteria that have more readily adapted.

Productivity, peak-rate, and mass extinction pose enormous challenges. Yet there exists an even more ominous threat—apathy on our part. The grand food bargain now spans multiple generations. Many see nearby restaurants and supermarkets as their source of food. How food got there is unimportant compared to price, selection, and individual preferences. When abundance foments apathy, living *without* learning takes over.

Always asking questions is one way to keep apathy at bay and avoid taking food for granted. For me, one such experience came on a hot summer day in Colorado. Standing in an un-air-conditioned concrete and metal building set up to slaughter sheep, I watched the procession of freshly killed lambs, suspended upside down, their blood still dripping onto the cement floor. Against the background of industrial machines and noise, knives clashed with steel as workers honed their blades razor sharp. Outfitted in stainless-steel-mesh aprons, rubber boots, and white clothing stained with blood and sweat, they stood next to each other executing precise cuts over and over without stopping. With each stab of their hooks and slice with their knives, perspiration poured down their arms and off their foreheads.

I was no stranger to viscera and blood, but the heat and unending line of gutted red carcasses was getting to me. Setting my gaze on the supervisor, I watched as he paced behind the workers, observing their actions and exhorting the slower ones to pick up their pace as the line of animals trudged by. Then I noticed it: clutched in his hand was a slab of fresh meat between two pieces of bread.

Raw animals, alive minutes ago, and a slaughterhouse boss haranguing workers to move faster, all the while eating a sandwich bursting with lamb meat: Was this what food was all about? Was volume all that mattered? If the workers maintained a higher pace, at some future date the line speed would be ratcheted up further and the cycle repeated. For the company, meat was about profitability. For consumers, it came down to price and sensory pleasure.

In the intervening years, simply raising questions about our relationship to food and the modern food system has sharpened my understanding and prompted other questions. Why do we ignore our reliance on other species, and our stewardship of resources? Why do we engage in an ongoing battle against nature, and exhibit such a cavalier outlook toward the environment? Why do we dismiss the welfare of the modern food system's workers? Why have such issues become secondary to profit and personal preference? At what point does this mindless drive for more turn against us?

Humans have appropriated up to 40 percent of the Earth's biological production potential. Through our efforts alone we have modified an estimated 50 percent of the Earth's surface. Taking into account the size and number of all animal species, the "biomass" of mammals that humans raise for food now exceeds the biomass of all mammalian wildlife on the planet.

But instead of learning from our past, society pawns off the most looming questions onto science and technology, and apathy allows us to go about life while we await solutions. Cellular agriculture, for example, with its "promise of solving enormous environmental, food-security, and economic challenges posed by our growing global population," is developing meat cultured in a laboratory, outside of an animal. Quantum dots, or nanoparticles (semiconducting materials several thousand times smaller in diameter than a single strand of hair), which biochemically react with bacteria when illuminated with light, are touted as a way to rejuvenate ineffective antibiotics. Identifying genes responsible for the evolution of biological processes, finding ways to capture more of the Sun's energy, and improving the efficiency of plants to remove carbon from carbon dioxide and turn it into carbohydrates are other moonshots that initially mesmerize our attention.

Indeed, coursing through America's bloodstream is a ready eagerness to green-light novel and exciting technologies while asking few if any questions as to their unforeseen consequences. But a brief look backward illustrates how apathy, combined with naiveté, allowed us to fall victim to cyberattacks, identity fraud, big data, and a decline in social civility. When evaluating the latest proposed scientific marvel, it is worth remembering Amara's law: *We tend to overestimate the effect of a technology in the short run and underestimate the effect in the long run.*

Ironically, we are less likely to embrace viable technologies that are closer at hand. They include perennial grasses and legumes to replace annuals like wheat, corn, and rice. Drip irrigation to conserve water.

Cover crops and buffer zones to reduce runoff and topsoil degradation. Greater diversity of species and crop rotation to boost nutrient ecology. The sustainability and reduced resource usage of circular production flows where by-products of one enterprise feed into another such as aquaculture and vegetable production. Or even more-localized farming, which reduces transportation and rewards the breeding of better-tasting plant varieties.

Such technologies lack the flash of quantum dots or the mystique of "clean meat." Their long-run emphasis is less attractive to venture capitalists seeking shorter-term profits. Their old-school versus new-magic approach embodies the kinds of practices I saw in Cuba two decades ago.

Off and on, I've checked in on Cuba's transition. By 2006, the peasant sector controlled a quarter of agricultural land, yet it produced close to two-thirds of the country's food. A year later, the United Nations estimated the number of calories available per person was higher in Cuba than in any other Latin American or Caribbean country.

But in the years since, part of Cuba's agriculture has reverted back to more resource-intensive production. The country has once again become dependent on importing petroleum and chemicals. The allure of higher profits from more volume was just too hard to pass up, even if it eventually returns Cubans to having to live and relearn all over again.

The standard of living that Americans take for granted partially explains why we avoid tough questions. But if we don't channel apathy into inquiry, that abundance will one day disappear. Going forward, we need to recognize the power we have as consumers. After all, it is our purchases that bankroll the modern food system. Stated another way, if the grand food bargain were made into a movie, consumers would be its executive producers. Without consumers, there would be no movie and certainly no grand food bargain.

Seeing ourselves as just an audience for food providers does not serve us well. Nor does reducing our role in making decisions to what we toss into shopping carts and order off menus. Food providers are fond of saying that consumers are in charge. They are correct: it is consumer demand that determines what food is supplied. Yet there is a huge difference between choosing from food that is already harvested, processed, and displayed, and choosing what kind of food should be produced in the first place. One approach confines consumer choice to the tail end of the modern food system. The other encourages us to step up and take leadership in resetting what the modern food system should be. As we'll explore in the final chapter, when it comes to living *and* learning, the most important question of all is whether consumers will choose to lead or be led.

Chapter 12

To Lead or Be Led?

Everyone thinks of changing the world, but no one thinks of changing himself.
— Leo Tolstoy

B efore Neil Armstrong could take his "one giant leap for mankind," the National Aeronautics and Space Administration (NASA) needed to confirm that a manned spacecraft could break free of the Earth's gravitational pull, orbit the Moon, and successfully return home. This was *Apollo 8*'s mission, and from launch to splashdown, NASA had meticulously planned every minute of flight.

On Christmas Eve 1968, as the spacecraft started circling the Moon, the three men aboard became the first humans to see the Moon's dark side with their own eyes. Per the detailed flight schedule, the crew would orbit the lunar surface nine more times before starting the long journey back. But just as *Apollo 8* emerged from the Moon's far side the fourth time, still outside radio contact with mission control, Commander Frank Borman unexpectedly noticed something not written down on the flight schedule—the Earth rising above the Moon's horizon.

Instantly, the men scrambled for cameras and color film to take pictures through a still-clear window before the moment and image were lost forever. The most famous photo they took is called *Earthrise*. In the foreground is the craggy, black-and-white lunar surface. In the background, surrounded by total darkness, is a round, bluish globe covered with swirls of white—quite miniature compared with the Moon. As astronaut Bill Anders later retold the moment: "We could see a very fragile-looking Earth, a very delicate-looking Earth. I was immediately almost overcome by the thought that here we came all the way to the Moon, and yet the most significant thing we're seeing is our own home planet, the Earth."

The images of Earth captured by the *Apollo 8* astronauts were not the first taken from space. Unmanned lunar probes and communication satellites had come before. But this occasion was different. Instead of impersonal circuitry and mechanical technology, three warm-blooded humans had boldly left the safety of Earth, traveled beyond its gravitational reach, and snapped the pictures. The vivid appearance of our planet, providing the only color in an otherwise black expanse of space, had been there all along.

From 240,000 miles away, *Earthrise* portrayed the precariousness of our own existence. As historian Robert Poole later wrote, "Looking back, it is possible to see that 'Earthrise' marked the tipping point, the moment when the sense of space age flipped from what it meant for space to what it meant for Earth."

This awakening spread worldwide; people began to see the Earth as a living dynamic organism. Words like *stewardship* and *sustainability* became meaningful. Looking after the planet's resources and environment took on importance. *Life* magazine declared, "Suddenly we are all conservationists." For a brief time, people caught a glimpse of how their own lives, those of other living beings, and a solitary planet were inextricably bound together.

For me, the tipping point came not from space but deep in the Kalahari Desert, though I would not realize its full impact until later. On that warm, sunny day when Paul and I accompanied a single Bushman in search of food, I saw that he had free rein to act with impunity. Had he acquiesced to our urging and carried back all of the eggs, he would have reinforced our Westernized beliefs; my memories of that day would have melted away and the event would have been forgotten. Instead, his behavior caught us off guard, teaching us what it meant to lead and not be led.

His actions transcended our understanding, limited as it was by our reliance on the modern food system. America's grand food bargain, begun in the nineteenth century, had maintained its lock on how we perceive our world well into the twenty-first. This insight was the missing piece I had been looking for—a glimpse of the fact that changes to the environment, brought about by humans' drive for food, still shape who we are and how we live. For the Bushman, ensuring harmony with the Kalahari forged who he was. For his people to survive some two thousand years in this desolate land, where we might have easily perished if left alone, they had to recognize the contribution of other living beings and care for the environment and its limited resources.

Americans, by contrast, live with the illusion of infinity. The story of how this came to be has two parts. The first was humankind's long passage to farming. The second, much more recent, was the transition to becoming a nation of consumers. As farmers, our lives were still subservient to food. As consumers, food became subservient to us.

It has been said that how we produce and consume food has a bigger impact on well-being than any other human activity. Indeed, until the grand food bargain came along, limits to food were an unchallenged fact of life. Coping with the scarcity of food structured daily living around the natural rhythms of seasons, plants, and animals. In geologic time, the transition from food scarcity to abundance was like flicking on a light switch.

The result is arguably the pinnacle of human accomplishment. What stands out is how food became readily available, more so than at any point in human history. What is less apparent, but more important, is how this growing glut of food has skewed our understanding of our surroundings and our perceptions of control.

Such an outlook started early. Colonial settlers, even while struggling to produce enough food, saw limitless bounties for the taking. To all appearances, America had won the resource lottery, inheriting unprecedented levels of ideal farmland and fresh water, not to mention a favorable climate. The sense of endless abundance only grew as the discovery of rich reserves of liquid fossil fuels intensified food production. There seemed to be no end to how much could be produced. Why would we bother to conserve resources when we could simply extract and consume more?

Today, the modern food system accommodates our schedules, not to mention our personal tastes. Convenience has been critical in reengineering our understanding. Food is no longer the means for society's survival, but instead a source of personal pleasure and expression of individual freedom and uniqueness. As food became ever more readily available, the easier it was to believe that we deserved more while being free of responsibilities—and the simpler it became to ignore the forces that made abundance possible.

Food producers have profited immeasurably from the new mindset of satisfying individual desires. So while people have been busy exploring their own wants, the modern food system keeps coming up with novel ways to infuse more calories while still delivering greater convenience. As the United States settled into being a nation of non-farmers, and food became a matter of personal preference, we assumed that this reshaping of society was neutral.

Yet food's effect on society was never neutral. Ramping up conveniences intensified food's broad reach over peoples' lives. The food system was shaping everything from consumer beliefs that yogurt improved health and digestion to advancing US interests abroad through more food aid. My recognition of food's influence was reinforced by Bernie Sanders— not the politician from Vermont, but the director of my department at Farmland Industries. A major reason for my joining Farmland had been their advanced analytical computing platform. The man behind it was Dr. Sanders, who, ironically, never used a computer.

Even more than his business acumen, I valued his insights about food and agriculture, often drawn from history. During one conversation, he talked about how food can be used as a means of control. A long-standing practice of the former Soviet Union was keeping prices of staple foods like bread artificially low, which indirectly tempered citizens' response to malfeasance on the part of its Communist leaders. Another example was when President Richard Nixon instructed the secretary of agriculture to make sure that food prices remained low, thus ensuring that food did not become a hot-button issue when reelection time rolled around. Today's continuation of farm subsidies, despite perpetual food surplus, stems from politicians' adept leveraging of the power of food.

In the name of food, wars have been launched, lands conquered, people enslaved, and freedoms lost. In 2011, rising food prices in Tunisia ignited demonstrations that spread to other countries in the region—what we know as the "Arab Spring." One country was Egypt, where artificially low prices had made bread an important part of their diet. When grain prices spiked in 2007–2008, and bread prices rose by 37 percent, the Egyptian government, the world's largest importer of wheat, did nothing. Its nonresponse amplified levels of hunger and helped catalyze revolt. Mass protests and the overthrow of the government followed.

When food is scarce, a cycle of unrest, protests, and instability follows. The use of lethal force to suppress a country's citizens—or even all-out civil war—is not uncommon. Such a cycle resulting from a scarcity of food is well recognized, but an overabundance of food has its own cycle, though it plays out on a longer time frame. America is in the midst of this cycle. We can see it happening already in the exploitation of finite resources, the disappearance of prime farmland and fossil water, the loss of governance and social norms, the erosion of public support to sustain sound science, and the unquestioned faith we put in markets.

The power of food is also evident at the individual level. I first saw it on display in my own backyard, over years of feeding cattle. Except for their first few weeks following their birth, I was present their entire lives. While some were docile, others were precocious, ready to break away at any opportunity. Each brought to the herd their own vibe, which together created a unique group identity. Yet despite differences in individual behavior, each morning and evening they all awaited food.

So twice each day, I trekked out to the barn. As they watched me walk up the lane, many stuck their heads through the feeding stalls in anticipation. A few signaled their impatience by bellowing. As I broke open fresh bales of hay and shoveled out much-desired fermented silage and milled grain, they settled in. As long as they had plenty to eat, they were under my control. Snow, cold, rain, or heat had no bearing.

As the months rolled by, they put on weight and filled out. When my father told me the date when the livestock truck would come, they were oblivious to what lay ahead. In their world, everything was as it should be. As the day drew near, I obliged them with as much food as they wanted. I also spent more time observing each while doing chores, locking away mental images of their presence.

The morning it happened began like any other. As I walked to the barn, they stuck their heads into the feeding stalls and prepared to eat. But this time I did not break open bales of hay or scoop out silage. Adjacent to the stalls was a loading chute, which had been there their entire lives. Backed up to it was the livestock carrier with its gates opened. As I looked at the cattle, they peered back at me, still waiting to be fed.

But instead of food, I pushed their heads out of the stalls while my father and brother surrounded them and herded them toward the loading chute. Confused and scared, a few searched for an opening to escape. But when the first one scampered up the loading ramp and into the truck, the others followed. While the driver closed the gates and secured his load, they huddled together in unfamiliar surroundings. As the truck slowly drove away, some stared back at me. This was the day they never could have seen coming. The abundance of food had ended the night before. Each time a load of cattle was dispatched to the slaughterhouse, similar sentiments of melancholy followed—as I knew that for them, this was the end of the line.

With the impersonal modern food system we support, cattle are there to fulfill a specific purpose—to transform energy that plants had previously captured from the Sun. On the farm, we harvested and fed this energy to them; they in turn converted and stored it as meat—muscle and fat. When consumers enter the supermarket and stop in the meat department, that muscle and fat is waiting for them in various cuts of meat and packages of ground beef.

At times, I have wondered: does the modern food system exist to serve consumers, or do consumers exist to serve the modern food system? Without people, the system is incomplete. The energy that begins with the Sun and is passed through plants and then into animals still needs to be converted into dollars. Plants have done their part. Animals have done their part. What remains is up to individual human consumers.

Through price and persuasion, the modern food system recruits each of us to carry out this final step that transforms food calories into money. The more calories we take in, the more money flows back to the food system. From the dollars-and-cents vantage point of the modern food system, what happens to consumers afterward is no more important than the fate of cattle destined for slaughter.

So long as people accept being just another step in a food system that transforms energy into somebody else's money, the power of the system over us grows, and our resilience to resist erodes. In extreme cases, food becomes a crutch, an opiate we use to endure desperate and unfulfilling lives. In his book *The Road to Wigan Pier*, George Orwell chronicled the coal-mining region of northern England during the depression times of the 1930s. Miners and their families lived on sugared tea, white bread and margarine, tins of fatty beef and potatoes. Dentists remarked that people over thirty who still had teeth were becoming an anomaly. Observers commented that the local diet made no sense when wholesome food would have served the community far better. Yet none of this mattered. These people had set up their relationship to food to provide them with "cheap luxuries."

Closer to home, a while back I visited with a family I have known for years. The parents asked about my recent projects, so I shared some thoughts about how, on our part, we have conformed our lives to the modern food system, forfeiting our understanding of the connections between food, life, and the environment.

The topic piqued the interest of their older children, who joined in and asked questions. No, building more dams did not increase the amount of water on a finite planet. Yes, boosting the yields of crops such as corn has relied on consuming more land, depleting reserves of underground water, and short-circuiting the Earth's natural nitrogen cycle. Yes, intensive food production requires additional water, which comes from drilling more wells and depleting existing aquifers, setting the stage for future shortages and land collapsing (subsidence).

More meat production has relied on the wide use of antimicrobials in concentrated animal-feeding operations. In return, as pathogen resistance in the environment increases, fewer treatment options for infection are available for humans. A similar pattern can be seen in expansive fields of monoculture crops. Constant application of the same chemicals increases resistance in pests such as weeds, spawning a vicious, unending cycle of applying more and more chemicals.

To increase profitability while compensating for differences in geography and climate, as well as labor expenses, more liquid fossil fuels are burned to ship and process foods and ingredients across the country and around the world. In return, unburned carbon is spewed into the atmosphere, where it further increases the susceptibility of plants to stress and disease. The same is occurring with water supplies, where excess animal waste and fertilizer runoff are destroying food habitat and polluting sources of drinking water.

As I explained how our acceding to the modern food system is kicking environmental problems down the road for future generations to deal with, I touched on how their lives and their children's lives will be different from ours. After hearing all this, the father let out a hearty laugh, and with a broad smile wished his kids the best, relieved by the thought that he would not be alive to face such consequences!

He was right. A lot of us will not be around—in person, that is. But our legacy will be, through the genes we've passed along to our offspring, the culture we've created, and the environment we've left behind. Looking at life generationally reinforces that we live in unprecedented times. Never before have anchors like food, culture, social norms, the environment, and factual understanding changed so quickly.

Carl Sagan said it best when, in 1995, he wrote,

> I have a foreboding of an America in my children's or grandchildren's time when the United States is a service and information economy; when nearly all the manufacturing industries have slipped away to other countries; when awesome technological powers are in the hands of a very few, and no one representing the public interest can even grasp the issues; when the people have lost the ability to set their own agendas or knowledgeably question those in authority; when, clutching our crystals and nervously consulting our horoscopes, our critical faculties in decline, unable to distinguish between what feels good and what's true, we slide, almost without noticing, back into superstition and darkness.

I fear that time has come. While I was writing this book, I asked individuals about their connection to food. Some offered valuable insights, but others questioned why I had chosen a topic that does not need fixing. For them, buying food when the urge strikes has become as natural as turning on a tap and filling a glass with water when they're thirsty.

Consumerism helps explain this attitude; it is the product of an artificial environment that we invented. The result has diminished our will to ask ourselves what is happening, or knowledgeably question and challenge those in authority. As the trend continues, we lose the ability to distinguish between what feels good and what is true. In the consumerist food world, abundance rules. Scarcity is an artifact of the past. And what were once conveniences have become nonnegotiable necessities.

This way of living tricks us into thinking that food will always be abundant. Everyone can have as much food as they like—so long as they bring money. The drawdown of finite resources is inconsequential. Government subsidies are free. Technology can overcome any obstacle. Markets are omniscient.

We got to this point by always wanting more and never questioning where more was leading us. A mindless drive for efficiency became the endgame where bigger was always better because food was being produced more efficiently. When efficiency became the goal, little else mattered. Extracting more resources took priority. Chemicals and anti-microbials were necessary to temporarily subdue nature. People were replaced by technology; those who remained were reduced to menial labor. Science, subsidies, and markets were methodically aligned to reward self-interest.

So how do we foster a different reality? It begins with greater awareness, followed by appreciation, and then increased understanding. The *Earthrise* photo gave humanity renewed perspective, reminding all of us that we and everything surrounding us are packed together on a lone planet hurtling through space at nearly 67,000 miles per hour, while spinning at some 1,000 miles per hour. A circling Moon stabilizes the Earth's axis, tempering extreme weather and making life habitable. The food that results is only possible because of Earth and its planetary orbit relative to the Sun. Five percent nearer or 15 percent farther away, and life and food as we know it could no longer exist. How marvelous and out of this world is that!

Our planet's trajectory also serves up different climates and seasons, the perfect backdrop to witness its harmonious interplay with the biology of nature. From freezing, snowy winters emerge the sweet smells and pastel colors of fruit-tree blossoms. A few short weeks later, what were seemingly cold, lifeless trunks and branches pointing skyward are now balls of vibrant life. As orchards come into full bloom, they beckon honeybees and other creations of nature to join in.

From this wonderland come fruits and vegetables that end up on grocery-store shelves and home kitchens. If we take the time to look closer, the simple banana is no longer a utilitarian source of calories but a biological marvel whose changing color is the perfect indicator of ripeness. Such marvels are not confined to bananas. Thick outer rinds protect the juicy cores of watermelons. Pliable skins of oranges and grapefruit keep microscopic invaders out while allowing the fruit inside to grow and mature. All are reminders of how nature protects our food supply. Yet nature is doing more.

If you can, instead of buying already shelled tree nuts, make the effort to crack open some walnuts or pecans. Take a moment to notice how the seed's hard shell accommodates the next generation of life inside. Or examine how kernels of wheat come with a built-in food source that bridges time until the Sun's rays and photosynthesis can take over and sustain the next generation.

Before plunging a fork into the next plateful of food, pause to admire the array of colors on display. Ask yourself how each ended up on your dinner table. Think about the journey that each one has traveled—how they competed for life, evolved to ward off predators, and adapted to changes in climate and temperature.

Take a moment to give thanks for an environment that nourishes and sustains your life. Consider the contributions of innumerable forces of energy that go unnoticed. The water that transports and filters nutrients through layers of sediment. The soil with microbes too numerous to count yet too essential to live without. And the millions of other species, each with its own unique fingerprint, that fulfill important niches in the grand tapestry of nature, without which we would not be here. Before that first bite, pause to contemplate how nightfall, sunshine, changing temperatures, and climate work in concert to support food production while providing you with a rhythm of life and a sense of normalcy.

As you eat, honor your food and the habitat it was harvested from by being more appreciative and less wasteful. Try to move beyond piling on additional salt, sugar, and fat, and feel the contributions of each food with its own texture, flavor, presentation, and color. Be mindful of the gift of each to not only provide pleasure but contribute to your health—not just from this meal but from future meals in the next month, the next decade—indeed, your entire lifetime.

Also, consider the number of human hands you will never see that came in contact with the food before you. Ponder what their lives are like as they walk up and down fields, bending over to cut heads of lettuce, climb up and down ladders to pick fruit, or carry out the same repetitive movements over and over in slaughterhouses and processing plants as their wrists throb with pain.

While enjoying your food, consider the uniqueness of this particular moment in time as it marks the history of humankind. Contemplate how your arrival on Earth fell within the .01 percent micro-slice of the Earth's history since humans first roamed the planet. Reflect on the 99.99 percent of humanity who came before you and how their entire time on Earth centered on securing enough food, while you spend your time worrying about putting on extra weight and how to lose it through exercise. For them, not having enough food was a fact of life. Taking food for granted was never an option. You, on the other hand, have the option to choose and act differently.

As you are contemplating your options, consider that you are the beneficiary of choices made by unknown relatives you will never meet. Think about what life would be like as a hunter and gatherer. Imagine yourself traveling the savannah plains of Africa following a season of plentiful rains. Off in the distance, you notice tall grass rustling. Your mind instantly registers the swaying stalks with other clues like pockets of wind swirls, unusual sounds of nature, recent tracks of predators, the location of the Sun along the horizon. As your hair stands up on the back of your neck, you stop.

Your survival and that of future generations hinges on your next move. Do the signs you just observed point to much-sought-after food, or are you about to become another creature's source of food? Did the rustling grass come from a momentary gust of wind, a lion on the prowl, or a game animal primed with fresh meat? The grass stalks are now still. Your memory of what you observed is elusive, making it hard to be sure. This is a time of day when lions are known to hunt. But it is also the time of day when game animals forage.

Your intuition tells you that encountering a lion is unlikely. Yet being wrong could mean the end of your life. Your choices are to advance forward, or retreat and detour around. Backtracking is safer, but requires more time and effort, and you are forgoing an opportunity to take down much-needed food. Which option do you choose?

You are the product of choices like these, when risk was pitted against reward and life hung in the balance. But you are different. You no longer have to make such choices. The "savannahs" we face have become supermarkets and restaurants. Unlike our antecedents, we have the benefit of history. We can make choices that they could not.

To guide our decisions, we possess more scientific knowledge and understanding of how intricately food, life, and nature are linked than any generation of people that ever lived on this planet. We know more about nutrition, health, and acute and chronic illness related to food than ever before. We can recognize the fragility of resources. We know the reality of how we can alter nature and the environment—but we cannot dictate what will happen afterward.

Compared with all those who came before us, we have everything stacked in our favor. Moreover, as humans, we possess something else that has eluded all other living beings from the beginning of time—*the ability to contemplate what the future might be, based on what we do in the present*. Unlike other creatures that have evolved and automatically respond to predator threats or changes in weather or events in the immediate future, our ability goes further, can be a conscious one, built from supreme cognitive abilities, understanding, and meaningful reflection.

Each time my thoughts return to life on the farm—planting and harvesting crops and feeding cattle—I have come to believe that this one ability—to exercise foresight—is what sets us apart from all other species. While other species can react, we can consciously *act*. So what has happened to us that refining this ability no longer seems necessary? As the grand food bargain made it easier to pleasure ourselves with food we desired on our terms, our skills to peer into the future, see what was happening, and change how we lived diminished accordingly.

The assumption of perpetual food abundance stepped in to replace it. The pursuit of food that had honed our foresight had dulled. Our lives no longer depended on it. Ready food availability became someone else's problem, not ours. The gift of food scarcity—to not take food for granted—was squandered.

While we do not always learn from the past, we are always bound by the future. Though the food-related decisions we make seldom carry the *immediate* life-or-death consequences of an earlier era, they still live on in the lives of those who follow us. This outlook is molded into our trajectory as the human race. The best side of humanity points the way forward when we first seek to understand, and then turn understanding into knowledge. From knowledge comes wisdom that guides individual actions. From individual actions emerge norms around acceptable behavior that enable societies to flourish.

This modus operandi puts into practice what it means to lead and not be led. At the core of the modern food system are individual behaviors, which collectively shape our America. Early in researching this book, I came across *The End of Overeating: Taking Control of the Insatiable American Appetite*, by Dr. David Kessler. After observing the growing obesity epidemic and how people—including himself—struggle with food and weight loss their entire lives, Kessler set out to uncover answers. As he put it, "I have lost weight, gained it back, and lost it again—over and over and over." In short, succinct chapters, he detailed how the modern food system is designed to stimulate reward pathways in the brain, conditioning people to crave more.

As I read each chapter, I anxiously awaited his recommendations. After all, Kessler was the commissioner of the Food and Drug Administration in the 1990s, serving under both Republican and Democratic administrations. During his tenure, FDA undertook several high-profile initiatives, including nutrition labeling of food, approval of AIDS drugs, and regulation of the tobacco industry. Kessler was never shy about pushing the boundaries of public health and marshaling all of FDA's powers in doing so.

In his last chapters, I expected specific strategies for quashing powerful self-serving interest groups and redirecting government to serve society's collective interests. Instead, he emphasized how the power of government is subservient to what people are no longer *willing to accept* as reasonable behavior. Governments do not lead, they follow. The power to change does not reside with self-serving legislators and profit-driven businesses. As he describes it, "the greatest power rests in our ability to change the definition of reasonable behavior."

Indeed, what we individually determine to be reasonable behavior is the primary catalyst for collective change. A current example is the consumption of sugary soft drinks. As people have realized that the constant anxiety of battling weight gain from consuming too many calories at every turn was too much, individual expectations of reasonable behavior changed—as did soft drink consumption. Year by year, sales of soda in the United States have been declining for over a decade.

As people link acute and chronic health and degradation of the environment to the forces driving the modern food system, an opportunity presents itself to reset what are reasonable behaviors. The same holds true for government policies that subsidize high levels of sugar, fat, and salt; the morass of food labels and health claims that trade away personal health for higher profits; or how politicians and businesses leverage the hunger of the most vulnerable to skirt around structural and economic inequities.

To lead begins with recognizing that food abundance, nutrition, and nature do not operate in different universes, and that treating them as such does not serve us well. To lead does not pretend that prime farmland, fresh water, and liquid fossil fuels are not closely tied to environmental consequences; that opportunity and independence for farmers are not coupled to competitive market conditions; or that science and technology can perpetually outmaneuver microbial resistance in pests and pathogens.

To lead is to challenge what the modern food system puts forward as serving our best interests, and to refuse to succumb to what others define as reasonable behavior on our behalf. By understanding the forces that drive the modern food system, we can see through the pretense that increasing meat-processing-line speeds, and handing over more food-safety responsibility to the same companies, will somehow cause foodborne disease outbreaks and acute illness to subside.

To lead is to not accept as unavoidable the multitude of pesticide residues found on foods like apples, apple sauces, blueberries, grapes, green beans, leafy greens, pears, peaches, potatoes, plums, spinach, strawberries, raisins, sweet peppers, tomatoes, and winter squashes. To lead is to recognize how foods like apple juice, avocados, bananas, beans, broccoli, cabbages, cantaloupes, carrots, cauliflower, celery, corn, eggplants, grapefruits, lentils, lettuce, onions, oranges, orange juice, peas, prunes, summer squashes, sweet potatoes, tomato sauces, and zucchini are being produced with far fewer residues—and sometimes none at all.

For more than two million years, the human race was driven to conquer and replace food scarcity with ready food availability. Perhaps more so than any other country, America first showed how it was possible. By 1880, scarcity of food was behind us: a new society of consumers had supplanted a nation of farmers. Sadly, since then, Americans have also shown our *inability* to live with abundance. From having turned scarcity into abundance, we converted abundance into glut, glut into waste and now waste into gutting the forces that made abundance possible. The path we are on is coming full circle, one individual decision at a time.

We have had our way with food long enough to build up resistance to any messages suggesting that individual actions still lead to collective outcomes. It has become summarily easy to fault the modern food system for all that is happening. It is not so much what the modern food system is doing to our health, natural resources, nature, and the environment, but what we are doing with the modern food system. More than anything else, this is the message I have wanted to convey with the examples of my own foibles and experiences, as well as those of others.

From experience comes reflection and occasional nuggets of insight. The most important for me is how food has been our greatest teacher. Through food we learned how well-being and finite resources were intertwined. How more nutrition advanced intellectual capacity and our ability to tame physical scarcity. How our survival relies on millions of other species we never see, not just the few we put into our mouths. Through food we could learn how harmony with the environment is far more important than our attempts to control it.

Because of food we learned how to cooperate with each other and live in communities. We learned social norms and basic expectations of decency. We learned how to work toward shared interests. And as a result, we discovered that collective well-being provides optimal ways to satisfy individual needs.

Food was our teacher in understanding the world around us. From what we learned we developed powers of observation as well as abilities to acquire more knowledge by separating personal beliefs and biases from bona fide evidence. From food we learned how to unlock the mysteries of nature, thereby making more food possible.

From our relationship with food came America's vision of prosperity. Food opened a new way of life and an economy built on opportunity that left behind a long global history of subsistence. From food came the ethics of work, perseverance, and personal responsibility. The meteoric rise in the human population since the nineteenth century, and the standards of living we've come to take for granted, all trace back to food.

Looking ahead, our well-being—as individuals, as a nation, and as a world—depends far less on the newest and greatest novel technology and far more on whether we can recapture this relationship to food. The most important question we can ask ourselves is: Are we still willing to learn from food—and to lead accordingly?

Acknowledgments

In the long list of things to do in life, writing a book—especially a book about food—was one of those things I never thought about or had a desire to pursue. Yet people change, and I came to realize how our relationship with food—not to be confused with what we actually put into our mouths—is as important to life itself as relying on clean air to breathe and fresh water to drink.

The seeds of this conversion were planted by Christopher Brown, my former boss and college dean—or, as he would introduce himself, "just an old horse doctor" who grew up on a farm in rural England. Working and traveling together afforded us with many opportunities to exchange our stories, including those we'd never told before. Then one day he put it out there: "You have a story about food that's important to share. I hope you'll consider writing a book." Catching me by surprise, that conversation and subsequent events launched me on a very different and unexpected journey.

Along the way, I have learned that, while it's my name that appears on the cover, books like this are the result of many people who share their ideas and their passion to further understanding and to better life for others, especially those who will follow us. At Michigan State University, from the start of this project until the finish, Professor Scott Winterstein has gone above and beyond, exemplifying the old-school norms of college professors whose unheralded contributions make lifelong differences. Despite his duties when I came on board to direct the National Food Safety and Toxicology Center, and later became department chair, he invested countless hours in discussion and review of draft chapters, always providing valuable insights and new ways of seeing things.

The W. K. Kellogg Foundation and its former Kellogg National Fellowship Program directed by Roger Sublett was also important. Its leadership program propelled me toward roads less traveled, in company with the most marvelous and diverse group of individuals imaginable, who, each in their own way, broadened my horizons and pushed me beyond my comfort zone. Martha Lee, director of the Kellogg Fellows Leadership Alliance, now carries on the tradition for all of us. Finally, Ricardo Salvador and Rick Foster, then with the W. K. Kellogg Foundation, provided important funding and support for separate food-related initiatives whose outcomes provided important stimulus to the development of this book's thesis.

Throughout my somewhat atypical career and travels, many of the experiences contained in the book were made possible or were enriched by the participation of colleagues, teachers, students, family, and dear friends from diverse nationalities and backgrounds. As time passes, my memory of names and details too often fails me, but your faces and influence live on—a sincere thank you.

In the actual writing of this book, key individuals have bestowed their time and attention to review early drafts, provide feedback, and offer insight. In particular, I want to acknowledge the valuable contributions of Bruce Dale, Arlene Friedland, Monty and Jeanice Harrison, Patricia Hatch, Jim Kliebenstein, João Magelhães, Jody Ranck, Andrea Saveri, Paul Terry, and Kris Van Wagoner. Also, in memoriam for their inspiration that I often draw upon, Charles Laughlin and Edward Mather.

From the onset, I wanted this book to reach a general audience, which meant finding a literary agent, Don Fehr, who saw the same potential in my initial proposal and made it happen. Through his efforts, landing with Island Press has been my good fortune. Working with Emily Turner Davis has been a joy that surpassed my expectations of what a developmental editor can so deftly and pleasantly accomplish. As copyeditor, Michael Fleming brought equal parts enthusiasm, expertise, and an eagle eye to elevate the manuscript to the next level. There are others at Island Press whom I do not know but want to thank for your dedication in bringing this book to fruition.

To parents who have passed away but taught me the value of work and provided opportunities to witness how life, nature, and the environment are intricately intertwined, I'll always be indebted. To my wife who has lived through the thick and thin of this book project, reading countless versions of chapters and taking on the important yet difficult task of whipping the endnotes into shape, your contribution has been immeasurable, as has been the encouragement of your family. To our two daughters, their husbands, and their families, your continued support, interest, and questions helped sustain this effort. This book was written for you, your generation, and your children's generation. May you have the wisdom to learn from the past, never take your relationship with food for granted, and be inspired to do better than we have.

NOTES

Chapter 1

1. **It is curious how seldom:** George Orwell, *The Road to Wigan Pier* (New York: Mariner Books, 1972), 83.

2. **forty-five miles per hour:** M. M. Shanawany and John Dingle, "Ostrich Production Systems," Food and Agriculture Organization of the United Nations, *Animal Production and Health Paper 144*, 1999, 6, http://www.fao .org/docrep/018/x2370e/x2370e.pdf.

3. **forty years in the wild:** Stephen Davies and B. Bertram, "Ostrich," in *Firefly Encyclopedia of Birds*, ed. Christopher Perrins (Buffalo, NY: Firefly Books, 2003), 34–37; Gerald Wood, *The Guinness Book of Animal Facts & Feats* (New York: Sterling Publishing, 1983); "Ostrich," *National Geographic*, accessed May 23, 2017, http://www.nationalgeographic.com/animals/birds/o /ostrich/.

4. **next 123 years:** Jean-Pierre Bocquet-Appel, "When the World's Population Took Off: The Springboard of the Neolithic Demographic Transition," *Science* 333, no. 6042 (July 2011): 560–61, https://doi.org/10.1126/science .1208880; US Census Bureau International Program, "Historical Estimates of World Population" and "World Population," accessed May 25, 2017, http: //www.census.gov/population/international/data/worldpop/table_history .php& http://www.census.gov /population/international/data/worldpop/table_population.php.

5. **aid for farmers:** Everett Edwards, "American Agriculture—The First 300 Years," in *Farmers in a Changing World: Yearbook of Agriculture, 1940*, US

Department of Agriculture (USDA), National Agricultural Library (NAL) Digital Collections, 246, http://naldc.nal.usda.gov/download/IND43893716 /PDF.

6. **good morals, and happiness:** Letter from Thomas Jefferson to George Washington, 14 August 1787, *National Archives*, accessed November 15, 2017, https://founders.archives.gov/documents/Jefferson/01-12-02-0040.

7. **labor force worked in farming:** D. M. Spielmaker, "History Timeline—Farmers & the Land," in *Growing a Nation: The Story of American Agriculture*, Utah State University, National Institute of Food Agriculture (NIFA) and USDA, 2006, accessed May 25, 2017, https://www.agclassroom.org/gan /timeline/farmers_land.htm.

8. **home to grow food:** Christopher Hamner, "Great Expectations for the Civil War," Teaching history.org, accessed May 25, 2017, http://teaching history.org/history-content/ask-a-historian/24413.

9. **railroad was built:** "An Act to Establish a Department of Agriculture," NAL, USDA, accessed May 25, 2017, https://www.nal.usda.gov/act-establish -department-agriculture; "The Homestead Act of 1862," *National Archives*, accessed May 25, 2017, https://www.archives.gov/education/lessons/homestead -act; "Pacific Railroad Act," *Our Documents*, accessed May 25, 2017, https://www .ourdocuments.gov/doc.php?doc=32; "Morrill Act," *Our Documents*, accessed May 25, 2017, https://www.ourdocuments.gov/doc.php?flash=true&doc=33.

10. **less than half the labor force:** Utah State University, NIFA, USDA, "History Timeline—Farmers & the Land."

11. **years of human existence:** Brian Villmoare et al., "Early *Homo* at 2.8 Ma from Ledi-Geraru, Afar, Ethiopia," *Science* 347, no. 6228 (March 2015): 1325–55, https://doi.org/10.1126/science.aaa1343; "Discovery of Jaw by ASU Team Sheds Light on Early Human Ancestor," *Discoveries*, Arizona State University, March 4, 2015, https://asunow.asu.edu/20150304-asu-human-fossil -discovery.

12. **eating bread and meat:** Stephen Kinzer, *The True Flag: Theodore Roosevelt, Mark Twain, and the Birth of American Empire* (New York: Henry Holt & Co., 2017), 45.

13. **plantations in Central America:** Stephen Kinzer, *The Brothers: John Foster Dulles, Allen Dulles, and Their Secret World War* (New York: Times Books / Henry Holt & Co., 2013).

14. **Europe's wartime demand:** Economic Research Service (ERS), "Chronological Landmarks in American Agriculture," AIB-425, November 1990, 45 (see entry for 1919), https://naldc.nal.usda.gov/download/CAT919495 57/PDF.

15. **benchmark for their own lives:** Timothy Snyder, *Black Earth: The Holocaust as History and Warning* (New York: Tim Duggan Books, 2015), Kindle edition, 398–400.

16. **to lead a life comparable:** Ibid., 416–18.

17. **German manufacturing industries:** Ibid., 398–400.

18. **The microwave oven:** John Gallawa, "A Brief History of Microwave Oven Development," in *The Complete Microwave Oven Service Handbook: Operation, Maintenance, Troubleshooting, and Repair* (New York: Pearson College Division, 2000).

19. **two moderately active adult:** USDA and US Health and Human Services, "Dietary Guidelines for Americans 2015–2020," 8th ed., December 2015, 78, https://health.gov/dietaryguidelines/2015/resources/2015-2020 _Dietary_Guidelines.pdf; Center for Nutrition Policy and Promotion, "Food Calories and Macronutrients per Capita per Day" in "Nutrient Content of the U.S. Food Supply, 1909–2010," USDA, accessed May 26, 2017, http://www .cnpp.usda.gov/USFoodSupply-1909-2010.

20. **role of nature fades:** Dylan Weese et al., "Long-Term Nitrogen Addition Causes the Evolution of Less-Cooperative Mutualists," *Evolution* 69, no. 3 (January 2015): 631–42, https://doi.org/10.1111/evo.12594.

21. **an already warming planet:** US Environmental Protection Agency, "Overview of Greenhouse Gases, Nitrous Oxide Emissions," accessed May 26, 2017, https://www3.epa.gov/climatechange/ghgemissions/gases/n2o.html.

22. **Seventy-nine percent of nitrous oxide:** Ibid.

23. **help farmers raise healthy:** Emily Aasand, "CHS Fertilizer Plant to Use Bakken Gas," *North American Shale*, September 9, 2014, http://north americanshalemagazine.com/articles/786/chs-fertilizer-plant-to-use-bakken -gas.

24. **discharging its runoff:** National Oceanic and Atmospheric Administration, "Gulf of Mexico 'Dead Zone' Is the Largest Ever Measured," August 2, 2017, http://www.noaa.gov/media-release/gulf-of-mexico-dead-zone-is -largest-ever-measured.

25. **thyroid problems, and birth defects:** Jonathan Patz et al., "Our Planet, Our Health, Our Future. Human Health and the Rio Conventions: Biological Diversity, Climate Change, and Desertification," World Health Organization, 2012, 38–39, http://www.who.int/globalchange/publications/ reports/health_rioconventions.pdf; "Nitrate in Drinking Water: A Public Health Concern for All Iowans, Executive Summary," Iowa Environmental Council, September 2016, http://www.iaenvironment.org/webres/File/Nitrate _in_Drinking_Water_Report_ES_Web.pdf.

26. **nitrates in water:** Stephen Kalkhoff et al., "Water Quality in the Eastern Iowa Basins, Iowa and Minnesota, 1996–98," US Geological Survey Circular 1210, 2000, https://pubs.usgs.gov/circ/circ1210/pdf/Circular1210.pdf.

27. **water quality was governed:** Donnelle Eller, "With Water Works' Lawsuit Dismissed, Water Quality Is the Legislature's Problem," *Des Moines Register*, last modified March 20, 2017, http://www.desmoinesregister.com /story/money/agriculture/2017/03/17/judge-dismisses-water-works-nitrates -lawsuit/99327928/.

28. **divided agricultural interests:** Donnelle Eller, "Will Water Works' Dismissed Lawsuit Lift Pressure on Iowa Farmers? No, Officials Say," *Des Moines Register*, last modified March 25, 2017, http://www.desmoinesregister .com/story/money/agriculture/2017/03/25/water-works-dismissed-lawsuit -lift-pressure-iowa-farmers-no-officials-say/99463452/.

29. **independence of water utilities:** MacKenzie Elmer, "Bill Would Mean Big Changes for Public Water Utilities. What Are They?" *Des Moines Register*, last modified March 2, 2017, http://www.desmoinesregister.com/story /news/politics/2017/03/02/bill-would-mean-big-changes-public-water -utilities-what-they/98628820/; MacKenzie Elmer, "Des Moines Council Supports Bill Dismantling Water Utilities," *Des Moines Register*, last modified March 21, 2017, http://www.desmoinesregister.com/story/news/2017/03/20/des -moines-council-supports-bill-dismantling-water-utilities/99317656/.

30. **won a Pulitzer Prize:** "Art Cullen of the *Storm Lake Times*, Storm Lake, IA," *The Pulitzer Prizes*, accessed May 29, 2017, http://www.pulitzer. org/winners/art-cullen.

31. **$282-million bill:** Mike Trautmann, "Iowa's Water Quality Problems Really Boil Down to This," *Des Moines Register*, last modified January 24, 2018, https://www.desmoinesregister.com/story/news/politics/2018/01/23/why -iowas-water-quality-problems-matter/1058266001/.

32. **On a campus of this size:** "Morrill Act."

33. **labor force in 1790:** ERS, "Agriculture and Its Related Industries Provide 11 Percent of the U.S. Employment" in "Ag and Food Sectors and the Economy," last modified October 18, 2017, https://www.ers.usda.gov /data-products/ag-and-food-statistics-charting-the-essentials/ag-and-food -sectors-and-the-economy/.

34. **food eaten outside the home:** ERS, "Table 1. Food and Alcoholic Beverages: Total Expenditures" in "Food Expenditures," last modified January 26, 2016, https://www.ers.usda.gov/data-products/food-expenditures.aspx.

35. **fate of recent generations:** Elizabeth Thomas, *The Old Way: A Story of the First People* (New York: Farrar, Straus and Giroux, 2006), 3.

Chapter 2

1. **King Kullen, first supermarket:** Nicholas Hirshon, "Rooms Above, Supermarket History Below at King Kullen Site," *New York Daily News*, September 8, 2008, http://www.nydailynews.com/new-york/queens/rooms-su permarket-history-king-kullen-site-article-1.322504.

2. **what is now Costa Rica:** Carl Sauer, *The Early Spanish Main* (Berkeley, CA: University of California Press, 1966), 138.

3. **all bananas are imported:** National Agricultural Statistics Service (NASS), "Noncitrus Fruits and Nuts 2014 Preliminary Summary," US Department of Agriculture (USDA), 2015, 64, http://usda.mannlib.cornell .edu/usda/nass/NoncFruiNu//2010s/2015/NoncFruiNu-01-23-2015.pdf; Economic Research Service (ERS), "Table B-10. Banana: Number of Farms, Acreage, Production, Price, Value, Hawaii, 1980 to Date," "Table G-36. Fresh Fruit: Per Capita Use, 1980 to Date," and "Table H-3. Imports As a Share of Domestic Fresh Fruit Consumption, 1975 to Date," in "Fruit and Tree Nut Yearbook 2014," USDA, 2014, http://usda.mannlib.cornell.edu/usda/ers /89022/2014/FTS2014.pdf; Food and Agricultural Organization (FAO) of the United Nations, "Figure 2. Distribution of Global Imports by Markets, 2012," in "Banana Market Review and Banana Statistics 2012–2013," FAO, 2014, http: //www.fao.org/docrep/019/i3627e/i3627e.pdf; FAO, "Production of Commodity by Country, 2013," FAOSTAT, accessed March 19, 2018, http://www .fao.org/faostat/en/#rankings/countries_by_commodity.

4. **Ingeniously packaged by nature:** "Gerber 1st Foods," Gerber, accessed March 19, 2018, https://www.gerber.com/products/baby-food-prod ucts/product/1st-foods-my-1st-fruits-starter-kit/20; Jennifer White, "Banana Nutrition for Babies," *Very Well Family* (blog), last modified September 18, 2017, https://www.verywellfamily.com/banana-nutrition-284428; James Martin, "Instant Banana Ice Cream," BBC, accessed March 19, 2018, https://www .bbc.co.uk/food/recipes/instantbananaicecrea_86115.

5. **second-largest exporter:** FAO, "Banana Market Review and Banana Statistics 2012–2013," 12.

6. **consume ten thousand bananas:** Dan Koeppel, *Banana: The Fate of the Fruit That Changed the World* (New York: Hudson Street Press, 2008), xi.

7. **Galileo a conviction of heresy:** Albert Van Helden, "Galileo," *Encyclopedia Britannica*, last modified, February 14, 2018, https://www.britannica. com/biography/Galileo-Galilei; Robert Westman, "Nicolaus Copernicus," *Encyclopedia Britannica*, last modified, March 21, 2018, https://www.britan nica.com/biography/Nicolaus-Copernicus.

8. **bulging oversized eyes:** Bruce Knecht, *Hooked: Pirates, Poaching, and the Perfect Fish* (New York: Rodale Books, 2007).

9. **old fish morphed into a new image:** "Chasing the Perfect Fish: The Chilean Sea Bass Craze Set Off a Seagoing Gold Rush, Tempting Toothfish Poachers," *Wall Street Journal*, last modified May 4, 2006, https://www.wsj.com /articles/SB114670694136643399.

10. **Catches of ten to twenty tons:** Ibid.

11. **"certified sustainable" label:** "Fish to Eat," Marine Stewardship Council, accessed March 19, 2018, https://www.msc.org/cook-eat-enjoy/fish -to-eat.

12. **helps ensure fish for tomorrow:** "What Does the Blue MSC Label Mean?" Marine Stewardship Council, accessed March 19, 2018, https://20 .msc.org/what-we-are-doing/our-approach/what-does-the-blue-msc-label -mean.

13. **people are willing to buy:** Florence Fabricant, "Chilean Sea Bass: More than an Identity Problem," *New York Times*, May 29, 2002, https://www .nytimes.com/2002/05/29/dining/chilean-sea-bass-more-than-an-identity -problem.html.

14. **nearly twenty-one thousand:** ERS, "New Products," last modified April 5, 2017, https://www.ers.usda.gov/topics/food-markets-prices/processing -marketing/new-products/.

15. **tossing bunches of bananas:** See, for example: Koeppel, *Banana*.

16. **word of a devastating fungus:** Nadia Ordonez et al., "Worse Comes to Worst: Bananas and Panama Disease—When Plant and Pathogen Clones Meet," *PLoS Pathogens* 11, no. 11 (November 2015): e1005197, http://journals.plos .org/plospathogens/article/file?id=10.1371/journal.ppat.1005197&type=print able.

17. **vast tracts of tropical rain forest:** Stephen Kinzer, *The Brothers: John Foster Dulles, Allen Dulles, and Their Secret World War* (New York: Times Books/ Henry Holt & Co., 2013).

18. **Panama disease started appearing:** Ordonez et al., "Worse Comes to Worst."

19. **TR4 has since spread:** Ibid.

20. **80 percent of bananas traded:** FAO, "Banana Market Review and Banana Statistics 2012–2013," 1.

21. **150 to 200 have been adopted:** "Women: Users, Preservers, and Mana-gers of Agro-biodiversity," FAO, 2018, accessed March 19, 2018, http://www.fao .org/docrep/x0171e/x0171e03.htm.

22. **less than 9 percent of total calories:** Jeanine Bentley, "US Trends in Food Availability and a Dietary Assessment of Loss-Adjusted Food Avail-

ability, 1970–2014," ERS, January 2017, EIB-166, 6, https://www.ers.usda.gov /webdocs/publications/82220/eib-166.pdf?v=42762.

23. **the space allocated is small:** Michael Ruhlman, *Grocery: The Buying and Selling of Food in America* (New York: Harry N. Abrams, 2017), Kindle edition, 215–16.

24. **one pound more per week:** "Data: Meat Consumption," Organisation for Economic Co-operation and Development (OECD), 2016, accessed March 19, 2018, https://data.oecd.org/agroutput/meat-consumption.htm.

25. **control of most meat animals:** James MacDonald, "Concentration, Contracting, and Competition Policy in U.S. Agribusiness," *Concurrences* no. 1 (2016):3–9,http://discovery.ucl.ac.uk/1478197/7/Lianos_03%20concurrences_1 -2016_on_topics_lianos_et_al.pdf.

26. **15 percent added slurry:** "Fact Sheet—Lean Finely Textured Beef," National Cattlemen's Beef Association, accessed March 19, 2018, http://www .beefusa.org/CMDocs/BeefUSA/Resources/LFTB%20Fact%20Sheet.pdf.

27. **Terms of the settlement:** Timothy Mclaughlin, "ABC TV Settles with Beef Product Maker in 'Pink Slime' Defamation Case," Reuters, June 28, 2017, https://www.reuters.com/article/us-abc-pinkslime-idUSKBN19 J1W9.

28. **inclusion is a minor cost:** Ed Yong, *I Contain Multitudes: The Microbes within Us and a Grander View of Life* (New York: ECCO, 2016), 224.

29. **rejected all of them:** Ibid.; M. B. Katan, "Why the European Food Safety Authority Was Right to Reject Health Claims for Probiotics," *Beneficial Microbes* 3, no. 2 (June 2012): 85–89, https://doi.org/10.3920/BM2012.0008.

30. **grew by only 2 percent:** NASS, "Milk Cows, Milk Productions," February 21, 2018, https://www.nass.usda.gov/Charts_and_Maps/Milk_Production _and_Milk_Cows/index.php.

31. **cows die or are culled:** Albert De Vries, "Cow Longevity Economics: The Cost Benefit of Keeping the Cow in the Herd," in *Proceedings of Cow Longevity Conference*, Hamra Farm/Tumba, Sweden, August 28–29, 2013, 23, http://www.milkproduction.com/Global/PDFs/Cow%20Longevity%20Con ference%20Proceedings%20.pdf.

32. **requiring certain nutrients:** USDA, "What Foods Are in the Grains Group?" ChooseMyPlate.gov, last modified November 3, 2017, https://www .choosemyplate.gov/grains.

33. **products made of mostly white flour:** Jeanine Bentley, "U.S. Trends in Food Availability and a Dietary Assessment of Loss-Adjusted Food Availability, 1790–2014," ERS, EIB-166.

34. **more extravagant the health claims:** Marion Nestle, *What to Eat* (New York: North Point Press, 2006), Kindle edition, 118.

35. **competing with restaurants:** ERS, "Table 10-Food Away from Home as a Share of Food Expenditures," in "Food Expenditure," last modified January 26, 2016, https://www.ers.usda.gov/data-products/food-expenditures .aspx.

36. **mass-produced ingredients:** ERS, "Food Dollar Series" application, last modified March 16, 2017, https://data.ers.usda.gov/reports.aspx?ID=17885.

37. **In his seminal book:** Adam Smith, *An Inquiry into the Nature and Causes of the Wealth of Nations* (Chicago: University of Chicago Press, 1977).

38. **maximize the country's wealth:** John Cassidy, *How Markets Fail: The Logic of Economic Calamities* (New York: Farrar, Straus and Giroux, 2009), chap. 2.

39. **led by an invisible hand:** Smith, *Wealth of Nations*, 364.

40. **income spent on food:** "Americans' Budget Shares Devoted to Food Have Flattened in Recent Years," and "Food Spending as a Share of Income Declines as Income Rises," ERS, last modified March 19, 2018, https://www .ers.usda.gov/data-products/ag-and-food-statistics-charting-the-essentials /food-prices-and-spending/.

41. **twice the number of calories:** USDA and US Department of Health and Human Services, "Dietary Guidelines for Americans 2015–2020," December 2015, Table A2-1, 78, https://health.gov/dietaryguidelines/2015/resources /2015-2020_Dietary_Guidelines.pdf.

Chapter 3

1. **When the Sun comes up:** Abe Gubegna (1934–1980), an Ethiopian novelist and playwright, is credited with this particular quotation. The original source is yet to be verified.

2. **Lest people feel too privileged:** Camilo Mora et al., "How Many Species Are There on Earth and in the Ocean?" *PLoS Biology* 9, no. 8 (August 2011): e1001127, https://doi.org/10.1371/journal.pbio.1001127.

3. **The losers go extinct:** "Mass Extinctions," American Museum of Natural History website, accessed November 13, 2017, https://www.amnh.org/ex hibitions/dinosaurs-ancient-fossils-new-discoveries/extinction/mass-extinction/; M. E. J. Newman, "A Model of Mass Extinction," *Journal of Theoretical Biology* 189, no. 3 (December 1997): 235–52, https://arxiv.org/pdf/ adap-org/9702003v1.pdf; David Raup, *Extinction: Bad Genes or Bad Luck?* (New York: W. W. Norton & Co., 1992).

4. **aphids into a vegetable patch:** Daniel Fairbanks, *Evolving: The Human Effect and Why It Matters* (Amherst, NY: Prometheus Books, 2012), 244.

5. **Ladybugs, those seemingly sweet:** Ibid.

6. **Starting the ball rolling:** Richard Wrangham, *Catching Fire: How Cooking Made Us Human* (New York: Basic Books, 2009).

7. **nutrients the human body could absorb:** "What's Cooking? The Evolutionary Role of Cookery," *The Economist*, February 19, 2009, http://www.economist.com/node/13139619; for more information, see: Suzana Herculano-Houzel, "The Remarkable, yet Not Extraordinary, Human Brain as a Scaled-Up Primate Brain and Its Associated Cost," *Proceedings of the National Academy of Sciences* 109, no. 1 (June 2012): 10661–68, http://www.pnas.org/content/109/Supplement_1/10661.full; Karina Fonseca-Azevedo and Suzana Herculano-Houzel, "Metabolic Constraint Imposes Tradeoff between Body Size and Number of Brain Neurons in Human Evolution," *PNAS* 109, no. 45 (November 2012): 18571–76, http://www.pnas.org/content/109/45/18571.full.

8. **neurons to rise dramatically:** Herculano-Houzel, "The Remarkable . . . Human Brain."

9. **more efficient digestive system:** Daniel Lieberman, *The Story of the Human Body: Evolution, Health, and Disease* (New York: Pantheon Books, 2013); Leslie Aiello and Peter Wheeler, "The Expensive-Tissue Hypothesis: The Brain and the Digestive System in Human and Primate Evolution," *Current Anthropology* 36, no. 2 (April 1995): 199–221, http://www.jstor.org/stable/2744104.

10. **mammals of similar mass:** Herculano-Houzel, "The Remarkable . . . Human Brain."

11. **a quarter of the energy consumed:** Fonseca-Azevedo and Herculano-Houzel, "Metabolic Constraint."

12. **Spring arrived a bit early:** William Klingaman and Nicholas Klingaman, *The Year without Summer: 1816 and the Volcano That Darkened the World and Changed History* (New York: St. Martin's Press, 2013), 30.

13. **thermometers had climbed:** Ibid., 39.

14. **forests were preventing the sunlight:** Ibid., 81–82.

15. **lowered ambient temperatures:** "Year without a Summer, 1816," *Celebrate Boston*, accessed November 13, 2017, http://www.celebrateboston.com/disasters/year-without-a-summer.htm.

16. **climatic shift to sunspots:** Klingaman and Klingaman, *The Year*, 17–30, 77–79; "Year Without," *Celebrate Boston*.

17. **the most fervent explanations:** Klingaman and Klingaman, *The Year*, 83.

18. **wheat yields plummeted and bread disappeared:** Ibid., chap. 8; Henry Stommel and Elizabeth Stommel, *Volcano Weather: The Story of 1816, The*

Year without a Summer (Newport, RI: Seven Seas Press, 1983); Patrick Webb, "Emergency Relief During Europe's Famine of 1817 Anticipated Crisis-Response Mechanisms of Today," *Journal of Nutrition* 132, no. 7 (July 2002): 2092S-2095S, http://jn.nutrition.org/content/132/7/2092S.long.

19. **In northern China:** Gillen Wood, "The Volcano That Changed the Course of History," *Slate*, April 9, 2014, http://www.slate.com/articles/health_and_science/science/2014/04/tambora_eruption_caused_the_year_without_a_summer_cholera_opium_famine_and.html; Michael Greshko, "201 Years Ago, This Volcano Caused a Climate Catastrophe," *National Geographic*, April 8, 2016, https://news.nationalgeographic.com/2016/04/160408-tambora-eruption-volcano-anniversary-indonesia-science/; Yang Yu-da, Man Zhimin, and Zheng Jingyun, "A Serious Famine in Yunnan (1815–1817) and the Eruption of Tambola Volcano," *Fudan Journal of Social Science* 1 (2005), http://en.cnki.com.cn/Article_en/CJFDTotal-FDDX200501011.htm; Klingaman and Klingaman, *The Year*, 275.

20. **Extreme monsoons and flooding:** Klingaman and Klingaman, *The Year*, 175; Michael Greshko, "201 Years Ago."

21. **started deep beneath the planet's crust:** "Temperatures at the Surface Reflect Temperatures below the Ground," US Geological Survey Volcano Hazards Program, last modified January 7, 2016, https://volcanoes.usgs.gov/vhp/thermal.html; "Magma," *National Geographic*, Education, accessed November 13, 2017, https://www.nationalgeographic.org/encyclopedia/magma/.

22. **eruption of Mount Tambora:** Bill Bryson, *A Short History of Nearly Everything* (New York: Broadway Books, 2004), 419; Richard Stothers, "The Great Tambora Eruption in 1815 and Its Aftermath," *Science* 224, no. 4654 (1984): 1191–98, http://doi.org/10.1126/science.224.4654.1191; Christopher Newhall and Stephen Self, "The Volcanic Explosivity Index (VEI): An Estimate of Explosive Magnitude for Historical Volcanism," *Journal of Geophysical Research* 87, no. C2 (1982): 1231–38, https://agupubs.onlinelibrary.wiley.com/doi/full/10.1029/JC087iC02p01231; "Mount Tambora," *Encyclopedia Britannica*, accessed November 13, 2017, https://www.britannica.com/place/Mount-Tambora.

23. **80 percent of the country's workforce:** Stanley Lebergott, "Labor Force and Employment, 1800–1960," in *Output, Employment, and Productivity in the United States after 1800*, ed. Dorothy Brady (Cambridge, MA: National Bureau of Economic Research, 1966), 117–204, http://www.nber.org/chapters/c1567.pdf.

24. **The year was dubbed:** Stommel and Stommel, *Volcano Weather*, chap. 2; Leah Shafer, "Eighteen Hundred and Froze to Death," *US Capital Historical Society*, July 11, 2013, https://uschs.wordpress.com/2013/07/11/eighteen

-hundred-and-froze-to-death/; Shirley Wajda, "Eighteen-Hundred-and-Froze-to-Death: 1816, The Year without a Summer," *Connecticut History*, http://connecticuthistory.org/eighteen-hundred-and-froze-to-death-1816-the-year-without-a-summer/; "Eighteen Hundred and Froze to Death: The Year There Was No Summer," *The Weather Doctor*, http://www.islandnet.com/~see/weather/history/1816.htm. All accessed November 13, 2017.

25. **Red River Valley:** Economic Research Service (ERS), *Chronology Landmarks in American Agriculture*, AIB-425, 1990, 9, https://naldc.nal.usda.gov/download/CAT91949557/PDF; J. R. Parker, "Grasshoppers," in the *Yearbook of Agriculture 1952* (Washington, DC: United States Government Printing Office, 1952), 595–604, https://naldc.nal.usda.gov/download/IND50000149/PDF.

26. **"hell from above":** Chuck Lyons, "1874: The Year of the Locust," *HISTORYNET*, February 5, 2017, http://www.historynet.com/1874-the-year-of-the-locust.htm; Chris Bennett, "Locust Swarms Bring Back Past for US Farmers," *Western Farm Press* (blog), March 7, 2013, http://westernfarmpress.com/blog/locust-swarms-bring-back-past-us-farmers.

27. **"everything but the mortgage":** Lyons, "1874"; Bennett, "Locust."

28. **largest swarm ever recorded:** Carol Yoon, "Looking Back at the Days of the Locust," *New York Times*, April 23, 2002, http://www.nytimes.com/2002/04/23/science/looking-back-at-the-days-of-the-locust.html.

29. **Fungi appeared in fruit orchards:** Murray Benedict, *Farm Policies of The United States, 1790–1950: A Study of Their Origins and Development* (New York: Twentieth Century Fund, 1953), 116.

30. **Boll weevil showed up:** Ibid.

31. **Seven of every ten acres planted:** National Agricultural Statistics Service (NASS), "Crop Production 2016 Summary," January 2017, 100, http://usda.mannlib.cornell.edu/usda/nass/CropProdSu//2010s/2017/CropProdSu-01-12-2017.pdf; Lance Honig, "Principal Crops Planted Acreage," in "Crop Production—Annual Grain Stocks, Rice Stocks, Cotton Ginnings, Winter Wheat and Canola Seedings, January Crop Production Executive Summary," NASS, January 12, 2018, 3, https://www.nass.usda.gov/Newsroom/Executive_Briefings/2018/01-12-2018.pdf.

32. **92 percent of all meat consumed:** ERS, "Red Meat, Poultry, and Fish, 1970 to 2015" in CSV format, in "Food Availability (Per Capita) Data System," last modified July 26, 2017, https://www.ers.usda.gov/webdocs/DataFiles/50472/redmeat.csv?v=42942.

33. **Some fifty thousand pesticides:** Eric Jorgensen, ed., *The Poisoned Well: New Strategies for Groundwater Protection* (Washington, DC: Island Press, 1989), 32, cited in: Andrew Smith, *Food in America: The Past, Present,*

and Future of Food, Farming, and the Family Meal, vol. 1 (Santa Barbara, CA: ABC-CLIO, 2017), 179.

34. **Eighty percent of all antibiotics:** Tracy Pham, "Drug Use Review," US Food and Drug Administration, April 5, 2012, 2, http://www.fda.gov /downloads/Drugs/DrugSafety/InformationbyDrugClass/UCM319435 .pdf; US Food and Drug Administration (FDA), "2013 Summary Report on Antimicrobials Sold or Distributed for Use in Food-Producing Animals," April 2015, 39, http://www.fda.gov/downloads/ForIndustry/UserFees/Animal DrugUserFeeActADUFA/UCM440584.pdf.

35. **military is in charge of food:** Hannah Dreier and Joshua Goodman, "Venezuela Military Trafficking Food as Country Goes Hungry," Associated Press, December 28, 2016, https://www.ap.org/explore/venezuela-undone /venezuela-military-trafficking-food-as-country-goes-hungry.html.

36. **We want everyone to have access:** Rachelle Krygier and Anthony Faiola, "Opposition Strike Paralyzes Parts of Venezuela as Fears of Violence Mount," *Washington Post*, July 20, 2017, https://www.washingtonpost.com /world/the_americas/opposition-strike-paralyzes-parts-of-venezuela-as -fears-of-violence-mount/2017/07/20/bd15120e-6cd0-11e7-abbc-a5348067 2286_story.html?utm_term=.3a7ff388c164.

37. **for the poorest Venezuelans:** Andreina Aponte, "For Poor Venezuelans, a Box of Food May Sway Vote for Maduro," Reuters, March 18, 2018, https: //www.reuters.com/article/us-venezuela-politics-food/for-poor-venezuelans -a-box-of-food-may-sway-vote-for-maduro-idUSKCN1GO173.

38. **Venezuela's economy has been in free fall:** For the World Bank's ranking of the world's national economies (measured by Gross Domestic Product in 2017), see: World Development Indicators database, World Bank, 1 July 2018, http://databank.worldbank.org/data/download/GDP.pdf.

39. **agriculture's financial contribution:** "Colombia," Observatory of Economic Complexity (OEC), accessed August 29, 2018, https://atlas.media.mit .edu/en/profile/country/col/; "Colombia," World Bank, accessed August 29, 2018, https://data.worldbank.org/country/colombia.

40. **livestock production still dominates:** Gert-Jan Stads et al., "Agricultural R&D Indicators Factsheet—Colombia," International Food Policy Research Institute, February 2016, http://ebrary.ifpri.org/utils/getfile/collection /p15738coll2/id/130293/filename/130504.pdf; "2014 Nutrition Country Profile -Colombia," IFPRI, accessed August 29, 2018, http://ebrary.ifpri.org/utils/get file/collection/p15738coll2/id/128523/filename/128734.pdf.

41. **longest-running insurgency:** Anthony Faiola, "Two Years After Colombia's Peace Accord, the Historic Pact Is in Jeopardy," *Washington Post*, June 16, 2018, https://www.washingtonpost.com/world/the_americas

/two-years-after-colombia-won-a-nobel-peace-prize-the-peace-is-in
-jeopardy/2018/06/15/c6030c9c-6d8b-11e8-b4d8-eaf78d4c544c_story.html?
utm_term=.ac36a9175025.

42. **the country exports more agricultural and food products:** "Colombia," OEC; "Colombia," World Bank.

43. **Pahom, an ambitious peasant:** Leo Tolstoy, "How Much Land Does
a Man Need?" *Literature Network*, accessed November 13, 2017, http://www.
online-literature.com/tolstoy/2738/; Leo Tolstoy, *What Men Live By and Other
Tales*, trans. L. and A. Maude (Project Gutenberg, EBook #6157, last modified
November 26, 2012), http://www.gutenberg.org/files/6157/6157-h/6157-h.htm.

Chapter 4

1. **burning the remains of humble creatures:** Carl Sagan, *Billions &
Billions: Thoughts on Life and Death at the Brink of the Millennium* (New York:
Random House, 1997).

2. **The formation of liquid energy:** David Montgomery, *Dirt: The Erosion of Civilizations* (Berkeley, CA: University of California Press, 2007),
199.

3. **returned a thousand barrels:** Charles Hall, Jessica Lambert, and Stephen Balogh, "EROI of Different Fuels and the Implications for Society,"
Energy Policy 64 (January 2014): 141–52, https://doi.org/10.1016/j.enpol.2013.05
.049.

4. **dirt is Earth's protective skin:** Montgomery, *Dirt*, 23.

5. **22,000 different soil types:** Ibid.

6. **Roots extending three to seventeen feet:** J. E. Weaver, "Classification
of Root Systems of Forbs of Grassland and a Consideration of Their Sig-
nificance," *Ecology* 39, no. 3 (July 1958): 393–401, http://digitalcommons.unl.edu
/cgi/viewcontent.cgi?article=1480&context=agronomyfacpub.

7. **patchwork of ill-conceived laws:** Murray Benedict, *Farm Policies of the
United States, 1790–1950: A Study of Their Origins and Development* (New York:
Octagon Books, 1966), chap. 1.

8. **moving farther inland:** Andrew Smith, *Food in America: The Past,
Present, and Future of Food, Farming, and the Family Meal*, vol. 1 (Santa Barbara, CA: ABC-CLIO, 2017), 15.

9. **unproductive to the practitioners:** Montgomery, *Dirt*, 123; George
Washington, *Letters from His Excellency George Washington to Arthur Young,
Esq., F.R.S., and Sir John Sinclair, Bart., M.P.: Containing an Account of His
Husbandry with His Opinions on Various Questions in Agriculture, and Many*

Particulars of the Rural Economy of the United States (Alexandria, VA: Cottom and Stewart, 1803), 6.

10. **how to promote soil improvements:** Montgomery, *Dirt*, 124.

11. **waste as we please:** Ibid., 125; Thomas Jefferson, *Notes on the State of Virginia*, ed. J. W. Randolph (Google Books, 1852), 94, https://books.google.com/books?id=DTWttRSMtbYC&printsec=frontcover&source=gbs_ge_summary_r&cad=0#v=onepage&q&f=false.

12. **"a miserable system of farming:** Andrew Downing, "A Blunt Warning about Unsustainable Farming Practices in America," in Smith, *Food in America*, 246–49.

13. **British capitulated their claim:** "The Caribbean and the British Empire," *British Empire Maproom*, accessed November 14, 2017, http://www.britishempire.co.uk/maproom/caribbean.htm.

14. **sold off the Louisiana Territory**: "Louisiana Purchase," Office of the Historian, accessed March 19, 2018, https://history.state.gov/milestones/1801-1829/louisiana-purchase.

15. **Alaska was bought from Russia:** "Alaska Purchase," *Encyclopedia Britannica*, accessed November 14, 2017, https://www.britannica.com/print/article/12326.

16. **tractors on farms had tripled:** Montgomery, *Dirt*, 146.

17. **nature was to blame:** Zeynep Hansen and Gary Libecap, "Small Farms, Externalities, and the Dust Bowl of the 1930s," *Journal of Political Economy* 112, no. 3 (June 2004): 665–94, http://www.nber.org/papers/w10055.pdf.

18. **programs began paying farmers:** Daniel Hellerstein, "The US Conservation Reserve Program: The Evolution of an Enrollment Mechanism," *Land Use Policy* 63 (April 2017): 601–10, https://doi.org/10.1016/j.landusepol.2015.07.017.

19. **higher profits were more important:** Alex Formuzis, "Here Today, Gone Tomorrow: USDA Conservation Program for Sensitive Cropland Wastes Billions of Tax Dollars," Environmental Working Group, June 7, 2017, https://www.ewg.org/release/here-today-gone-tomorrow-usda-conservation-program-sensitive-cropland-wastes-billions-tax.

20. **fast enough to sustain industrial agriculture:** Montgomery, *Dirt*, 3.

21. **being depleted eighteen times faster:** Natural Resources Conservation Service, "Soil Erosion," US Department of Agriculture, accessed November 14, 2017, https://www.nrcs.usda.gov/Internet/FSE_DOCUMENTS/nrcs142p2_010152.pdf.

22. **3,200 football fields each day:** "Farms Under Threat—The State of America's Farmland," American Farmland Trust, May 9, 2018, https://www

.farmlandinfo.org/sites/default/files/AFT_Farms_Under_Threat_May2018
%20maps%20B_0.pdf.

23. **a mass genocide:** "Rwanda Genocide of 1994," *Encyclopedia Britannica*, accessed June 6, 2018, https://www.britannica.com/event/Rwanda-genocide-of -1994.

24. **"rain follows the plow":** Matt Simon, "Fantastically Wrong: American Greed and the Harebrained Theory of 'Rain Follows the Plow'," *Wired Science*, June 25, 2014, https://www.wired.com/2014/06/fantastically-wrong -rain-follows-the-plow/; Marc Reisner, *Cadillac Desert: The American West and Its Disappearing Water* (New York: Penguin Books, 1993), 35.

25. **Timber Culture Act in 1873:** Smith, *Food in America*, vol. 1, 35; Barron McIntosh, "Use and Abuse of the Timber Culture Act," *Annuals of the Association of American Geographers* 65, no. 3 (September 1975): 347–62, http://doi .org/10.1111/j.1467-8306.1975.tb01044.x.

26. **center-pivot irrigation systems:** Robert Glennon, *Water Follies: Groundwater Pumping and the Fate of America's Fresh Waters* (Washington, DC: Island Press, 2012), 26.

27. **estimated at several trillions of gallons:** Ibid.

28. **forty-four of every one hundred acres:** Michael Cohen, Juliet Christian-Smith, and John Berggren, "Water to Supply the Land: Irrigated Agriculture in the Colorado River Basin," *Pacific Institute*, May 9, 2013, http: //pacinst.org/wp-content/uploads/2013/05/pacinst-crb-ag.pdf.

29. **one in six gallons stored in reservoirs:** "Colorado River Basin: Consumptive Uses and Losses Report 1996–2000," Bureau of Reclamation (Revised August 2012), 15, https://www.usbr.gov/uc/library/envdocs/reports/crs /pdfs/cul-1996-2000.pdf.

30. **farms became so reliant on Colorado River:** David Owen, *Where the Water Goes: Life and Death along the Colorado River* (New York: Riverhead Books, 2017), chap. 14, 173–84.

31. **due to unprecedented temperatures:** Bradley Udall and Jonathan Overpeck, "The Twenty-First Century Colorado River Hot Drought and Implications for the Future," *Water Resources Research* 53, no. 3 (February 2017): 2404–18, http://doi.org/10.1002/2016WR019638.

32. **In the East, surface-water laws:** "Riparian Doctrine," Legal Information Institute, Cornell University Law School, accessed November 14, 2017, https://www.law.cornell.edu/wex/riparian_doctrine.

33. **In the West, surface rights:** "Prior Appropriation Doctrine," Legal Information Institute, Cornell University Law School, accessed November 14, 2017, https://www.law.cornell.edu/wex/prior_appropriation_doctrine.

34. **more scientifically wrong:** Glennon, *Water Follies*, 29–30.

35. **overall level began plummeting:** Ibid., 26; Virginia McGuire, US Geological Survey, "Water-Level Changes and Change in Water in Storage in the High Plains Aquifer, Predevelopment to 2013 and 2011–13," Scientific Investigations Report 2014-5218, 2014, https://pubs.usgs.gov/sir/2014/5218/pdf /sir2014_5218.pdf.

36. **equivalent to Lake Erie:** David Steward et al., "Tapping Unsustainable Groundwater Stores for Agricultural Production in the High Plains Aquifer of Kansas, Projections to 2110," *Proceedings of the National Academy of Sciences* (*PNAS*) 110, no. 37 (September 2013): E3477–86, http://www.pnas.org /content/pnas/110/37/E3477.full.pdf; Bruno Basso, Anthony Kendall, and David Hyndman, "The Future of Agriculture over the Ogallala Aquifer: Solutions to Grow Crops More Efficiently with Limited Water," *Earth's Future* 1, no. 1 (December 2013): 39–41, http://onlinelibrary.wiley.com/doi/10.1002 /2013EF000107/epdf.

37. **70 percent will be drained:** Steward et al., "Tapping Unsustainable Groundwater."

38. **seven thousand dams:** National Agricultural Statistics Service, "Market Value of Agricultural Products Sold Including Direct Sales" in Census of Agriculture reports from year 1987 to 2012, USDA, https://www.agcensus .usda.gov/Publications/; example for 2012 report, 9, https://www.agcensus.usda .gov/Publications/2012/Full_Report/Volume_1,_Chapter_1_US/usv1.pdf.

39. **grow by 80 percent:** Texas Water Development Board, "Water for Texas 2012 State Water Plan," January 2012, http://www.twdb.texas.gov/publi cations/state_water_plan/2012/2012_SWP.pdf.

40. **primary solution: build more reservoirs:** Ibid.

41. **agriculture uses some 80 percent:** Economic Research Service (ERS), "Irrigation & Water Use," last modified April 30, 2018, https://www.ers.usda. gov/topics/farm-practices-management/irrigation-water-use/.

42. **In many western states, it's over 90 percent:** Ibid.

43. **the self-imposed deadline:** "Sustainable Groundwater Management Act," Division of Agriculture and Natural Resources, University of California, accessed March 25, 2018, http://groundwater.ucdavis.edu/SGMA/.

44. **from infrastructure to rights of usage:** Theodore Grantham and Joshua Viers, "100 Years of California's Water Rights System: Patterns, Trends, and Uncertainty," *Environmental Research Letters* 9 (August 2014): 084012–22, http://iopscience.iop.org/article/10.1088/1748-9326/9/8/084012/pdf.

45. **Groundwater is not regulated:** "California Overspends Water Rights by 300 Million Acre Feet," University of California–Merced, August 19, 2014, http://www.ucmerced.edu/news/2014/california-overspends-water-rights -300-million-acre-feet.

46. **newly drilled wells exploded:** Justin Gillis and Matt Richtel, "Beneath California Crops, Groundwater Crisis Grows," *New York Times*, April 5, 2015, https://www.nytimes.com/2015/04/06/science/beneath-california-crops -groundwater-crisis-grows.html.

47. **It Just Went Underground:** Mark Grossi, "The California Drought Isn't Over, It Just Went Underground," *Water Deeply*, July 5, 2017, https:// www.newsdeeply.com/water/articles/2017/07/05/the-california-drought-isnt -over-it-just-went-underground.

48. **"Why move to Nebraska?":** Grant Gerlock, "Nebraska Recruiting California Dairies to Pump Up Rural Economy," Nebraska Educational Telecommunications Commission, December 18, 2014, http://netnebraska.org /article/news/951441/nebraska-recruiting-california-dairies-pump-rural -economy.

49. **"All the water there will be, is.":** "Rivers & Streams," Foothills Conservancy of North Carolina, accessed March 25, 2018, https://foothillsconser vancy.org/places-we-protect/rivers-streams/.

50. **sugarcane is king:** "Brazil: Food Balance Sheets_Production Quantity _All Items," FAOSTAT, last modified February 13, 2017, http://www.fao.org /faostat/en/#data/FBS.

51. **eight barrels of energy:** Joel Bourne, "Green Dreams," Biofuels, *National Geographic*, October 2007, http://ngm.nationalgeographic.com/2007 /10/biofuels/biofuels-text; Government of the State of São Paulo, "Assessment of Greenhouse Gas Emissions in the Production and Use of Fuel Ethanol in Brazil," March 2004, https://www.wilsoncenter.org/sites/default/files/brazil .unicamp.macedo.greenhousegas.pdf.

52. **ratio less than 3:1 required subsidies:** Charles Hall, Stephen Balogh and David Murphy, "What Is the Minimum EROI That a Sustainable Society Must Have?" *Energies* 2, no. 1 (2009): 25–47, http://www.mdpi.com/1996 -1073/2/1/25; Hall et al., "EROI . . . for Society."

53. **between 0.87 to 1.27 barrels were returned:** David Murphy, Charles Hall, and Bobby Powers, "New Perspectives on the Energy Return on (Energy) Investment (EROI) of Corn Ethanol," *Environment, Development, and Sustainability* 13, no. 1 (February 2011): 179–202, https://doi.org/10.1007/s10668 -010-9255-7.

54. **all came from landfill gas:** US Environmental Protection Agency, "2016 Renewable Fuel Standard Data," data are current as of March 10, 2018, https://www.epa.gov/fuels-registration-reporting-and-compliance-help /2016-renewable-fuel-standard-data.

55. **What was left was destined for:** ERS, "U.S. Domestic Corn Use" graph, accessed May 22, 2015, https://www.ers.usda.gov/topics/crops/corn

-and-other-feedgrains/background/; ERS, "Feed Grains Data-All Years," Table 1, 4, last modified November 15, 2017, https://www.ers.usda.gov/data -products/feed-grains-database/feed-grains-yearbook-tables/.

56. **biofuel from corn had not lived up:** National Research Council, *Renewable Fuel Standard: Potential Economic and Environmental Effects of U.S. Biofuel Policy* (Washington, DC: National Academies Press, 2011), https:// www.nap.edu/read/13105/chapter/1.

57. **exporting 1.1 million barrels of oil a day:** US Energy Information Administration (EIA), "U.S. Crude Oil Exports Increased and Reached More Destinations in 2017," March 15, 2018, https://www.eia.gov/todayinenergy /detail.php?id=35352.

58. **requires immense quantities of water:** Andrew Kondash and Avner Vengosh, "Water Footprint of Hydraulic Fracturing," *Environment Science & Technology Letters* 2, no. 10 (2015): 276–80, http://pubs.acs.org/doi/full/10.1021 /acs.estlett.5b00211; Bobby Magill, "Water Use Rises as Fracking Expands," *Scientific American*, July 1, 2015, https://www.scientificamerican.com/article /water-use-rises-as-fracking-expands/.

59. **one-half of soil loss:** Montgomery, *Dirt*, 200.

60. **unbridled access to farmland:** Bureau of Transportation Statistics, "Table 1-6: Estimated U.S. Roadway Lane-Miles by Functional System (a)," last modified May 20, 2017, https://www.bts.gov/content/estimated-us-road way-lane-miles-functional-system; National Aeronautics and Space Administration, "Earth: By the Numbers-Equatorial Circumference," accessed March 25, 2018, https://solarsystem.nasa.gov/planets/earth/by-the-numbers/.

61. **3.5 million miles of rivers:** National Wild and Scenic Rivers System, "A National System," National Park Service, accessed November 14, 2017, https://www.rivers.gov/national-system.php; US Army Corps of Engineers, "National Inventory of Dams," accessed January 19, 2015, http://nid.usace .army.mil/cm_apex/f?p=838:5:0::NO.

62. **on-demand availability of liquid energy:** Pipeline and Hazardous Materials Safety Administration, "Annual Report Mileage for Hazardous Liquid or Carbon Dioxide Systems," "Annual Report Mileage for Natural Gas Transmission & Gathering Systems," and "Annual Report Mileage for Gas Distribution Systems," US Department of Transportation, last modified March 5, 2018, https://www.phmsa.dot.gov/data-and-statistics/pipeline/an nual-report-mileage-hazardous-liquid-or-carbon-dioxide-systems.

63. **don't need to think about the energy:** "Enabling Everyday Progress: Egg" (short), Energy Lives Here_Exxon Mobil, *YouTube*, released November 25, 2014, https://www.youtube.com/watch?v=ihjRqd9NkDc; "Enabling Everyday Progress: Egg," ExxonMobil Commercial (2014–15), *Popisms.com*,

posted December 9, 2014, https://www.popisms.com/TelevisionCommercial
/105859/ExxonMobil-Commercial-2014-2015.aspx.

64. **latest forecasts only extend:** EIA, "Do We Have Enough Oil Worldwide to Meet Our Future Needs?" last modified September 15, 2017, http://www
.eia.gov/tools/faqs/faq.cfm?id=38&t=6.

65. **estimated reserves are much smaller:** Howard Frumkin, Jeremy Hess,
and Stephen Vindigni, "Energy and Public Health: The Challenge of Peak
Petroleum," *Public Health Reports* 124, no. 1 (January-February 2009): 5–19,
https:/www.ncbi.nlm.nih.gov/pmc/articles/PMC2602925/.

66. **percentage would have been even higher:** "Statistical Review of
World Energy-Underpinning Data, 1965–2016," British Petroleum, https://
www.bp.com/en/global/corporate/energy-economics/statistical-review
-of-world-energy.html; for production until 2009, see: Table 7.3 (conversion
factors), p. 437, and Table 7.6 (cumulative production), p. 440, in Thomas
Johansson et al., eds., *Global Energy Assessment—Toward a Sustainable Future*
(New York: Cambridge University Press, 2012), http: //www.iiasa.ac.at/web
/home/research/Flagship-Projects/Global-Energy-Assessment/GEA_Chap
ter7_resources_lowres.pdf.

Chapter 5

1. **were Incan descendants:** Alfred Bingham, "Raiders of the Lost City,"
American Heritage 38, no. 5 (July/August 1987), http://www.americanheritage.
com/content/raiders-lost-city; Ruth Wright and Alfredo Zegarra, eds., *The
Machu Picchu Guidebook: A Self-Guided Tour* (Englewood, NJ: Westcliffe Pub-
lishers, 2001), ix.

2. **Rather than accept despair:** "Elinor Ostrom," *The Economist*, June 30,
2012, http://www.economist.com/node/21557717.

3. **"The Tragedy of the Commons":** Garrett Hardin, "The Tragedy of
the Commons," *Science* 162, no. 3859 (December 1968): 1243–48, http://science
.sciencemag.org/content/sci/162/3859/1243.full.pdf.

4. **Nobel Prize in Economics:** "Elinor Ostrom Biographical," Nobel
Prize citation, accessed September 2, 2018, https://www.nobelprize.org/prizes
/economics/2009/ostrom/auto-biography/; "Oliver E. Williamson Biographical," Nobel Prize citation, accessed September 2, 2018, https://www.nobelprize
.org/prizes/economics/2009/williamson/auto-biography/.

5. **Her studies in Nepal:** Elinor Ostrom, "How Farmer Managed Irrigation Systems Build Social Capital to Outperform Agency Managed Systems That Rely Primarily on Physical Capital," in P. Pradhan and U. Gautam,

eds., *Proceedings of the 2nd International Seminar, Held on 18–19 April 2002, Kathmandu, Nepal*, accessed March 25, 2018, http://citeseerx.ist.psu.edu/view doc/download;jsessionid=8F434FFFF9C192D93DD0A1E402A21269? doi=10.1.1.539.3262&rep=rep1&type=pdf; Elinor Ostrom et al., "Revisiting the Commons: Local Lessons, Global Challenges," *Science* 28 4, no. 5412 (April 1999): 278–82, http://www.sciencemag.org/content/284/5412/278.full; "Elinor Ostrom," *The Economist*.

6. **replace five antiquated canals:** Elinor Ostrom, "Social Capital, Self-Organization, and Development," Workshop in Political Theory and Policy Analysis, Indiana University, December 1994, https://pdf.usaid.gov/pdf_docs/PNABT618.pdf; Ostrom, "How Farmer Managed"; Ostrom et al., "Revisiting." For more information, see: Casper Sorensen, "Social Capital and Rural Development: A Discussion of Issues," Social Capital Initiative Working Paper no. 10., The World Bank, October 2000, http://citeseerx.ist.psu.edu/viewdoc/download?doi=10.1.1.104.9767&rep=rep1&type=pdf; Wai Fung Lam, *Governing Irrigation Systems in Nepal: Institutions, Infrastructure, and Collective Action* (Oakland, CA: ICS Press, 1998).

7. **Instead of higher yields:** Ostrom et al., "Revisiting."

8. **proposals for a federal department:** Everett Edwards, "American Agriculture—The First 300 Years," in *Farmers in a Changing World: Yearbook of Agriculture 1940*, National Agricultural Library (NAL) Digital Collections, US Department of Agriculture, 246, http://naldc.nal.usda.gov/download/IND 43893716/PDF.

9. **petitioning Congress for support:** Swann Harding, *Two Blades of Grass: A History of Scientific Development in the US Department of Agriculture* (Norman, OK: University of Oklahoma Press, 1947), 14.

10. **"spirit of discovery and improvement":** Edwards, "American Agriculture," 246.

11. **provide farmers with weather reports:** Economic Research Service (ERS), "Chronological Landmarks in American Agriculture," USDA, AIB-425, November 1990, 24 (under the year 1872), https://naldc.nal.usda.gov/download/CAT91949557/PDF.

12. **federal financial system for agriculture:** US Department of the Treasury, "The Federal Farm Loan Act," Federal Reserve Archival System for Economic Research (FRASER), Federal Reserve Bank of St. Louis, October 13, 1916, https://fraser.stlouisfed.org/scribd/?title_id=1102&filepath=/files/docs/historical/congressional/federal-farm-loan-act.pdf.

13. **12 percent of all farms:** National Agricultural Statistics Service, "Table 2. Market Value of Agricultural Products Sold Including Landlord's Share

and Direct Sales: 2012 and 2007," in USDA, *2012 Census of Agriculture*, vol. 1, chap. 1, https://www.agcensus.usda.gov/Publications/2012/Full_Report /Volume_1,_Chapter_1_US/st99_1_002_002.pdf.

14. **corn received 30 percent of farm subsidies:** Environmental Working Group (EWG), "The United States Farm Subsidy Information," accessed November 15, 2017, https://farm.ewg.org/region.php?fips=00000.

15. **"It is precisely the people's Department:** Wayne Rasmussen, "Lincoln's Agricultural Legacy," NAL, USDA, accessed March 25, 2018, https:// www.nal.usda.gov/lincolns-agricultural-legacy.

16. **Only a last minute intervention:** Warren Belasco, *Meals to Come: A History of the Future of Food* (Berkeley, CA: University of California Press, 2006), figure 16.

17. **"dialing for dollars":** Norah O'Donnell, "Are Members of Congress Becoming Telemarketers?" CBS *60 Minutes*, April 24, 2016, https:// www.cbsnews.com/news/60-minutes-are-members-of-congress-becoming -telemarketers/; David Graham, "The Humiliating Fundraising Existence of a Member of Congress," *The Atlantic*, June 25, 2013, https://www.theatlantic. com/politics/archive/2013/06/the-humiliating-fundraising-existence-of-a -member-of-congress/277227/; David DeWitt, "Former Congressman Rails Against Gerrymandering and Money in Politics," *Athens* (Ohio) *News*, April 30, 2017, https://www.athensnews.com/news/local/former-congressman-rails -against-gerrymandering-and-money-in-politics/article_99eea9fe-2dbd-11e7 -a595-efb5580c316c.html.

18. **fourth-highest number of political slots:** Zach Paiker, "Help Wanted: 4,000 Presidential Appointees," Center for Presidential Transition, March 16, 2016, http://presidentialtransition.org/blog/posts/160316_help-wanted-4000 -appointees.php.

19. **"How else could companies overlook:** Michael Porter and Mark Kramer, "Creating Shared Value: How to Reinvent Capitalism—And Unleash a Wave of Innovation and Growth," *Harvard Business Review* 89 (January/February 2011), 62–77, http://www.nuovavista.com/SharedValuePorterHar vardBusinessReview.PDF.

20. **"Bring it on":** Daryll Ray and Harwood Schaffer, "The 1996 'Freedom to Farm' Farm Bill," Agricultural Policy Analysis Center, University of Tennessee, no. 703, originally published in *MidAmerica Farmer Grower* 35, no. 3 (January 17, 2014), http://www.agpolicy.org/weekpdf/703.pdf.

21. **After two years of lobbying:** Peggy Lowe, "Lobbyists of All Kinds Flock to Farm Bill," *Harvest Public Media*, July 14, 2014, http://investigate midwest.org/2014/07/14/lobbyists-of-all-kinds-flock-to-farm-bill/.

22. **The 1993 Farm Bill was 24 pages:** "1933 Farm Bill—Agricultural Adjustment Act of 1933," National Agricultural Law Center, accessed March 25, 2018, http://nationalaglawcenter.org/farmbills/.

23. **2014 Farm Bill came in at 609 pages:** "Agricultural Act of 2014," US Government Publishing Office (GPO), accessed June 11, 2018, https://www.gpo.gov/fdsys/pkg/BILLS-113hr2642enr/pdf/BILLS-113hr2642enr.pdf.

24. **$800 million per page:** ERS, "Projected Spending Under the 2014 Farm Bill," last modified January 16, 2018, https://www.ers.usda.gov/topics/farm-economy/farm-commodity-policy/projected-spending-under-the-2014-farm-bill/.

25. **better off giving farmers free insurance:** Bruce Babcock, "Impact of Scaling Back: Crop Insurance Premium Subsidies," EWG, July 11, 2012, https://www.ewg.org/research/impact-scaling-back; Bruce Babcock, "Giving It Away Free: Free Crop Insurance Can Save Money and Strengthen the Farm Safety Net," EWG, April 1, 2012, https://www.ewg.org/research/giving-it-away-free.

26. **rate of return on retained premiums:** US Government Accountability Office (GAO), "Crop Insurance: Opportunities Exist to Improve Program Delivery and Reduce Costs (Table 1)," GAO-17-501, July 2017, 25, https://www.gao.gov/assets/690/686145.pdf.

27. **Insurance policies were authorized:** Dennis Shields, "Crop Insurance Provisions in the 2014 Farm Bill (P.L. 113-79)," Congressional Research Service (CRS), April 22, 2014, 2, http://nationalaglawcenter.org/wp-content/uploads//assets/crs/R43494.pdf.

28. **prohibited the release of information:** Nancy Watzman, "Farm Bill Allows Congress to Keep Crop Subsidies Secret," Sunlight Foundation, February 7, 2014, https://sunlightfoundation.com/2014/02/07/farm-bill-allows-congress-to-keep-crop-subsidies-secret/; "Agriculture Risk Protection Act of 2000," GPO, June 20, 2000, Title I (B), Sec. 122, https://www.gpo.gov/fdsys/pkg/PLAW-106publ224/pdf/PLAW-106publ224.pdf; GPO, "Agricultural Act of 2014," Title XI, Secs. 11001, 11002; Ralph Chite, "The 2014 Farm Bill (P.L. 113-79): Summary and Sideby-Side," CRS, February 12, 2014, 206, http://nationalaglawcenter.org/wp-content/uploads/2014/02/R43076.pdf.

29. **the government pays 62 percent:** GAO, "Crop Insurance Opportunities," 10.

30. **figured out how to be compensated twice:** Anne Schechinger and Craig Cox, "Double Dipping: How Taxpayers Subsidize Farmers Twice for Crop Losses," EWG, November 2017, https://cdn3.ewg.org/sites/default/files/u352/EWG_SubsidyDoubleDippingReport_C03-min.pdf.

31. **stop subsidizing the wrong things.":** "Editorial: To Clean Up Our Water, Go 'Nuts' Like This Iowa Farmer," *Des Moines Register*, June 30, 2017, http://www.desmoinesregister.com/story/opinion/columnists/iowa-view/2017/06/30/editorial-clean-up-our-water-go-nuts-like-iowa-farmer/438843001/.

32. **familiar phrases from the past:** Kaush Arha et al., eds., *U.S. Agricultural Policy and the 2007 Farm Bill*, Woods Institute for The Environment, Stanford University, 2006, 16, accessed November 15, 2017, https://woods.stanford.edu/sites/default/files/files/Farm-Bill-Workshop-Book-200602_BThompson.pdf.

33. **"a win for farmers and consumers":** Dianne Feinstein, US Senator for California, "Feinstein: Farm Bill Passage Big Win for California Farmers, Consumers," press release, February 4, 2014, https://www.feinstein.senate.gov/public/index.cfm/press-releases?ID=C81B79F9-1D1D-4120-8110-A85E5897609B; Debbie Stabenow, US Senator for Michigan, "Farm Bill Resources Center," accessed November 11, 2015, http://www.stabenow.senate.gov/farmbill/.

34. **an additional 60 percent:** Ryan Alexander, "Farming Bigger Losses for Taxpayers," *U.S. News*, March 31, 2016, https://www.usnews.com/opinion/economic-intelligence/articles/2016-03-31/farm-bill-costs-are-exploding.

35. **"If angels were to govern men:** James Madison, "Federalist Paper no. 51 (1788)," Bill of Rights Institute, https://www.billofrightsinstitute.org/founding-documents/primary-source-documents/the-federalist-papers/federalist-papers-no-51/.

36. **"it's the right thing to do.":** Skip Schulz, "Western UP Helps Kansas Fire Victims," *Daily Mining Gazette*, March 24, 2017, http://www.mininggazette.com/news/2017/03/western-up-helps-kansas-fire-victims/; Von Lozon, "A Michigan Group Is Raising Donations for Farmers Affected by Wildfires," *MLive*, March 21, 2017, http://www.mlive.com/news/saginaw/index.ssf/2017/03/michigan_group_raising_donatio.html.

37. **majorities can become minorities:** Steven Levitsky and Daniel Ziblatt, *How Democracies Die* (New York: Crown Publishing Group, 2018).

38. **the power which knowledge gives:** "Celebrating James Madison and the Freedom of Information Act," FOIA Post, US Department of Justice, last modified August 6, 2014, https://www.justice.gov/oip/blog/foia-post-2008-celebrating-james-madison-and-freedom-information-act.

Chapter 6

1. **the Pan American Highway:** "Fastest Journey on Foot—Pan-American Highway," Guinness World Records, accessed June 18, 2018, http://www

.guinnessworldrecords.com/world-records/fastest-journey-on-foot-pan
-american-highway; "A Gap in the Andes," Earth Observatory, National
Aeronautics and Space Administration, June 27, 2016, https://earthobserva
tory.nasa.gov/IOTD/view.php?id=88271.

2. **there were six million people:** Jean-Pierre Bocquet-Appel, "When
the World's Population Took Off: The Springboard of the Neolithic Demographic Transition," *Science* 333, no. 6042 (July 2011): 560–61, https://doi.org/10
.1126/science.1208880.

3. **pass the one billion mark:** US Census Bureau International Program, "Historical Estimates of World Population" and "World Population,"
accessed November 15, 2017, https://www.census.gov/data/tables/time-series
/demo/international-programs/historical-est-worldpop.html & http://www
.census.gov/population/international/data/worldpop/table_population.php;
United Nations Population Fund (UNFPA), "World Population Milestones,"
accessed June 12, 2018, http://www.unesco.org/education/tlsf/mods/theme_c
/popups/mod13t01s03.html; UN Department of Economic and Social Affairs
Population Division, "The World at Six Billion," October 12, 1999, http://www
.un.org/esa/population/publications/sixbillion/sixbilpart1.pdf.

4. **shortchanging the power of science:** Thomas Malthus, *An Essay on
the Principle of Population* (London: J. Johnson Publisher, 1798), I.17, accessed
via Library of Economics and Liberty, http://www.econlib.org/library/Mal
thus/malPop.html.

5. **Earth surpassed two billion:** US Census Bureau, "World Population."

6. **not have enough to eat:** Gordon Conway, *The Doubly Green Revolution: Food for All in the Twenty-First Century* (New York: Penguin Books,
1997), 44.

7. **the food shortfall was "so great:** "Green Revolution: Curse or Bless-
ing?" International Food Policy Research Institute (IFPRI), accessed November 15, 2017, http://ebrary.ifpri.org/utils/getfile/collection/p15738coll2/id/64639
/filename/64640.pdf.

8. **hired a scientist named Norman Borlaug:** John Perkins, "The
Rockefeller Foundation and the Green Revolution, 1941–1956," *Agriculture and
Human Values* 7, no. 3–4 (June 1990): 6–18, https://doi.org/10.1007/BF01557305.

9. **so-called developing countries doubled:** "Africa's Turn—A New
Green Revolution for the 21st Century," Rockefeller Foundation, July 2006,
https://assets.rockefellerfoundation.org/app/uploads/20060701123216/dc
8aefda-bc49-4246-9e92-9026bc0eed04-africas_turn.pdf; Conway, *The Doubly
Green Revolution*, 44.

10. **population swelled by 60 percent:** US Census Bureau, "Historical
Estimates of World Population."

11. **daily supply of calories increased:** Paul Davies, "An Historical Perspective from the Green Revolution to the Gene Evolution," *Nutrition Reviews* 61, no. 6 (June 2003): S124–34, https://doi.org/10.1301/nr.2003.jun.S124-S134.

12. **impending doom awaiting hundreds of millions:** Paul Sabin, *The Bet: Paul Ehrlich, Julian Simon, and Our Gamble Over Earth's Future* (New Haven, CT: Yale University Press, 2013), 1.

13. **science and technology would overcome:** Julian Simon and David M. Gardner, "World Food Needs and 'New Proteins,'" 520–21, cited in: Sabin, *The Bet*, 2.

14. **gentleman farmer from Vermont:** Coy Cross II, *Justin Smith Morrill: Father of the Land-Grant Colleges* (East Lansing, MI: Michigan State University Press, 1999), 13.

15. **deficient agricultural knowledge and skills:** Cross, *Justin Smith Morrill*, 79.

16. **Europe was investing in agricultural colleges:** Coy Cross II, "Democracy, the West, and Land-Grant Colleges," 8, in Daniel Fogel and Elizabeth Maison-Huddle, eds., *Precipice or Crossroads? Where America's Great Public Universities Stand and Where They Are Going Midway through Their Second Century* (New York: State University of New York Press, 2012).

17. **"We want no fancy farmers":** Christopher Lucas, *American Higher Education: A History*, 2nd ed. (Basingstoke, UK: Palgrave Macmillan, 2006), 154.

18. **"an unconstitutional robbing of the Treasury:** Cross, *Justin Smith Morrill*, 82.

19. **know is the Bible and figgers:** Allan Nevins, *The State Universities and Democracy* (Urbana, IL: University of Illinois Press, 1962), 38, https://archive.org/details/stateuniversitieoonevi.

20. **character of both Governments:** Gerhard Peters and John Woolley, "James Buchanan: Veto Message," American Presidency Project, February 24, 1859, http://www.presidency.ucsb.edu/ws/?pid=68368.

21. **"The method of science:** Carl Sagan and Ann Druyan, *The Demon-Haunted World: Science as a Candle in the Dark* (New York: Ballantine Books, 1997), 26.

22. **The discovery of vitamins:** Richard Semba, "The Discovery of the Vitamins," *International Journal for Vitamin and Nutrition Research* 82, no. 5 (October 2012): 310–15, https://doi.org/10.1024/0300-9831/a000124.

23. **population boomed by over 110 million:** US Census Bureau, "POP Culture: 1860" and "POP Culture: 1940," last modified July 18, 2017, https://www.census.gov/history/www/through_the_decades/fast_facts/1860_fast_facts.html.

24. **Prior to World War II:** Daniel Kleinman, *Politics on the Endless Frontier: Postwar Research Policy in the United States* (Durham, NC: Duke University Press, 1995), 28–29.

25. **up to the 1950s:** Philip Pardey, Julian Alston, and Connie Chan-Kang, "Public Food and Agricultural Research in the United States: The Rise and Decline of Public Investments, and Policies for Renewal," AGree Transforming Food & Ag Policy, April 2013, vi, 13 (Table 2), http://www.foodandag policy.org/sites/default/files/AGree-Public%20Food%20and%20Ag%20 Research%20in%20US-Apr%202013.pdf.

26. **President Roosevelt commissioned Bush:** Roger Pielke Jr., "In Retrospect: Science—The Endless Frontier," *Nature* 466 (August 2010): 922–23, https://www.nature.com/articles/466922a.pdf.

27. **"purest realms of science.":** Vannevar Bush, *Science—The Endless Frontier, A Report to the President on a Program for Postwar Scientific Research* (Washington, DC: National Science Foundation, 1960), chap. 3, https://ar chive.org/details/scienceendlessfroounit.

28. **Such research was driven by curiosity:** Ibid.

29. **basic research meant uncovering "practical applications":** Ibid.

30. **Speaking of agriculture:** Ibid., chap. 1.

31. **"embedded in commercial possibility.":** Don Lotter, "The Genetic Engineering of Food and the Failure of Science—Part 2: Academic Capitalism and the Loss of Scientific Integrity," *International Journal of Sociology of Agriculture and Food* 16, no. 1 (2009), 50–68, http://www.ijsaf.org/archive/16/1 /lotter2.pdf.

32. **other agencies soon leap-frogged:** Pielke Jr., "In Retrospect."

33. **USDA received less than 2 percent:** "Figure 4-19: Federal Obligations for R&D, by Agency and Character of Work: FY 2011," *Science and Engineering Indicators 2014* (Arlington, VA: National Science Foundation, NSB14-01), 4–36, https://www.nsf.gov/statistics/seind14/content/etc/nsb1401.pdf.

34. **legislation that tied up loose ends:** Pardey et al., "Public Food," 42, fn. 39.

35. **"the patent system to promote:** US Government Publishing Office, "Public Law 96-517," accessed November 16, 2017, https://www.gpo.gov/fdsys /pkg/STATUTE-94/pdf/STATUTE-94-Pg3015.pdf.

36. **the most inspired piece of legislation**: "Innovation's Golden Goose," *The Economist*, December 12, 2002, http://www.economist.com/node/1476 653.

37. **behave more like businesses than neutral arbiters:** "Bayhing for Blood or Doling Out Cash?" *The Economist*, December 20, 2005, 115, http: //www.economist.com/node/5327661.

38. **accelerate licensing, startup ventures, and patent applications:** National Research Council, *Spurring Innovation in Food and Agriculture: A Review of the USDA Agriculture and Food Research Initiative Program* (Washington, DC: National Academies Press, 2014), 16, http://wssa.net/wp-content/uploads/Spurring-Innovation-in-Food-and-Ag_A-Review-of-USDA-AFRI-by-NAS.

39. **"measurable societal impacts.":** Ibid.

40. **The number-one challenge:** Bradford Barham, Jeremy Foltz, and Daniel Prager, "Making Time for Science," *Research Policy* 43, no. 1 (February 2014): 21–31, https://doi.org/10.1016/j.respol.2013.08.007.

41. **$454 billion spent on research:** "Table 4-1, U.S. R&D Expenditures, by Performing Sector and Source of Funds: 2008–15," in "Science & Engineering Indicators 2018," National Science Board, chap. 4, 4–10, https://www.nsf.gov/statistics/2018/nsb20181/assets/1038/research-and-development-u-s-trends-and-international-comparisons.pdf.

42. **Of that amount, 0.6 percent:** Matthew Clancy, Keith Fuglie, and Paul Heisey, "U.S. Agricultural R&D in an Era of Falling Public Funding," Economic Research Service (ERS), November 10, 2016, https://www.ers.usda.gov/amber-waves/2016/november/us-agricultural-rd-in-an-era-of-falling-public-funding/.

43. **society's larger withdrawal from public universities:** ERS, "Projected Spending Under the 2014 Farm Bill," last modified January 16, 2018, https://www.ers.usda.gov/topics/farm-economy/farm-commodity-policy/projected-spending-under-the-2014-farm-bill/.

44. **college tuition and fees skyrocketed**: Ilan Kolet, "College Tuition's 1,120 Percent Increase," *Bloomberg Businessweek*, August 23, 2012, https://www.bloomberg.com/news/articles/2012-08-23/college-tuitions-1-120-percent-increase.

45. **more than half of all states:** Michael Mitchell, Michael Leachman, and Kathleen Masterson, "A Lost Decade in Higher Education Funding," Figure 8, Center on Budget and Policy Priorities, August 23, 2017, https://www.cbpp.org/sites/default/files/atoms/files/2017_higher_ed_8-22-17_final.pdf.

46. **At Michigan State University:** "Michigan State University Proposed 2001–2002 Budgets," Michigan State University, accessed June 18, 2018, https://opb.msu.edu/functions/budget/documents/2001-02Budgets.pdf; and "Michigan State University 2017–2018 Budgets," accessed June 18, 2018, https://opb.msu.edu/functions/budget/documents/2017-18Budgets.pdf.

47. **71 percent of the general operating budget:** "FY17 and FY18 Budget Overview," Michigan State University, accessed June 18, 2018, https://opb.msu.

edu/functions/budget/documents/FY1718CompleteBudgetGuidelinesFinal
.pdf.

48. **universities are in a bind:** Jon Marcus, "The Decline of the Midwest's Public Universities Threatens to Wreck Its Most Vibrant Economies," *The Atlantic*, October 15, 2017, https://www.theatlantic.com/business/archive/2017/10/midwestern-public-research-universities-funding/542889/.

49. **Those guided by different priorities:** Those here refers to anyone who has tried to bend the science platform to serve their own vested interests. This includes legislators who withhold funding or attempt to discredit scientific findings; lobbyists, trade associations, agribusinesses, etc., who try to invalidate or misdirect scientific results that threaten to raise costs or lower profits; and consumers who fear that their standards of living could be jeopardized by science-based outcomes. These are all examples of direct attempts to steer the scientific platform in self-serving ways. Indirectly, all of us are guilty when we believe that the role of science is to make our lives better rather than help us become more knowledgeable about how all life (not just our own), nature, and the Earth are intimately intertwined.

50. **States have pared back their commitment:** Christopher Newfield, *The Great Mistake: How We Wrecked Public Universities and How We Can Fix Them* (Baltimore, MD: Johns Hopkins University Press, 2016), 133–38.

51. **research results that benefit the funder:** José Massougbodji et al., "Reviews Examining Sugar-Sweetened Beverages and Body Weight: Correlates of Their Quality and Conclusions," *American Journal of Clinical Nutrition* 99, no. 5 (May 2014): 1096–1104, https://doi.org/10.3945/ajcn.113.063776; Thomas Bodenheimer, "Uneasy Alliance—Clinical Investigators and the Pharmaceutical Industry," *New England Journal of Medicine* 342, no. 20 (May 2000): 1539–44, http://doi.org/10.1056/NEJM200005183422024; Joel Lexchin et al., "Pharmaceutical Industry Sponsorship and Research Outcome and Quality: Systematic Review," *BMJ* 326 (May 2003): 11 67–70, https://doi.org/10.11 36/bmj.326.7400.11 67; Lenard Lesser et al., "Relationship between Funding Source and Conclusion among Nutrition-Related Scientific Articles," *PLoS Medicine* 4, no. 1 (January 2007):0041–46, https://doi.org/10.1371/journal.pmed.0040005.

52. **nothing to do with advancing knowledge:** Marion Nestle, "Corporate Funding of Food and Nutrition Research: Science or Marketing?" *JAMA Internal Medicine* 176, no. 1 (January 2016): 13–14, http://doi.org/10.1001/jamainternmed.2015.6667.

53. **agricultural production increased 169 percent:** Clancy et al., "U.S. Agricultural R&D."

54. **$16.2 billion spent on food and agricultural research:** Ibid.

55. **declining productivity gains in major crops:** Julian Alston, Jason Beddow, and Philip Pardey, "Agricultural Research, Productivity, and Food Prices in the Long Run," *Science* 325, no. 5945 (September 2009): 1209–10, http://doi.org/10.1126/science.1170451.

56. **Rachel Carson has been under attack by revisionists:** Naomi Oreskes and Erik Conway, *Merchants of Doubt: How a Handful of Scientists Obscured the Truth on Issues from Tobacco Smoke to Global Warming* (New York: Bloomsbury Press, 2010).

57. **98 percent of climate scientists:** William Anderegg et al., "Expert Credibility in Climate Change," *Proceedings of the National Academy of Sciences* 107, no. 27 (July 2010): 12107–9, http://www.pnas.org/content/107/27/12107 .full.pdf.

58. **Despite its glaring errors:** John Bohannon, "Who's Afraid of Peer Review?" *Science* 342, no. 6154 (October 2013): 60–65, http://doi.org/10.1126/science .342.6154.60.

59. **wide use of antibiotics in animal feeds:** US General Accounting Office, "Food and Drug Administration's Regulation of Antibiotics Used in Animal Feeds," September 19, 1977, http://www.gao.gov/assets/100/98536.pdf.

60. **Great Britain had already banned:** Ibid.

61. **Today, 80 percent of all antibiotics consumed:** Tracy Pham, "Drug Use Review," US Food & Drug Administration, April 5, 2012, 2, http://www .fda.gov/downloads/Drugs/DrugSafety/InformationbyDrugClass/UCM 319435.pdf; FDA, "2013 Summary Report on Antimicrobials Sold or Distributed for Use in Food-Producing Animals," April 2015, 39, http://www.fda .gov/downloads/ForIndustry/UserFees/AnimalDrugUserFeeActADUFA /UCM440584.pdf.

62. **purging scientists from its Scientific Board:** Chris Mooney and Juliet Eilperin, "EPA Just Gave Notice to Dozens of Scientific Advisory Board Members That Their Time Is Up," *Washington Post*, June 20, 2017, https: //www.washingtonpost.com/news/energy-environment/wp/2017/06/20 /trump-administration-to-decline-to-renew-dozens-of-scientists-for-key -epa-advisory-board/?utm_term=.fa283cfoce3d; Aria Bendix, "EPA Says Goodbye to Half Its Scientific Board," *The Atlantic*, May 9, 2017, https://www .theatlantic.com/news/archive/2017/05/epa-dismisses-half-the-scientists -on-its-review-board/525909/.

63. **hardly anyone knows anything:** Carl Sagan, "Why We Need to Understand Science," *Skeptical Inquirer* 14, no. 3 (Spring, 1990), https://www.csi cop.org/si/show/why_we_need_to_understand_science.

64. **argue about the rules of geometry:** Steven Shapin, *A Social History of Truth: Civility and Science in Seventeenth-Century England* (Chicago: Uni-

versity of Chicago Press, 1994), 224. Cited by: Naomi Oreskes, "Science and Public Policy: What's Proof Got to Do With It?" *Environmental Science & Policy* 7 (2004): 369–83, http://sciencepolicy.colorado.edu/publications/special /oreskes_science_and_public_policy.pdf.

Chapter 7

1. *Today, the logic of buying and selling:* Michael Sandel, *What Money Can't Buy: The Moral Limits of Markets* (New York: Farrar, Straus and Giroux, 2012), Kindle edition, 93–94.

2. **Adolf Hitler ordered his forces:** Alexis Peri, *The War Within: Diaries from the Siege of Leningrad* (Cambridge, MA: Harvard University Press, 2017), Kindle edition, 349.

3. **most of the 800,000 who perished:** Ibid.

4. **the museum's director launched a daring plan:** Gary Nabhan, *Where Our Food Comes From: Retracing Nikolay Vavilov's Quest to End Famine* (Washington, DC: Island Press, 2008), 2.

5. **hinterlands of Russia:** Ibid.

6. **Seven weeks later:** Ibid., 2.

7. **the Research Institute of Plant Industry:** Ibid., 9.

8. **2,500 species of food crops:** Ibid., 3.

9. **the Third Reich's future use:** Ibid., 8.

10. **simply cold-treating seeds:** James Crow, "N. I. Vavilov, Martyr to Genetic Truth," *Genetics* 134, no. 1 (May 1993): 1–4, https://www.ncbi.nlm.nih .gov/pmc/articles/PMC1205417/pdf/ge1341r.pdf.

11. **The official press release:** Nabhan, *Where Our Food Comes From*, 7.

12. **most dedicated coworkers slowly starved to death:** Ibid., 8.

13. **excluded products of nature:** "The Patent Act of 1790, chap. 7, 1 stat. 109–12 (April 10, 1790)—The First United States Patent Statute," chap. VII, IP Mall, University of New Hampshire School of Law, accessed September 3, 2018, http://www.ipmall.info/sites/default/files/hosted_resources/lipa/patents /Patent_Act_of_1790.pdf.

14. **It was Thomas Jefferson:** "Summary of Public Service, [After 2 September 1800]," *Founders Online, National Archives*, https://founders.archives .gov/documents/Jefferson/01-32-02-0080.

15. **directed overseas consuls to collect rare seeds:** A. Pieters, "Seed Distribution by the United States Department of Agriculture," *The Plant World* 13, no. 12 (December 1910): 292–96, https://www.jstor.org/stable/pdf/43476829 .pdf; A. Pieters, "The Business of Seed and Plant Introduction and Dis-

tribution," in *Yearbook of the Department of Agriculture—1905* (Washington, DC: US Government Printing Office [GPO], 1906), 291, https://naldc.nal.usda.gov/download/IND43646995/PDF.

16. **the country was all in on:** "The Patent Act of 1790," IP Mall.

17. **one billion packages of seed:** Debbie Barker, "History of Seed in the U.S.: The Untold American Revolution," Center for Food Safety, August 2012, https://www.centerforfoodsafety.org/files/seed-report-for-print-final_25743.pdf.

18. **Small fledgling seed companies:** Jorge Fernandez-Cornejo, "The Seed Industry in U.S. Agriculture: An Exploration of Data and Information on Crop Seed Markets, Regulation, Industry Structure, and Research and Development," Economic Research Service (ERS), AIB-786, February 1, 2004, 25, https://www.ers.usda.gov/publications/pub-details/?pubid=42531.

19. **control prices, limit supply, and increase profits:** Jack Kloppenburg, *First the Seed: The Political Economy of Plant Biotechnology* (Madison, WI: University of Wisconsin Press, 2004), 147.

20. **sexually propagated plants:** Ibid., 132–33; Debbie Barker, "Seed Giants vs. U.S. Farmers," Center for Food Safety, February 13, 2013, https://www.centerforfoodsafety.org/files/seed-giants_final_04424.pdf.

21. **patents as a threat to the food supply:** "Chapter 57—Plant Variety Protection," GPO, accessed December 10, 2017, https://www.gpo.gov/fdsys/pkg/USCODE-2010-title7/pdf/USCODE-2010-title7-chap57-subchapI-partA-sec2321.pdf; Barker, "Seed Giants vs. U.S. Farmers."

22. **When the bill was enacted:** Philip Howard, *Concentration and Power in the Food System: Who Controls What We Eat* (New York: Bloomsbury Academic, 2016), 106.

23. **the smaller ones were gone:** ERS, "The Seed Industry," 26.

24. **fewer than a hundred remained:** Ibid., 106.

25. **a perfect herbicide:** Stephen Duck and Stephen Powles, "Glyphosate: A Once-in-a-Century Herbicide," *Pest Management Science* 64, no. 4 (2008): 319–25, http://naldc.nal.usda.gov/download/17918/PDF.

26. **once-in-a-century blockbuster:** Duck and Powles, "Glyphosate"; for more information see: John Franz, Michael Mao, and James Sikorski, *Glyphosate: A Unique Global Herbicide*, ACS Monograph Series no. 189 (Washington DC: American Chemical Society, 1997).

27. **a bacterium cell was patentable:** "Diamond v. Chakrabarty, 447 U.S. 303 (1980)," JUSTIA, US Supreme Court, accessed December 10, 2017, https://supreme.justia.com/cases/federal/us/447/303/case.html.

28. **no longer save and replant seeds:** "1985 Pat. App. Lexis 11,227 U.S.P.Q. BNA 443," *Yumpu.com*, accessed December 10, 2017, https://www.yumpu.

com/en/document/view/52362808/1985-pat-app-lexis-11-227-uspq-bna-443
-schmeiser-; Barker, "Seed Giants vs. U.S. Farmers," 15.

29. **the farmer agreed to pay all costs:** "2017 Monsanto Technology /
Stewardship Agreement (Limited Use License)," in "Monsanto 2017 Technology Use Guide," Monsanto, accessed March 29, 2018, https://monsanto.com
/app/uploads/2017/05/2017_tug.010617final.pdf.

30. **Patent holders now determined:** "Do Seed Companies Control GM
Crop Research?" (editorial), *Scientific American*, August 1, 2009, https://www
.scientificamerican.com/article/do-seed-companies-control-gm-crop-
research/; Nathanael Johnson, "Genetically Modified Seed Research: What's
Locked and What Isn't," *Grist*, August 5, 2013, http://grist.org/food/geneti
cally-modified-seed-research-whats-locked-and-what-isnt/.

31. **partial access for research:** "Academic Research Agreements,"
Monsanto, April 7, 2017, https://monsanto.com/company/media/statements
/academic-research-agreements/; Barker, "Seed Giants vs. U.S. Farmers," 19.

32. **dominated by three companies:** Wayne Ma, "Five Things to Know
about ChemChina," *Wall Street Journal*, February 3, 2016, https://blogs.wsj
.com/briefly/2016/02/03/5-things-to-know-about-chemchina/.

33. **none had absolute control:** Jeremy Rifkin, *The Zero Marginal Cost
Society: The Internet of Things, The Collaborative Commons, and the Eclipse of
Capitalism* (New York: St. Martin's Griffin, 2015), 30; Richard Schlatter, *Pri-
vate Property: The History of an Idea* (New York: A. M. Kelley, 1968), 1.

34. **families starved and watched helplessly:** Rifkin, *The Zero Marginal
Cost Society*, 29–33.

35. **the rich against the poor:** Ibid., 31.

36. **return to aristocratic control:** "Government Land Policy (Issue),"
Gale Encyclopedia of U.S. Economic History, *Encyclopedia.com*, accessed November 10, 2017, http://www.encyclopedia.com/history/encyclopedias-alma
nacs-transcripts-and-maps/government-land-policy-issue; "American Agriculture and the Development of a Nation's Land Policy," Center for Agricultural History and Rural Studies, Iowa State University, accessed November 10, 2017, http://rickwoten.com/LandPolicy.html.

37. **web of loyalties and insider connections:** Barry Lynn, *Cornered: The
New Monopoly Capitalism and the Economics of Destruction* (Hoboken, NJ:
Wiley, 2011), Kindle edition, 2287–89.

38. **"the farm is a factory.":** Robert Moulton, "Is This the Biggest Farm
in the World?" *Scientific American* 121, no. 8 (August 23, 1919), 183, cited in:
Andrew Smith, *Food in America: The Past, Present, and Future of Food, Farming, and the Family Meal* (Santa Barbara, CA: ABC-CLIO, 2017), v. 3.

39. **Wanting a larger factory:** Moulton, "Is This the Biggest Farm?"

40. **farms peaked near seven million:** "Agriculture 1950. Changes in Agriculture, 1900 to 1950," in "U.S. Census of Agriculture—1950, A Graphic Summary," vol. V, part 6, US Department of Agriculture, accessed November 10, 2017, http://usda.mannlib.cornell.edu/usda/AgCensusImages/1950/05/06 /1820/41667073v5p6ch4.pdf.

41. **powerful banks and railroads:** Howard, *Concentration and Power*, 18.

42. **Ninety-five percent of farm implements:** W. Neuman, "Negotiated Meanings and State Transformation: The Trust Issue in the Progressive Era," *Social Problems* 45, no. 3 (August 1998): 315–35, https://doi.org/10.2307/3097189.

43. **Ironically, breaking up the trusts:** Ibid.

44. **the whaling fleet doubled in size:** "How the Oil Industry Saved the Whales," *San Joaquin Valley Geology*, last modified October 12, 2015, http: //www.sjvgeology.org/history/whales.html; for more information see: "The History of the Oil Industry," *San Joaquin Valley Geology*, last modified January 11, 2017, http://www.sjvgeology.org/history/index.html; "History of the Oil and Gas Industry," Business Reference Services, *BERA* 5/6, 2005/2006, last modified February 16, 2018, http://www.loc.gov/rr/business/BERA/issue5 /history.html; Samuel Pees, "Whale Oil," Petroleum History Institute, accessed November 10, 2017, http://www.petroleumhistory.org/OilHistory/pages /Whale/whale.html; Bennett Wall, "Oil Industry," *History*, accessed March 29, 2018, https://www.history.com/topics/oil-industry.

45. **Mergers and acquisitions benefited:** Howard, *Concentration and Power*, 18–19.

46. **When Bill Clinton took over:** Lynn, *Cornered*, 270.

47. **monopoly is the best friend:** Ibid., chap. 5.

48. **"deadly combination.":** Neil Harl, "The Structural Transformation of Agriculture," presented at the 2003 Master Farmer Awards Ceremony, West Des Moines, Iowa, March 20, 2003, http://www2.econ.iastate.edu/faculty /harl/Structural TransformationofAg.pdf; Neil Harl, "Antitrust Issues in the New Food System," presented at American Agricultural Economics Association Workshop, Tampa, Florida, July 29, 2000, http://www.farmfoundation. org/news/articlefiles/94-harl.pdf; Neil Harl, "The Age of Contract Agriculture: Consequences of Concentration in Input Supply," *Journal of Agribusiness* 18, no. 1 (March 2000): 115–27, http://ageconsearch.umn.edu/bitstream /14701/1/18010115.pdf.

49. **Formed on the eve of the Great Depression:** Donald Barnes et al., "The Capper-Volstead Act: Opportunity Today and Tomorrow," presented at the National Council of Farmer Cooperatives' National Institute on Cooperative Education, Annual Conference, Pittsburgh, PA, August 5, 1997, http: //www.uwcc.wisc.edu/info/capper.html.

50. **farms producing hogs fell by almost three-quarters:** James Mac-Donald, "Concentration, Contracting, and Competition Policy in U.S. Agribusiness," *Concurrences,* no. 1 (2016): 3–9, http://discovery.ucl.ac.uk/1478197/7 /Lianos_03%20concurrences_1-2016_on_topics_lianos_et_al.pdf.

51. **control nearly two-thirds of all hogs:** Ibid.

52. **95 percent of all hogs marketed:** Howard, *Concentration and Power,* 82.

53. **rural labor with few opportunities:** Christopher Leonard, *The Meat Racket: The Secret Takeover of America's Food Business* (New York: Simon & Schuster, 2014).

54. **living below the poverty line:** "The Business of Broilers: Hidden Costs of Putting a Chicken on Every Grill," Pew Charitable Trusts, December 20, 2013, http://www.pewtrusts.org/-/media/legacy/uploadedfiles/peg/publications/report/businessofbroilersreportthepewcharitabletrustspdf.pdf.

55. **so toxic it can kill humans and the pigs:** Kevin Schulz, "Hydrogen Sulfide—the Invisible Killer in Hog Manure," *National Hog Farmer,* September 18, 2015, http://www.nationalhogfarmer.com/facilities/hydrogen -sulfide-invisible-killer-hog-manure.

56. **a victory for America's cattle and beef producers:** Larry Dreiling, "USDA Withdraws GIPSA Rule," *High Plains Journal,* October 17, 2017, http: //www.hpj.com/livestock/usda-withdraws-gipsa-rule/article_3531a6dc-b36f -11e7-8ef0-73108b90a059.html.

57. **increased consumer prices for meat:** Ibid.

58. **market dominance exceeds 70 percent:** MacDonald, "Concentration."

59. **control more than half of each market:** Keith Fuglie et al., "Rising Concentration in Agricultural Input Industries Influences New Farm Technologies," ERS, December 3, 2012, https://www.ers.usda.gov/amber-waves/2012 /december/rising-concentration-in-agricultural-input-industries-influences -new-technologies/.

60. **Walmart controlling one-third:** Stephanie Clifford, "Wal-Mart Tests Service for Buying Food Online," *New York Times,* April 24, 2011, http:// www.nytimes.com/2011/04/25/business/25walmart.html; "Grocery Goliaths: How Food Monopolies Impact Consumers," *Food & Water Watch,* December 2013, https://www.foodandwaterwatch.org/sites/default/files/Grocery%20 Goliaths%20Report%20Dec%202013.pdf.

61. **Tyson Foods owns thirty-eight brands:** "Our Brands," Tyson Foods, accessed March 29, 2018, https://www.tysonfoods.com/our-brands; "Trusted Brands," Smithfield Foods, accessed March 29, 2018, https://www.smith fieldfoods.com/our-brands.

62. **Smithfield now controls 27 percent:** "Estimated Daily U.S. Slaughter Capacity by Plant (head per day)," *Pork Checkoff,* National Pork Board, last

modified August 9, 2017, https://www.porkcdn.com/sites/porkorg/library /2015/12/estimated_daily_u.s._slaughter_capacity_by_plant_hpd.pdf.

63. **shares in Shuanghui were revealed:** Sharon Terlep, "Goldman Left Out of Smithfield Deal," *Wall Street Journal*, June 20, 2013, https://www.wsj .com/articles/SB10001424127887323893504578555953698195268.

64. **conflicts in the securities business were a fact of life:** Ibid.

65. **To minimize financial risk:** Markus Henn, "The Speculator's Bread— What Is behind Rising Food Prices?" *European Molecular Biology Organization* (EMBO) reports, 12, no. 4 (April 2011): 296–301, https://doi.org/10.1038/embor .2011.38.

66. **"virtual hoarding:** "Testimony of Michael W. Masters, Managing Member Portfolio Manager Masters Capital Management, LLC Before the Committee on Homeland Security and Governmental Affairs United States Senate," US Senate, June 24, 2008, 7, http://hsgac.senate.gov/public/ _files/052008Masters.pdf; Sophia Murphy, David Burch, and Jennifer Clapp, "Cereal Secrets: The World's Largest Grain Traders and Global Agriculture," *Oxfam*, August 2012, https://www.oxfamamerica.org/static/oa4/cereal-secrets .pdf.

67. **pushed into poverty and malnutrition:** "The Global Social Crisis: Report on the World Social Situation 2011," United Nations, 2011, 63, http: //www.un.org/esa/socdev/rwss/docs/2011/rwss2011.pdf; "Global Economic Prospects: Commodities in the Crossroads 2009," World Bank, 2009, xii, 119, http://siteresources.worldbank.org/INTGEP2009/Resources/10363_Web PDF-w47.pdf.

68. **not responsible for what happened:** Frederick Kaufman, "How Goldman Sachs Created the Food Crisis," *Foreign Policy*, April 27, 2011, http: //foreignpolicy.com/2011/04/27/how-goldman-sachs-created-the-food-crisis /; Deborah Doane, "What Goldman Sachs Should Admit: It Drives Up the Cost of Food," *The Guardian*, May 23, 2013, https://www.theguardian.com /commentisfree/2013/may/23/goldman-sachs-agm-drive-food-prices-up.

69. **We were wrong to believe:** Henn, "The Speculator's Bread"; "Bill Clinton: 'We Blew It' on Global Food," CBS News, October 23, 2008, https: //www.cbsnews.com/news/bill-clinton-we-blew-it-on-global-food/.

70. **The only place you see a free market:** Dan Carney, "Dwayne's World," *Mother Jones*, July/August 1995 Issue, http://www.motherjones.com /politics/1995/07/dwaynes-world/.

71. **rationalize away once-important values:** Sandel, *What Money Can't Buy*, chap. 1.

72. **higher rate of suicide:** Wendy McIntosh et al., "Suicide Rates by Occupational Group—17 States, 2012," Centers for Disease Control and Pre-

vention, *Morbidity and Mortality Weekly Report (MMWR)* 65, no. 25: 641–45, July 1, 2016, https://www.cdc.gov/mmwr/volumes/65/wr/mm6525a1.htm.

Chapter 8

1. **the American Southwest:** "Zachary Taylor," Miller Center, University of Virginia, accessed January 2, 2018, https://millercenter.org/president/taylor; Holman Hamilton, *Zachary Taylor, Soldier in the White House* (Indianapolis, IN: Bobbs-Merrill, 1951).

2. **Old Rough and Ready was dead:** Hamilton, *Zachary Taylor*, 387–93.

3. **poisonous preservatives:** Swann Harding, *Two Blades of Grass: A History of Scientific Development in the U.S. Department of Agriculture* (Norman, OK: University of Oklahoma Press, 1947), 313.

4. **"embalmed meat":** Andrew Smith, *Eating History: Thirty Turning Points in the Making of American Cuisine* (New York: Columbia University Press, 2009), 158.

5. **questionable additives were actually preservatives:** Ibid., 160.

6. **The "Beef Trust":** Maureen Ogle, *In Meat We Trust: An Unexpected History of Carnivore America* (Boston: Houghton Mifflin Harcourt, 2013), 63–89.

7. **press seized on germ theory:** Ibid., 74.

8. **The agency in charge was:** US Food and Drug Administration (FDA), "Part I: The 1906 Food and Drugs Act and Its Enforcement," last modified February 1, 2018, https://www.fda.gov/AboutFDA/History/FOrgsHistory/EvolvingPowers/ucm054819.htm; Wallace Janssen, "The Story of the Laws Behind the Labels," FDA, last modified March 11, 2014, https://www.fda.gov/AboutFDA/WhatWeDo/History/Overviews/ucm056044.htm.

9. **unfit for human food:** Federal Meat Inspection Act (FMIA) of 1906, "An Act Making Appropriations for the Department of Agriculture for the Fiscal Year Ending June Thirtieth, Nineteen Hundred and Seven," March 5, 1906, Legis Works, http://legisworks.org/congress/59/session-1/publaw-382.pdf.

10. **companies off the hook:** Marion Nestle, *Safe Food: The Politics of Food Safety* (Berkeley, CA: University of California Press, 2010), 53.

11. **The agency in charge became:** Food Safety and Inspection Service (FSIS), "FSIS History," USDA, last modified February 21, 2018, https://www.fsis.usda.gov/wps/portal/informational/aboutfsis/history.

12. **the disease would land on American shores:** Kevin Walker et al., "Comparison of Bovine Spongiform Encephalopathy Risk Factors in the

United States and Great Britain," *Journal American Veterinary Association* 199, no. 11 (December 1991): 1554–61, https://www.ncbi.nlm.nih.gov/pubmed/17787 35; "Qualitative Analysis of BSE Risk Factors in the United States," Centers for Epidemiology and Animal Health, Animal and Plant Health Inspection Service, Veterinary Services, USDA, Fort Collins, CO, 1991, http://agris.fao .org/agris-search/search.do?recordID=US201300040862.

13. **daughter eating hamburgers:** "1990: Gummer Enlists Daughter in BSE Fight," BBC, May 16, 1990, http://news.bbc.co.uk/onthisday/hi/dates /stories/may/16/newsid_2913000/2913807.stm; Adrian Lee, "What Became of Cordelia Gummer, the MadCow Girl?" *Express*, May 16, 2015, https://www .express.co.uk/news/uk/577667/Cordelia-Gummer-Mad-Cow-disease-BSE -scandal-25-years.

14. **231 individuals in twelve countries:** Centers for Disease Control and Prevention (CDC), "Variant Creutzfeldt-Jakob Disease (vCJD), Risk for Travelers," last modified March 20, 2017, https://www.cdc.gov/prions/vcjd/risk -travelers.html.

15. **seven hundred people were affected:** Rogers Lois, "Killer in Beef Spreads Alarm," *Sunday* (London) *Times*, April 16, 1995, accessed via Lexis Nexis Academic; Elise Golan et al., "A Closer Look at Food Safety Drivers in the Meat Industry—The 1993 Jack in the Box Restaurant *E. coli* O157:H7 Outbreak," in *Food Safety Innovation in the United States*, ERS, AER-831, April 2004, 10, https://www.ers.usda.gov/webdocs/publications/41634/18038 _aer831d.pdf?v=42265; Jeff Benedict, *Poisoned: The True Story of the Deadly E. coli Outbreak That Changed the Way Americans Eat* (Buena Vista, VA: Inspire Books, 2011).

16. **The bacteria tore apart cells:** Madeline Drexler, *Secret Agents: The Menace of Emerging Infections* (Washington, DC: Joseph Henry Press, 2002), chap. 4.

17. **we have customer complaints:** Bill Marler, "Jack in the Box *E. coli* Outbreak: Lessons Learned the Hard Way," *Marler Clark* (law firm blog), January 22, 2013, http://wwwmarlerblog.com/legal-cases/jack-in-the-box-e-coli -outbreak-lessons-learned-the-hard-way/.

18. **"So good, it's scary!":** Emily Green, "The Bug That Ate the Burger," *Los Angeles Times*, June 6, 2001, http://articles.latimes.com/2001/jun/06/food /fo-6863.

19. **restaurant chain was McDonald's:** Lee Riley et al., "Hemorrhagic Colitis Associated with a Rare *Escherichia coli* Serotype," *New England Journal of Medicine* 308, no. 12 (March 1983): 681–85, https://www.marlerblog.com /uploads/image/nejm198303243081203.pdf; Bill Marler, "Publisher's Platform: McDonald's and *E. coli*, 30 Years Later," *Food Safety News*, March 31, 2013, http:

//www.foodsafetynews.com/2013/03/publishers-platform-mcdonalds-and-e
-coli-30-years-later/.

20. **As we prepared our report:** *"Escherichia coli* O157:H7 Issues and Rami-
fication,"Center for Epidemiology and Animal Health, APHIS, USDA, March
1994, https://www.aphis.usda.gov/animal_health/emergingissues/downloads
/ecosumps.pdf.

21. **In the aptly titled:** FDA, *Bad Bug Book—Foodborne Pathogenic Micro-
organisms and Natural Toxins,* 2nd ed., 2012, https://www.fda.gov/Food/Food
borneIllnessContaminants/CausesOfIllnessBadBugBook/.

22. **ten to one hundred organisms:** See: ibid., "Cronobacter Species—2.
Disease. Infective Dose."

23. *Salmonella* **cases exceed all others:** Stacy Crim et al., "Incidence
and Trends of Infection with Pathogens Transmitted Commonly Through
Food—Foodborne Diseases Active Surveillance Network, 10 US Sites, 2006–
2013," CDC, *Morbidity and Mortality Weekly Report (MMWR)* 63, no. 15: 328–
32, April 18, 2014, http://www.cdc.gov/mmwr/preview/mmwrhtml/mm6315a3
.htm.

24. **its latest residence:** "Viral Gastroenteritis (Stomach Flu)," National
Library of Medicine, National Institutes of Health, last modified March 5,
2018, https://medlineplus.gov/ency/article/000252.htm.

25. **twenty-one million people:** CDC, "Burden of Norovirus Illness and
Outbreaks—Norovirus Illness," last modified July 10, 2017, http://www.cdc
.gov/norovirus/php/illness-outbreaks.html.

26. **Of those infected:** CDC, "Estimates of Foodborne Illnesses in the
United States—Burden of Foodborne Illness: Findings," last modified July
15, 2016, https://www.cdc.gov/foodborneburden/2011-foodborne-estimates
.html#modalIdString_CDCTable_0; CDC, "Estimates of Foodborne Illnesses in the United States—Burden of Foodborne Illness: Overview," last
modified July 15, 2016, https://www.cdc.gov/foodborneburden/estimates-over
view.html.

27. **as Marion Nestle describes:** Nestle, *Safe Food,* 55.

28. **it is cobbled together:** Renée Johnson, "The Federal Food Safety System: A Primer," Congressional Research Service, December 16, 2016, 1, http:
//fas.org/sgp/crs/misc/RS22600.pdf; Nestle, *Safe Food,* 55.

29. **requires extraordinary efforts:** Nestle, *Safe Food,* 15.

30. **FDA is responsible for:** Johnson, "The Federal Food System," 9.

31. **Over a ten-year period:** Caroline DeWaal et al., "All Over the Map:
A 10-Year Review of State Outbreak Reporting," Center for Science in the
Public Interest, June 2015, 35 & 55, https://cspinet.org/sites/default/files/attach
ment/all-over-the-map-report-2015.pdf.

32. **fifteen million lines of products:** An imported line of product is a distinct product within a shipment. A shipment may include multiple lines.

33. **had increased to forty million:** FDA, "Total Lines of Products Imported into the U.S. per Fiscal Year," last updated January 24, 2018, https://www.fda.gov/ForIndustry/ImportProgram/.

34. **egregious criminal fraud:** William Neuman, "An Iowa Egg Farmer and a History of Salmonella," *New York Times*, September 21, 2010, http://www.nytimes.com/2010/09/22/business/22eggs.html?pagewanted=print.

35. **knowingly shipped to forty-six states:** Helena Bottemiller, "Safe at the Plate?" *Columbia Journalism Review*, January/February 2013, http://www.cjr.org/cover_story/safe_at_the_plate.php.

36. **"The time had come to modernize:** Robert B. Wallace and Maria Oria, eds., *Enhancing Food Safety: The Role of the Food and Drug Administration* (Washington, DC: National Academies Press, 2010), xii.

37. **a single food safety agency:** Ibid., 17.

38. **"a sea change for food safety:** Margaret Hamburg, "Food Safety Modernization Act: Putting the Focus on Prevention," *Foodsafety.gov*, accessed January 3, 2018, http://www.foodsafety.gov/news/fsma.html.

39. **overhauled top to bottom:** Michael Taylor, "The FDA Food Safety Modernization Act: Putting Ideas into Action," FDA, January 27, 2011, http://wayback.archive-it.org/7993/20171115133532/https://www.fda.gov/AboutFDA/CentersOffices/OfficeofFoods/ucm241192.htm.

40. **FDA finally has all the tools:** US Senator Dick Durbin, "Durbin's Food Safety Bill Signed into Law," US Senator Dick Durbin website, January 4, 2011, https://www.durbin.senate.gov/newsroom/press-releases/durbins-food-safety-bill-signed-into-law.

41. **an additional $1.4 billion:** Johnson, "The Federal Food Safety System," 9.

42. **food-related problems and outbreaks emerged:** FDA, "Operational Strategy for Implementing the FDA Food Safety Modernization Act (FSMA)," May 2, 2014, http://www.fda.gov/Food/GuidanceRegulation/FSMA/ucm395105.htm.

43. **rely on voluntary compliance:** Ibid.

44. **most dangerous jobs:** US Government Accountability Office (GAO), "Workplace Safety and Health, Additional Data Needed to Address Continued Hazards in the Meat and Poultry Industry," GAO-16-337, April 2016, https://www.gao.gov/assets/680/676796.pdf.

45. **FSIS's mandate includes:** "21 U.S.C. 602: Congressional Statement of Findings," US Government Publishing Office (GPO), accessed January 4,

2018, https://www.gpo.gov/fdsys/pkg/USCODE-2010-title21/pdf/USCODE
-2010-title21-chap12-subchapI-sec602.pdf.

46. **not meeting the public's expectations:** Helena Bottemiller, "Looking Back: The Story Behind Banning *E. coli* O157:H7," *Food Safety News*, September 14, 2011, http://www.foodsafetynews.com/2011/09/looking-back-in-time-the-story-behind-banning-ecoli-0157h7/.

47. **10,500 poultry birds:** "Modernization of Poultry Slaughter Inspection," *Federal Register* 79, no. 162 (August 21, 2014): 49570, https://www.federal register.gov/documents/2014/08/21/2014-18526/modernization-of-poultry -slaughter-inspection.

48. **1,300 hogs:** FSIS, "Evaluation of HACCP Inspection Models Project (HIMP) for Market Hogs," November 2014, 12, http://www.fsis.usda.gov/wps /wcm/connect/f7be3e74-552f-4239-ac4c-59a024fd0ec2/Evaluation-HIMP -Market-Hogs.pdf?MOD=AJPERES.

49. **390 cattle per hour:** "§ 310.1 Extent and Time of Post-Mortem Inspection; Post-Mortem Inspection Staffing Standards," GPO, 9 CFR Ch. III, January 1, 2012, 125, https://www.gpo.gov/fdsys/pkg/CFR-2012-title9-vol2/pdf /CFR-2012-title9-vol2-sec310-1.pdf.

50. **Inspector General took a closer look:** Office of Inspector General (OIG), "What OIG Found," in "Food Safety and Inspection Service—Inspection and Enforcement Activities at Swine Slaughter Plants," Audit Report no. 24601-0001-41, May 2013, https://www.usda.gov/oig/webdocs/24601-0001-41. pdf.

51. **becoming repeat violators:** FSIS, "Evaluation of HACCP Inspection Models Project (HIMP) for Market Hogs," 12.

52. **150.7 million livestock carcasses:** FSIS, "Strategic Plan Fiscal Year 2011–2016: Key Accomplishments," June 2017, 4, https://www.fsis.usda.gov /wps/wcm/connect/60c74c0c-4000-478b-b249-a67b3e3bc555/Strategic-Plan -2011-2016-Key-Accomplishments.pdf?MOD=AJPERES.

53. *Salmonella* **was found in:** European Centre for Disease Prevention and Control, "The European Union Summary Report on Trends and Sources of Zoonoses, Zoonotic Agents, and Food-Borne Outbreaks in 2016," *EFSA Journal* 15, no. 12, November 2017, 29–32, https://efsa.onlinelibrary.wiley.com /doi/epdf/10.2903/j.efsa.2017.5077.

54. **For packaged poultry parts:** "81 FR 7285—New Performance Standards for Salmonella and Campylobacter in Not-Ready-to-Eat Comminuted Chicken and Turkey Products and Raw Chicken Parts and Changes to Related Agency Verification Procedures: Response to Comments and Announcement of Implementation Schedule," *Federal Register* 81, no. 28 (February 11, 2016): 7286, https://www.gpo.gov/fdsys/pkg/FR-2016-02-11/pdf/2016-02586

.pdf; FSIS, "Pathogen Reduction—*Salmonella* and *Campylobacter* Performance Standards Verification Testing," April 18, 2017, 26-9, https://www.fsis.usda. gov/wps/wcm/connect/b0790997-2e74-48bf-9799-85814bac9ceb/28_IM_PR _Sal_Campy.pdf?MOD=AJPERES.

55. **For ground poultry:** FSIS, "Pathogen Reduction," 26-6, 26-9.

56. **FSIS advises consumers:** FSIS, "Washing Food: Does It Promote Food Safety?" last modified July 1, 2013, https://www.fsis.usda.gov/wps/portal /fsis/topics/food-safety-education/get-answers/food-safety-fact-sheets/safe -food-handling/washing-food-does-it-promote-food-safety/washing-food.

57. **Calls for a single food-safety agency:** GAO, "Food Safety—A National Strategy Is Needed to Address Fragmentation in Federal Oversight," GAO 17-74, January 2017, https://www.gao.gov/assets/690/682095.pdf.

58. **Acme [Meat] Packing Company:** Alexandra Silver, "Top 10 Things You Didn't Know About the Green Bay Packers," *TIME*, February 4, 2011, http://content.time.com/time/specials/packages/article/0,28804,2046390 _2046393_2046466,00.html.

59. **higher line speeds with few complaints:** Ted Genoways, *The Chain: Farm, Factory, and the Fate of Our Food* (New York: HarperCollins, 2014).

60. **cut hourly compensation:** Bureau of Labor Statistics (BLS), "Employment and Earnings December 1983," vol. 30, no. 12, December 1983, 84, https://fraser.stlouisfed.org/files/docs/publications/employment/1980s/empl _121983.pdf; BLS, "Employment and Earnings December 1984," vol. 31, no. 12, December 1984, 88, https://fraser.stlouisfed.org/files/docs/publications/em ployment/1980s/empl_121984.pdf.

61. **Over 90 percent of the seafood:** National Oceanic and Atmospheric Administration, "Fisheries of the United States, 2016 Fact Sheet," October 31, 2017, 4, https://www.fisheries.noaa.gov/resource/outreach-and-education/fish eries-united-states-2016-fact-sheet.

62. **cut by half through mostly immigrant labor:** BLS, "Occupational Employment and Wages, May 2016, 51-3023 Slaughterers and Meat Packers," last modified March 31, 2017, https://www.bls.gov/oes/2016/may/oes513023.htm.

63. **hourly compensation in China:** "'Made in China' Isn't So Cheap Anymore, and That Could Spell Headache for Beijing," *CNBC*, February 27, 2017, https://www.cnbc.com/2017/02/27chinese-wages-rise-made-in-china -isnt-so-cheap-anymore.html; Tim Worstall, "Chinese Wages Are Showing Paul Krugman Is Right Once Again," *Forbes*, March 1, 2017, https://www.forbes .com/sites/timworstall/2017/03/01/chinese-wages-are-showing-paul-krug man-is-right-once-gain/#7bd81a353fea.

64. **Chinese plants were equivalent to United States standards:** FSIS, "Final Report of an Audit Conducted in the People's Republic of China,

March 4–19, 2013," December 13, 2013, http://www.fsis.usda.gov/wps/wcm /connect/ed782de3-82e1-4298-aac9-14da84d1ebd2/2013_China_Poultry _Slaughter_FAR.pdf?MOD=AJPERES.

65. **it doesn't make much sense:** Claudia Feldman, "Food Activist Goes to the Mat Again—This Time over a Chicken-in-China Tempest," *Houston Chronicle*, February 22, 2014, http://www.houstonchronicle.com/life/food /article/Food-activist-goes-to-the-mat-again-this-time-5253155.php.

66. **In 2016, FSIS ruled that:** FSIS, "Frequently Asked Questions— Equivalence of China's Poultry Processing and Slaughter Inspection Systems," last modified June 16, 2017, https://www.fsis.usda.gov/wps/portal/fsis /newsroom/news-releases-statements-transcripts/news-release-archives-by -year/archive/2016/faq-china-030416.

67. **privately owned chicken companies in China:** Dan Flynn, "Deal On: USDA Gives Green Light to China's Poultry Inspections," *Food Safety News*, September 14, 2017, http://www.foodsafetynews.com/2017/09/deal-on -usda-gives-green-light-to-chinas-poultry-inspections.

68. **"measures necessary for the protection:** World Trade Organization (WTO), "The WTO Agreement on the Application of Sanitary and Phytosanitary Measures (SPS Agreement)," accessed June 27, 2018, https://www.wto .org/english/tratop_e/sps_e/spsagr_e.htm.

69. *Salmonella* **started on the West Coast:** CDC, "Multistate Outbreak of Multidrug-Resistant Salmonella Heidelberg Infections Linked to Foster Farms Brand Chicken (Final Update)," July 31, 2014, https://www.cdc.gov /salmonella/heidelberg-10-13/.

70. **a genetic match was found:** CDC, "Multistate Outbreak of Multidrug-Resistant Salmonella Heidelberg"; CDC, "Table 2. Estimated Annual Number of Episodes of Domestically Acquired Foodborne Illnesses Caused by 31 Pathogens, United States," last modified December 20, 2011, https://wwwnc.cdc.gov/eid/article/17/1/p1-1101-t2.

71. **export chickens, ducks, and turkeys** *it* **raises:** "Eligibility of the People's Republic of China (PRC) to Export to the United States Poultry Products from Birds Slaughtered in the PRC," *Federal Register* 82, no. 115 (June 16, 2017): 27625–29, https://www.federalregister.gov/documents/2017/06/16/2017 -12554/eligibility-of-the-peoples-republic-of-china-prc-to-export-to-the -united-states-poultry-products.

72. **To no one's surprise:** Flynn, "Deal On."

73. **establishments to choose what they want:** Amy Mayer, "Citing Food Safety, USDA Proposes New Hog-Slaughter Rules That Give Industry More Control," *Harvest Public Media*, January 23, 2018, http://harvestpublic

media.org/post/citing-food-safety-usda-proposes-new-hog-slaughter-rules
-give-industry-more-control.

74. **whatever line speed they wanted:** "Modernization of Swine Slaughter Inspection,"*Federal Register* 83, no. 22 (February 1, 2018): 4780–823, https://www
.fsis.usda.gov/wps/wcm/connect/c17775a2-fd1f-4c11-b9d2-5992741b0e94
/2016-0017.pdf?MOD=AJPERES.

75. **chronic funding and staffing shortages:** FDA, "2018 FDA Justification of Estimates for Appropriations Committees—Browse by Section. Narrative by Activity—Foods," last modified March 26, 2018, https://www.fda.gov
/downloads/AboutFDA/ReportsManualsForms/Reports/BudgetReports
/UCM566331.pdf.

76. **making millions of decisions every day:** FDA, "Operational Strategy."

77. **two hundred different countries:** FDA, "President's FY 2017 Budget Request: Key Investments for Implementing the FDA Food Safety Modernization Act: Implementing the New FSMA Import Safety System," 1, accessed March 31, 2018, https://www.fda.gov/downloads/Food/GuidanceRegulation
/FSMA/UCM436623.pdf.

78. **70 percent are processed food products:** Economic Research Service (ERS), "Summary—Import Share of the Volume of U.S. Food Consumption," (Excel Table) in "U.S. Export Share of Production, Import Share of Consumption (2008–2014)," accessed March 12, 2015.

79. **1 percent of imported food is examined:** GAO, "Imported Food Safety—FDA's Targeting Tool Has Enhanced Screening, but Further Improvements Are Possible," GAO-16-399, May 2016, Highlights, https://www
.gao.gov/assets/680/677538.pdf.

80. **Sampling thirty recalls:** OIG, "The Food and Drug Administration's Food-Recall Process Did Not Always Ensure the Safety of the Nation's Food Supply," US Department of Health and Human Services, A-01-16-01502, December 2017, https://oig.hhs.gov/oas/reports/region1/11601502.pdf.

81. **one of the safest in the world:** CDC, "Update on Multistate Outbreak of Listeria Associated with Cantaloupes," last modified September 30, 2011, https://www.cdc.gov/media/releases/2011/t0928_listeria_outbreak.html; Rachael Rettner, "Sure You Want to Eat That? Some Foodborne Illnesses Rising," *Live Science*, April 18, 2013, https://www.livescience.com/36940-food
borne-illness-united-states-trends.html; "FDA, USDA, NOAA Statements on Food Safety," *FDA News & Events*, last modified March 23, 2011, http:
//wayback.archive-it.org/7993/20161022183206/http://www.fda.gov/News
Events/PublicHealthFocus/ucm248257.htm.

82. **the number had jumped to thirty-eight:** CDC, "National Outbreak Reporting System (NORS)," accessed June 27, 2018, https://wwwn.cdc.gov/nors dashboard/.

83. **just over two billion dollars:** Johnson, "The Federal Food Safety System," 9.

84. **three hundred times less:** Johnson, "The Federal Food Safety System," 10; Office of Management and Budget, "Table 3.2—Outlays by Function and Subfunction: 1962–2023," accessed January 10, 2018, https://www.white house.gov/omb/historical-tables/.

85. **fifteen cents for food safety:** ERS, "Table 1—Food and Alcoholic Beverages: Total Expenditures 1," last modified January 26, 2016, https://www .ers.usda.gov/data-products/food-expenditures.aspx#26634.

Chapter 9

1. *one-sidedness of our agricultural production:* W. O. Atwater, "The Food-Supply of the Future," *Century Illustrated Monthly Magazine,* November 1891–April 1892, vol. 43, 1891, 101–12. Cited in Andrew Smith, *Food in America: The Past, Present, and Future of Food, Farming, and the Family Meal,* vol. 3 (Santa Barbara, CA: ABC-CLIO, 2017), 254–60.

2. **dietary guidelines needed to appeal:** Marion Nestle, *Food Politics: How the Food Industry Influences Nutrition and Health* (Berkeley, CA: University of California Press, 2013), 55; "Case Study 5: The Politics of the Pyramid," in Laura Sims, *The Politics of Fat: Food and Nutrition Policy in America* (Armonk, NY: M. E. Sharpe, 1998).

3. **already muzzled messages:** US Department of Agriculture (USDA) and US Department of Health and Human Services (HHS), "Dietary Guidelines for Americans, 1980," February 1980, https://health.gov/dietaryguide lines/1980thin.pdf; Elizabeth Frazão, "America's Eating Habits: Changes and Consequences," ERS, AIB-750, May 1999, 45, https://naldc.nal.usda.gov/down load/22976/PDF.

4. **politically palatable version:** Sims, *The Politics of Fat,* Case Study 5; Nestle, *Food Politics,* 51–52; for a more complete history of events that unfolded, see Nestle, *Food Politics,* chap. 2.

5. **compared with sixteen peer countries:** National Research Council, *U.S. Health in International Perspective: Shorter Lives, Poorer Health* (Washington, DC: National Academies Press, 2013), http://nap.edu/13497.

6. **spend more on health care:** Ibid.; Economic Research Service (ERS), "Percent of Consumer Expenditures Spent on Food, Alcoholic Beverages,

and Tobacco That Were Consumed at Home, by Selected Countries, 2013,"
last modified October 11, 2017, http://www.ers.usda.gov/data-products/food
-expenditures.aspx.

7. **dead last in chronic maladies:** HHS, "Health, United States, 2014,"
no. 2015-1232, May 2015, 97, http://www.cdc.gov/nchs/data/hus/hus14.pdf.

8. **more than half obese:** Ibid., 215.

9. **high-risk cholesterol levels:** Ibid., 201.

10. **one of three cancer deaths:** "Does Body Weight Affect Cancer Risk?"
American Cancer Society, last modified January 4, 2018, http://www.cancer
.org/cancer/cancercauses/dietandphysicalactivity/bodyweightandcancerrisk
/body-weight-and-cancer-risk-effects.

11. **Caucasian, college-educated:** National Research Council, *U.S. Health
in International Perspective.*

12. **1894 dietary recommendations:** Frazão, "America's Eating Habits,"
33.

13. **importance of minerals:** Ibid., 33–34; Derek Yach et al., "Preventive Nu-
trition and the Food Industry: Perspectives on History, Present, and Future
Directions," in Adrianne Bendich and Richard Deckelbaum, eds., *Preventive
Nutrition: The Comprehensive Guide for Health Professionals*, 4th ed. (New York:
Humana Press, 2010), 778–80; Centers for Disease Control and Prevention
(CDC), "Achievements in Public Health, 1900–1999: Safer and Healthier
Foods," *MMWR* 48, no. 40 (October 15, 1999): 905–13, http://www.cdc.gov/mmwr
/preview/mmwrhtml/mm4840a1.htm.

14. **basic food groupings:** Frazão, "America's Eating Habits," 35–36.

15. **more food of greater variety:** Nestle, *Food Politics*, chap. 1.

16. **number of servings and serving sizes:** Frazão, "America's Eating Habits," 36–38; Nestle, *Food Politics*, 40.

17. **To reduce backlash:** USDA and HHS, "Dietary Guidelines for Americans, 1980."

18. **cheaper per calorie than the fresh fruits and vegetables:** Andrea
Carlson and Elizabeth Frazão, "Are Healthy Foods Really More Expensive?
It Depends on How You Measure the Price," ERS, EIB-96, May 2012, https:
//www.ers.usda.gov/webdocs/publications/44678/19980_eib96.pdf?v=42321.

19. **open-heart bypass surgery:** "Statistical Abstract of the United States:
2011," US Census Bureau, Table 102, 76, ftp://ftp.census.gov/library/publications
/2010/compendia/statab/130ed/tables/11s0103.pdf.

20. **surgeon general officially acknowledge:** Kelly Brownell and Kather-
ine Horgen, *Food Fight: The Inside Story of the Food Industry, America's Obesity
Crisis, and What We Can Do about It* (New York: McGraw-Hill, 2004), 14;
Office of Disease Prevention and Health Promotion, "The Surgeon General's

Call to Action to Prevent and Decrease Overweight and Obesity, 2001," HHS, 2001, http://www.cdc.gov/nccdphp/dnpa/pdf/CalltoAction.pdf.

21. **a new cultural norm:** "What Is Nutrition Transition?" Carolina Population Center, accessed March 5, 2018, http://www.cpc.unc.edu/projects/nu trans/whatis. For more information, see: Daniel Ervin, David López-Carr, Anna López-Carr, *The Nutrition Transition, Oxford Bibliographies*, last modified June 25, 2013, http://www.oxfordbibliographies.com/view/document/obo -9780199874002/obo-9780199874002-0078.xml.

22. **all too happy to oblige:** Michael Moyer, "Why Does Food Taste So Delicious?" *Scientific American*, September 1, 2013, https://www.scientificameri can.com/article/why-does-food-taste-so-delicious/; Shirlee Wohl, "The Experience of Eating," *Yale Scientific*, April 3, 2011, http://www.yalescientific.org /2011/04/the-experience-of-eating/.

23. **chemicals like endorphins and dopamine:** Paul Kenny, "Is Obesity an Addiction?" *Scientific American*, September 1, 2013, https://www.scientific american.com/article/is-obesity-an-addiction/; David Kessler, *The End of Overeating: Taking Control of the Insatiable American Appetite* (New York: Rodale, 2009).

24. **cannot get through the day:** "The Hartman Group's Food & Beverage Culture Year in Review, 2017," Hartman Group, accessed March 5, 2018, https: //www.hartman-group.com/acumenPdfs/year-in-review-2017.pdf.

25. **rotten bones of his children:** George Orwell, *The Road to Wigan Pier* (New York: Mariner Books, 1972), 83.

26. **stood at 120 pounds:** George Bray and Barry Popkin, "Dietary Sugar and Body Weight: Have We Reached a Crisis in the Epidemic of Obesity and Diabetes?" *Diabetes Care* 37, no. 4 (2014), 950–56, https://doi.org/10.2337/dc13 -2085.

27. **new record for meat and poultry consumption:** Mildred Haley, "U.S. Red Meat and Poultry Forecasts," in "Livestock, Dairy, and Poultry Outlook," ERS, LDP-M-282, December 18, 2017, 21, https://www.ers.usda.gov /webdocs/publications/85473/ldp-m-280.pdf?v=43026.

28. **double the recommended amount:** USDA and HHS, "Dietary Guidelines for Americans, 2015–2020," eighth edition, Table A3-1, December 2015, 81, https://health.gov/dietaryguidelines/2015/resources/2015-2020_Diet ary_Guidelines.pdf.

29. **human being is primarily a bag:** Orwell, *The Road to Wigan Pier*, 83.

30. **food products rolled out each year:** ERS, "New Food and Beverage Product Introductions, By Product Type, 2008–16," last modified April 5, 2017, https://www.ers.usda.gov/topics/food-markets-prices/processing-mar keting/new-products/.

31. **consumers coming back for more:** Michael Moss, *Salt Sugar Fat: How the Food Giants Hooked Us* (New York: Random House, 2013), Introduction.

32. **tinkering with fat globules:** Ibid.

33. **three-quarters of products:** Barry Popkin and Corinna Hawkes, "Sweetening of the Global Diet, Particularly Beverages: Patterns, Trends, and Policy Responses," *The Lancet* 4, no. 2 (February 2016): 174–86, https://doi .org/10.1016/S2213-587(15)00419-2.

34. **three-quarters of dietary salt:** Loren Cordain et al., "Origins and Evolution of the Western Diet: Health Implications for the 21st Century," *American Journal of Clinical Nutrition* 81, no. 2 (February 1, 2005): 341–54, https: //www.ncbi.nlm.nih.gov/pubmed/15699220.

35. **300,000 edible species of plants:** Food and Agriculture Organization of the United Nations, "Women: Users, Preservers and Managers of Agrobiodiversity," 1999, http://citeseerx.ist.psu.edu/viewdoc/download;jsessionid =2BB791DFD15ED4EF10EAE1AC83D930E3?doi=10.1.1.395.2601&rep=rep1 &type=pdf.

36. **each went their separate ways:** Moss, *Salt Sugar Fat,* Introduction.

37. **the CEO was replaced:** Ibid., chap. 11.

38. **adding salt back into soup:** Ibid., chap. 13.

39. **"Taste is king.":** Annie Gasparro, "A Spoonful of Sugar Helps the Sales Go Up: Cereal Makers Return to the Sweet Stuff," *Wall Street Journal,* April 5, 2018, https://www.wsj.com/articles/a-spoonful-of-sugar-helps-the -sales-go-up-cereal-makers-return-to-the-sweet-stuff-1522937066.

40. **food consumers as confused:** Jennifer Reingold, "PepsiCo CEO: We've Never Seen Consumers So Confused," *Fortune,* April 23, 2015, http://fortune.com/2015/04/23/pepsico-ceo-weve-never-seen-consumers-so-confused/.

41. **renewed interest in labels:** Sims, *The Politics of Fat,* 241–42.

42. **All Bran cereal:** Ibid.

43. **FDA is mostly hands-off:** US Food and Drug Administration (FDA), "'Natural' on Food Labeling," last modified November 11, 2017, https://www .fda.gov/Food/GuidanceRegulation/GuidanceDocumentsRegulatoryInfor mation/LabelingNutrition/ucm456090.htm.

44. **admitted no wrongdoing:** Elaine Watson, "Settlement Fund in Stevia Deceptive Marketing Lawsuit Alleging Truvia Is Not 'Natural' Rises to $6.1m," *Food Navigator-USA,* last modified December 2, 2014, https://www .foodnavigator-usa.com/Article/2014/12/02/Cargill-agrees-to-6.1m-settle ment-in-Truvia-stevia-naturallawsuit.

45. **eat the entire contents:** FDA, "Food Serving Sizes Get a Reality Check," last modified August 18, 2016, https://www.fda.gov/ForConsumers /ConsumerUpdates/ucm386203.htm.

46. **two grams per serving:** Center for Food Safety and Applied Nutrition, "A Food Labeling Guide: Guidance for Industry," FDA, January 2013, 80, https://www.fda.gov/downloads/Food/GuidanceRegulation/GuidanceDocumentsRegulatoryInformation/UCM265446.pdf.

47. **yogurt with probiotics:** FDA, "Label Claims for Conventional Foods and Dietary Supplements," last modified January 3, 2018, https://www.fda.gov/Food/LabelingNutrition/ucm111447.htm.

48. **AHA now offers its own endorsement:** Marion Nestle, *What to Eat* (New York: Farrar, Straus and Giroux, 2007), Kindle edition, 353; "Heart-Check Food Certification Program Nutrition Requirements," American Heart Association, last modified February 27, 2018, http://www.heart.org/HEARTORG/HealthyLiving/HealthyEating/Heart-CheckMarkCertification/Heart-Check-Food-Certification-Program-Nutrition-Requirements_UCM_300914_Article.jsp.

49. **The AHA believes:** "Heart-Check Food Certification Program Certified Products Listed by Food Category," AHA, last modified April 4, 2018, https://www.heart.org/idc/groups/heart-public/@wcm/@fc/documents/downloadable/ucm_474830.pdf.

50. **Congress prohibited adding substances:** "Public Law 85-929," United States Code, Office of the Law Revision Counsel, House of Representatives, September 6, 1958, http://uscode.house.gov/statutes/pl/85/929.pdf.

51. **some eight hundred ingredients:** "Fixing the Oversight of Chemicals Added to Our Food," Pew Charitable Trusts, November 7, 2013, 3, http://www.pewtrusts.org/~/media/legacy/uploadedfiles/phg/content_level_pages/reports/FoodAdditivesCapstoneReportpdf.pdf.

52. **ten thousand substances:** Ibid., 3.

53. **similar approaches in other countries:** US Government Accountability Office, "FDA Should Strengthen Its Oversight of Food Ingredients Determined to Be GRAS," GAO-10-246, February 2010, 13, https://www.gao.gov/new.items/d10246.pdf.

54. **no obligation to even notify:** Pew Trusts, "Fixing the Oversight," 3.

55. **substances were introduced into food:** Ibid., 5.

56. **free of conflicts of interests:** Bernard Lo and Marilyn Field, eds., *Conflict of Interest in Medical Research, Education, and Practice* (Washington, DC: National Academies Press, 2009), The National Academies, https://www.nap.edu/catalog/12598/conflict-of-interest-in-medical-research-education-and-practice.

57. **trans fat be phased out:** "Final Determination Regarding Partially Hydrogenated Oils," *Federal Register*, June 17, 2015, https://www.federalreg

ister.gov/documents/2015/06/17/2015-14883/final-determination-regarding
-partially-hydrogenated-oils.

58. **non-interstate commerce:** Information was provided by Mical Honig-fort, Supervisory Consumer Safety, FDA, in an e-mail response on June 24, 2015.

59. **gelatin from bones and skins:** Daniel Marti, Rachel Johnson, and Kenneth Mathews Jr., "Where's the (Not) Meat? Byproducts from Beef and Pork Production," ERS, LDP-M-209-01, November 2011, https://www.ers.usda.gov/webdocs/publications/37427/8801_ldpm20901.pdf?v=41056.

60. **cell cultures grown:** "Frequently Asked Questions—Bovine Serum," International Serum Industry Association, May 11, 2011, http://www.serumindustry.org/documents/sera20110511_000.pdf.

61. **Colony Collapse Disorder:** Agricultural Research Service, "ARS Honey Bee Health and Colony Collapse Disorder," USDA, last modified October 26, 2017, https://www.ars.usda.gov/oc/br/ccd/index/.

62. **honey production per colony:** Stephanie Riche et al., "Table 5—Selected US Honey Market Statistics," in "Sugar and Sweetener Outlook," ERS, SSS-M-314, October 17, 2014, 12, https://www.ers.usda.gov/webdocs/publications/39403/49326_sss_m_314.pdf?v=41960.

63. **honey imports are skyrocketing:** Ronald Ward, "Honey Demand and the Impact of the National Honey Board's Generic Promotion Programs," National Honey Board, March 2014, 6, http://www.natureplica.com/wp-content/uploads/2014/06/National-Honey-Board-on-Honey-Demand.pdf.

64. **imports now supply two-thirds:** Riche et al., "Sugar and Sweetener Outlook," 11.

65. **sugars are added to foods:** Julia Belluz and Javier Zarracina, "Sugar, Explained. Sugar Is the Dietary Villain of Our Day. But the Science Is Complicated," *Vox*, December 24, 2017, https://www.vox.com/science-and-health/2017/1/13/14219606/sugar-intake-dietary-nutrition-science.

66. **Chinese production continued to increase:** Honey data were from FAOSTAT under Production and Trade domains, accessed March 5, 2018, http://www.fao.org/faostat/en/#data; Jessica Leeder, "Honey Laundering: The Sour Side of Nature's Golden Sweetener," *The Globe and Mail*, last modified April 29, 2018, https://www.theglobeandmail.com/technology/science/honey-laundering-the-sour-side-of-natures-golden-sweetener/article562759/.

67. **doubled in a twelve-year period:** Ward, "Honey Demand and the Impact," 6–7.

68. **sticky substance may still taste sweet:** FDA, "Proper Labeling of Honey and Honey Products: Guidance for Industry," February 2018, https:

//www.fda.gov/downloads/Food/GuidanceRegulation/GuidanceDocuments
RegulatoryInformation/UCM595961.pdf.

69. **German food conglomerate:** Leeder, "Honey Laundering"; "Two Companies and Five Individuals Charged with Roles in Illegal Honey Imports; Avoided $180 Million In Anti-Dumping Duties," US Attorney's Office, Northern District of Illinois, last modified July 27, 2015, https://www.justice
.gov/usao-ndil/pr/two-companies-and-five-individuals-charged-roles-illegal
-honey-imports-avoided-180.

70. **evade $180 million in duties:** US Attorney's Office, Northern District of Illinois, "Two Companies and Five Individuals."

71. **Chinese honey was seized:** US Immigration and Customs Enforcement, "ICE, CBP in Houston Seize Illegally Imported Honey Valued at $2.45 Million," last modified February 11, 2015, https://www.ice.gov/news
/releases/ice-cbp-houston-seize-illegally-imported-honey-valued-245
-million.

72. **countries with little history of exports:** Susan Berfield, "The Honey Launderers: Uncovering the Largest Food Fraud in U.S. History," Bloomberg, September 20, 2013, http://www.bloomberg.com/bw/articles/2013-09-19
/how-germany-s-alw-got-busted-for-the-largest-food-fraud-in-u-dot-s-dot
-history.

73. **antibiotic given to bees but not approved:** Berfield, "The Honey Launderers"; for more information about chloramphenicol dangers to adults and children, see: HHS, "Chloramphenicol. CAS No. 56-75-7" in "The 13th Report on Carcinogens," October 2, 2014, https://ntp.niehs.nih.gov/ntp/roc
/content/profiles/chloramphenicol.pdf; Mike Isildar et al., "DNA Damage in Intact Cells Induced by Bacterial Metabolites of Chloramphenicol," *American Journal of Hematology* 28, no. 1 (May 1988), 40–46, http://doi.org/10.1002/ajh
.2830280109.

74. **marker for illegal Chinese honey:** FDA, "FDA Import Alert 36-04," February 8, 2018, https://www.accessdata.fda.gov/cms_ia/importalert_111.
html.

75. **issued six import alerts:** Ibid.

76. **anti-inflammatory drugs used in horses:** "EU Tests Identify Horsemeat in Almost Five Percent of Beef Products," *DW Akademie*, April 16, 2013, http://www.dw.de/eu-tests-identify-horsemeat-in-almost-five-percent-of
-beef-products/a-16748554.

77. **tone down its findings:** Felicity Lawrence, "Horsemeat Scandal Report Calls for Urgent and Comprehensive Reforms," *The Guardian*, September 4, 2014, http://www.theguardian.com/uk-news/2014/sep/04/horsemeat-scandal
-report-urgent-comprehensive-reforms.

78. **food fraud was not a random:** Chris Elliott, "Elliott Review into the Integrity and Assurance of Food Supply Networks—Final Report," HM Government, July 2014, https://www.gov.uk/government/uploads/system/up loads/attachment_data/file/350726/elliot-review-final-report-july2014.pdf.

79. **falsification of official health documents:** AFP, "European Police Crack Massive Horsemeat Trafficking Ring," *Telegraph*, April 25, 2015, http://www.telegraph.co.uk/news/worldnews/europe/eu/11563295/European-police-crack-massive-horsemeat-trafficking-ring.html.

80. **Heinz ketchup bottles:** Daniel Distant, "Fake Ketchup Factory Discovered in NJ after Hundreds of Bottles Explode," *Christian Post*, October 23, 2012, http://global.christianpost.com/news/fake-ketchup-factory-discovered-in-nj-after-hundreds-of-bottles-explode-83777/.

81. **Poultry meat covered in feces:** Felicity Lawrence, "Horsemeat Scandal: Probe Failure by Authorities Dates Back to 1998," *The Guardian*, January 21, 2014, http://www.theguardian.com/uk-news/2014/jan/21/horsemeat-scandal-probe-failure-authorities-dates-back-1998-rotherham.

82. **"100% pure olive oil.":** Stephanie Strom, "Trade Group Lawsuit Challenges Olive Oil Labeling," *New York Times*, February 6, 2013, http://www.nytimes.com/2013/02/07/business/trade-group-lawsuit-challenges-olive-oil-labeling.html.

83. **Meat made from rats:** "China Cracks Down on Fake Meat Made from Rats and Foxes," *RT*, May 3, 2013, http://rt.com/news/china-meat-crimes-crackdown-766/.

84. **Melamine (an industrial toxin):** Richard Spencer, "Two Sentenced to Death over China Melamine Milk Scandal," *Telegraph*, January 22, 2009, https://www.telegraph.co.uk/news/worldnews/asia/china/4315627/Two-sentenced-to-death-over-China-melamine-milk-scandal.html; Jessie Jiang, "China: Tainted Pork Renews Food Safety Fears," *TIME*, March 23, 2011, http://content.time.com/time/world/article/0,8599,2060741,00.html; Cliff White, "Gel-Injected Shrimp a Growing Problem in China," *Seafood Source*, October 7, 2016, https://www.seafoodsource.com/news/food-safety-health/gel-injected-shrimp-agrowing-problem-in-china; Juliet Song, "In China, the Curious Case of the Gel-Injected Shrimp," *The Epoch Times*, last modified November 14, 2017, https://www.theepochtimes.com/in-china-the-curious-case-of-the-gel-injected-shrimp_1934980.html; "Chinese Alarm over Formaldehyde-Tainted Cabbages," BBC News, May 7, 2012, http://www.bbc.com/news/world-south-asia-17981323. For more information, see: "China Food Safety," *South China Morning Post*, accessed April 8, 2018, http://www.scmp.com/topics/china-food-safety; "Food Scandals in China," *Timetoast*, accessed April 8, 2018, http://www.timetoast.com/timelines/food-scandals-in-china.

85. **"gutter oil":** David Barboza, "Recycled Cooking Oil Found to Be Latest Hazard in China," *New York Times*, March 31, 2010, http://www.ny times.com/2010/04/01/world/asia/01shanghai.html; Michael Riggs, "China's Frightening, Unpleasant Cooking-Oil Scandal," *The Atlantic*, October 30, 2013, http://www.theatlantic.com/china/archive/2013/10/chinas-frightening -unpleasant-cooking-oil-scandal/281000/; Editorial Board, "Taiwan's 'Gutter Oil' Scandal," *New York Times*, September 18, 2014, https://www.nytimes.com /2014/09/19/opinion/taiwans-gutter-oil-scandal.html.

86. **thirty different medical conditions:** Brownell and Horgen, *Food Fight*, 43; "The Impact of Obesity on Your Body and Health," American Society for Metabolic and Bariatric Surgery, accessed March 5, 2018, https://as mbs.org/patients/impact-of-obesity.

87. **cheaper to fill up on unhealthy foods:** Carlson and Frazão, "Are Healthy Foods Really More Expensive?"

88. **burn off a slice of pizza:** Penny Klatell, "Seven Ways to Cut Down on Pizza Calories," *Eat Out Eat Well*, March 11, 2015, http://www.eatouteatwell .com/seven-ways-to-cut-down-on-pizza-calories/.

89. **attempts to lose weight:** "Nudge, Nudge," *The Economist*, December 15, 2012, https://www.economist.com/node/21568072/print.

90. **metabolisms had slowed down:** Erin Fothergill et al., "Persistent Metabolic Adaptation 6 Years After 'The Biggest Loser' Competition," *Obesity* 24, no. 8 (August 2016), 1612–19, http://doi.org/10.1002/oby.21538; Gina Kolata, "After 'The Biggest Loser,' Their Bodies Fought to Regain Weight," *New York Times*, May 2, 2016, https://www.nytimes.com/2016/05/02/health /biggest-loser-weight-loss.html.

91. **best dietary advice:** Frazão, "America's Eating Habits," 34.

92. **evils of overeating:** Ibid.

Chapter 10

1. *engineered* **to resist pesticides:** The term *pesticide* customarily includes herbicides, fungicides, insecticides, repellants, and other control agents.

2. **For thousands of years:** Paul Kriwaczek, *Babylon: Mesopotamia and the Birth of Civilization* (New York: Thomas Dunne Books, 2012), Kindle edition; "Ancient Mesopotamia: The History, Our History," Oriental Institute Museum, University of Chicago, accessed March 5, 2018, http://chnm. gmu.edu/worldhistorysources/d/355/whm.html.

3. **Silt particles too small to see:** Thorkild Jacobsen and Robert Adams, "Salt and Silt in Ancient Mesopotamian Agriculture," *Science* 128, no. 3334

(November 21, 1958): 1251–58, http://science.sciencemag.org/content/128/3334/1251.

4. **potatoes provided:** Charles Mann, *1493: Uncovering the New World Columbus Created* (New York: Vintage, 2011), Kindle edition, 209.

5. **mostly milk and potatoes:** Ibid., 211.

6. **But along with the guano:** Ibid., 226.

7. **famine claimed one million lives:** Joseph O'Neill, *The Irish Potato Famine* (Minneapolis, MN: Abdo Group, 2009), 7.

8. **"Suitcase farmers,":** Morris Cooke, *Report of the Great Plains Drought Area Committee (to the President)*, August 27, 1936, *Hathi Trust Digital Library*, https://babel.hathitrust.org/cgi/pt?id=coo.31924000933956;view=1up;seq=1.

9. **Total land cultivated:** Ibid., 6.

10. **In the Southern Plains:** Andrew Smith, *Food in America: The Past, Present, and Future of Food, Farming, and the Family Meal*, vol. 1 (Santa Barbara, CA: ABC-CLIO, 2017), 35–36.

11. **some stage of erosion:** Cooke, *Report of the Great Plains Drought*, 5.

12. **Farmers placed the blame:** Zeynep Hansen and Gary Libecap, "Small Farms, Externalities, and the Dust Bowl of the 1930s," *Journal of Political Economy* 112, no. 3 (2004): 665–94, http://www2.bren.ucsb.edu/~glibecap/DustBowl JPE.pdf.

13. **close the book on infectious disease:** Bill Bryson, *A Short History of Nearly Everything* (New York: Broadway Books 2003), 315; James Surowiecki, "No Profit, No Cure," *New Yorker*, November 5, 2001, https://www.newyorker.com/magazine/2001/11/05/no-profit-no-cure.

14. **immunity to penicillin:** Centers for Disease Control and Prevention (CDC), "Antibiotic Resistance Threats in the United States, 2013," 2013, 28, https://www.cdc.gov/drugresistance/pdf/ar-threats-2013-508.pdf.

15. **adding antibiotics to livestock feed:** Maureen Ogle, "Riots, Rage, and Resistance: A Brief History of How Antibiotics Arrived on the Farm," *Scientific American*, September 3, 2013, https://blogs.scientificamerican.com/guest-blog/riots-rage-and-resistance-a-brief-history-of-how-antibiotics-arrived-on-the-farm/.

16. **promote growth is a mystery:** Vikram Krishnasamy, Joachim Otte, and Ellen Silbergeld, "Antimicrobial Use in Chinese Swine and Broiler Poultry Production," *Antimicrobial Resistance and Infection Control* 4, no. 17 (2015): 1–9, http://www.aricjournal.com/content/pdf/s13756-015-0050-y.pdf.

17. **bacteria thwarting the drugs:** Ogle, "Riots, Rage and Resistance."

18. **FDA tried to rein in usage:** Ibid.

19. **80 percent of all antibiotics consumed:** Tracy Pham, "Drug Use Review," US Food and Drug Administration (FDA), April 5, 2012, 2, http://www.fda.

gov/downloads/Drugs/DrugSafety/InformationbyDrugClass/UCM319435
.pdf; FDA, "2013 Summary Report on Antimicrobials Sold or Distributed for
Use in Food-Producing Animals," April 2015, 39, http://www.fda.gov/down
loads/ForIndustry/UserFees/AnimalDrugUserFeeActADUFA/UCM440584
.pdf.

20. **an average of 355 chickens:** Krishnasamy et al., "Antimicrobial Use in
Chinese Swine and Broiler"; Steve Martinez, "Vertical Coordination in the
Pork and Broiler Industries: Implications for Pork and Chicken Products," Economic Research Service, AER-777, April, 1999, https://www.ers.usda.gov/web
docs/publications/40999/17966_aer777_1_.pdf?v=41063; "Big Chicken: Pollution and Industrial Poultry Production in America," Pew Charitable Trusts
Environment Group, July 27, 2011, http://www.pewtrusts.org/~/media/legacy
/uploadedfiles/peg/publications/report/pegbigchickenjuly2011pdf.

21. **less than fifty days:** Krishnasamy et al., "Antimicrobial Use in Chinese
Swine and Broiler."

22. **thirteen new classes of antibiotics:** Brian Vastag, "NIH Superbug Outbreak Highlights Lack of New Antibiotics," *Washington Post*, August
24, 2012, http://www.washingtonpost.com/national/health-science/nih-super
bug-outbreak-highlights-lack-of-new-antibiotics/2012/08/24/ec33doc8-ee24
-11e1-boeb-dac6b50187ad_print.html; "Reviving the Pipeline of Life-Saving
Antibiotics: Exploring Solutions to Spur Innovation," Pew Trusts, April 12,
2012, http://www.pewtrusts.org/en/research-and-analysis/issue-briefs/2012
/04/12/reviving-the-pipeline-of-lifesaving-antibiotics.

23. **In the last half century:** Vastag, "NIH Superbug Outbreak."

24. **MRSA accounts for:** CDC, "Antibiotic Resistance Threats," 16.

25. **ominous threat is called CRE:** CDC, "CDC: Action Needed Now
to Halt Spread of Deadly Bacteria," March 5, 2013, https://www.cdc.gov/media
/releases/2013/p0305_deadly_bacteria.html.

26. **"nightmare bacteria,":** CDC, "CDC: Action Needed Now."

27. *pass along* **their resistance:** CDC, "Carbapenem-Resistant Entero-
bacteriaceae in Healthcare Settings," last modified February 23, 2018, https:
//www.cdc.gov/hai/organisms/cre/index.html.

28. **antibiotic-resistant infections:** CDC, "Antibiotic Resistance Threats."

29. **annual usage is forecast to grow:** Thomas Van Boeckel et al., "Global
Trends in Antimicrobial Use in Food Animals," *Proceedings of the National
Academy of Sciences* 112, no. 18 (May 5, 2015): 5649–54, http://www.pnas.org/content
/pnas/112/18/5649.full.pdf.

30. **nonbinding recommendations:** FDA, "#209 Guidance for Industry—
The Judicious Use of Medically Important Antimicrobial Drugs in Food-
Producing Animals," April 13, 2012, https://www.fda.gov/downloads/Animal

Veterinary/GuidanceComplianceEnforcement/GuidanceforIndustry/UCM 216936.pdf.

31. **first time since 2009:** FDA, "2016 Summary Report on Antimicrobials Sold or Distributed for Use in Food-Producing Animals," December 2017, https://www.fda.gov/downloads/ForIndustry/UserFees/AnimalDrugUser FeeActADUFA/UCM588085.pdf.

32. **five times higher:** "Comparison of UK and US Antibiotic Use by Farm-Animal Species," Alliance to Save Our Antibiotics, February 8, 2018, http://www.saveourantibiotics.org/media/1789/us-and-uk-antibiotic-use-compari son-calculations-080218.pdf.

33. **substances like nicotine sulfate:** Smith, *Food in America*, vol. 1, 28.

34. **fifty thousand different pesticides:** Ibid.

35. **playing under a shower of DDT:** Daniel Fairbanks, *Evolving: The Human Effect and Why It Matters* (Amherst, NY: Prometheus Books, May 2012), chap. 9, Kindle edition.

36. **Believed to be safe:** Smith, *Food in America*, vol. 1, 28.

37. **DDT soon found other uses:** Ibid., 97.

38. **warned in 1947 not to use DDT:** Ibid., 28–29.

39. **safe enough to drink:** Carey Gillam, *Whitewash: The Story of a Weed Killer, Cancer, and the Corruption of Science* (Washington, DC: Island Press), 27.

40. **company wrote in its application:** "Petition for Determination of Non-regulated Status: Soybeans with a Roundup-Ready Gene, Monsanto #93-089U," Animal and Plant Health Inspection Service, September 14, 1993, 56, http://www.aphis.usda.gov/brs/aphisdocs/93_25801p.pdf.

41. **refuge-crops requirements:** Dominic Reisig, "Factors Associated with Willingness to Plant Non-Bt Maize Refuge and Suggestions for Increasing Refuge Compliance," *Journal of Integrated Pest Management* 8, no. 1 (January 1, 2017), 1–10, https://doi.org/10.1093/jipm/pmx002.

42. **glyphosate-resistant weed species:** "Glyphosate Resistance in Weeds in North America," DuPont Pioneer, accessed March 20, 2018, https://www.pio neer.com/home/site/us/agronomy/library/glyphosate-resistance-in-weeds/.

43. **"restricted use.":** US Environmental Protection Agency (EPA), "Restricted Use Products (RUP) Report," accessed March 20, 2018, https://www .epa.gov/pesticide-worker-safety/restricted-use-products-rup-report.

44. **over three million acres were affected:** Dan Charles, "Monsanto Attacks Scientists after Studies Show Trouble for Weedkiller Dicamba," *The Salt*, National Public Radio, October 26, 2017, https://www.npr.org/sections /thesalt/2017/10/26/559733837/monsanto-and-the-weed-scientists-not-a-love -story.

45. **Missouri's largest peach farm:** Tom Philpott, "Farmers Say Monsanto's Pesticide Drifted from Nearby Farms and Killed Their Crops. Now They Need Monsanto Seeds to Fix Them," *Mother Jones*, October 5, 2017, https://www.motherjones.com/food/2017/10/farmers-say-monsantos-pesticide-drifted-from-nearby-farms-and-killed-their-crops-now-they-need-monsanto-seeds-to-fix-them/.

46. **farmers were to blame:** Charles, "Monsanto Attacks Scientists."

47. **full-blown resistance to dicamba:** Chris Bennett, "First Signs of Dicamba Resistance?" *Ag Web*, March 6, 2017, https://www.agweb.com/article/first-signs-of-dicamba-resistance-naa-chris-bennett/.

48. **Fields should not be entered:** EPA, "Chlorpyrifos," accessed March 19, 2018, https://www.epa.gov/ingredients-used-pesticide-products/chlorpyrifos.

49. **impaired cognitive functioning:** Virginia Rauh et al., "Brain Anomalies in Children Exposed Prenatally to a Common Organophosphate Pesticide," *PNAS* 109, no. 20 (May 2012): 7871–76, https://doi.org/10.1073/pnas.1203396109; "Prenatal Exposure to Common Insecticide Linked to Decreases in Cognitive Functioning at Age Seven," Mailman School of Public Health, Columbia University, April 18, 2011, https://www.mailman.columbia.edu/public-health-now/news/prenatal-exposure-common-insecticide-linked-decreases-cognitive-functioning.

50. **Studies of juvenile salmon:** Cathy Laetz et al., "The Synergistic Toxicity of Pesticide Mixtures: Implications for Risk Assessment and the Conservation of Endangered Pacific Salmon," *Environmental Health Perspectives* 117, no. 3 (March 2009): 348–53, https://doi.org/10.1289/ehp.0800096.

51. **EPA's own biological evaluation:** Michael Biesecker, "AP Exclusive: Pesticide Maker Tries to Kill Risk Study," Associated Press, April 20, 2017, https://apnews.com/a29073ecef9b4841b2e6cca07202bb67.

52. **zero tolerance for chlorpyrifos:** EPA, "Proposal to Revoke Chlorpyrifos Food Residue Tolerances," accessed March 19, 2018, https://archive.epa.gov/epa/ingredients-used-pesticide-products/proposal-revoke-chlorpyrifos-food-residue-tolerances.html.

53. **exceed allowable standards:** EPA, "Revised Human Health Risk Assessment on Chlorpyrifos," accessed March 19, 2018, https://www.epa.gov/ingredients-used-pesticide-products/revised-human-health-risk-assessment-chlorpyrifos.

54. **full respect for human health:** Biesecker, "AP Exclusive: Pesticide Maker."

55. **rejecting its own science:** Eric Lipton, "EPA Chief, Rejecting Agency's Science, Chooses Not to Ban Insecticide," *New York Times*, March 29, 2017,

https://www.nytimes.com/2017/03/29/us/politics/epa-insecticide-chlor
pyrifos.html.

56. **vested interests will once again triumph:** Dan Flynn, "9th Circuit Orders EPA to Stop 'Stalling' and Ban Ag Use of Popular Pesticide," *Food Safety News*, August 10, 2018, https://www.foodsafetynews.com/2018/08/9th -circuit-orders-epa-to-stop-stalling-and-ban-ag-use-of-popular-pesticide/#.

57. **long-term effects remain unknown:** CDC, "Dichlorodiphenyltrich-loroethane (DDT) Factsheet," last modified April 7, 2017, https://www.cdc.gov /biomonitoring/pdf/ddt_factsheet.pdf.

58. **Amazon rain forest:** Jerry Shields, *The Invisible Billionaire: Daniel Ludwig* (Boston: Houghton Mifflin, 1986), 12.

59. **paid three million dollars:** Ibid., 295.

60. **plant trees like rows of corn:** Ibid., 287.

61. **plastic in soil:** Sileshi Nugusu et al., "Studies on Foreign Body Inges-tion and their Related Complications in Ruminants Associated with In-appropriate Solid Waste Disposal in Gondar Town, North West Ethiopia," *International Journal of Animal and Veterinary Advances* 5, no. 2 (2013): 67–74, http://maxwellsci.com/print/ijava/v5-67-74.pdf.

62. **How carbon dioxide can retain heat:** Naomi Oreskes and Erik Con-way, *Merchants of Doubt: How a Handful of Scientists Obscured the Truth on Issues from Tobacco Smoke to Global Warming* (New York: Bloomsbury Press, 2010), chap. 6.

63. **humans are most responsible:** William Anderegg et al., "Expert Credi-bility in Climate Change," *PNAS* 107, no. 27 (July 2010): 12107–9, https://doi.org /10.1073/pnas.1003187107.

64. **This is the site:** EPA, "Learn about Dioxin," accessed March 19, 2018, https://www.epa.gov/dioxin/learn-about-dioxin.

65. **The contamination extended:** EPA, "Tittabawassee River, Saginaw River & Bay, Midland, MI, Cleanup Activities," accessed March 19, 2018, https: //cumulis.epa.gov/supercpad/SiteProfiles/index.cfm?fuseaction=second .cleanup&id=0503250.

66. **physiologically tolerable limits:** Bryson, *A Short History*, 246.

Chapter 11

1. **deadliest Atlantic hurricane:** Neal Lott et al., "Hurricane Mitch: The Deadliest Atlantic Hurricane since 1780," National Climatic Data Center, Na-tional Oceanic and Atmospheric Administration, accessed March 20, 2018,

ftp://ftp.ncdc.noaa.gov/pub/data/extremeevents/specialreports/Hurri
cane-Mitch-1998.pdf; "Hurricane Mitch," *Encyclopedia Britannica*, accessed
March 20, 2018, http://www.britannica.com/event/Hurricane-Mitch.

2. **Staple crops like beans:** Ibid.

3. **tractors sat idle:** Raj Patel, "What Cuba Can Teach Us about Food
and Climate Change," *Slate*, April 5, 2012, http://www.slate.com/articles/
health_and_science/future_tense/2012/04/agro_ecology_lessons_from_cuba
_on_agriculture_food_and_climate_change_.html; Miguel Altieri and Fer-
nando Funes-Monzote, "The Paradox of Cuban Agriculture," *Monthly Review* 63, no. 8 (January 2012), http://monthlyreview.org/2012/01/01/the-para
dox-of-cuban-agriculture/.

4. **average Cuban lost twenty pounds:** Patel, "What Cuba Can Teach
Us."

5. *to feed a growing population:* Charles Godfray et al., "Food Security:
The Challenge of Feeding 9 Billion People," *Science* 327, no. 5967 (February
2010): 812–18, http://science.sciencemag.org/content/327/5967/812.full; Nikos
Alexandratos et al., "World Agriculture: Towards 2030/2050," Food and Agriculture Organization of the United Nations (FAO), June 2006, http://www
.fao.org/fileadmin/user_upload/esag/docs/Interim_report_AT2050web.pdf.

6. **reach 9.8 billion people:** Department of Economic and Social Affairs, "World Population Projected to Reach 9.8 Billion in 2050, and 11.2 Billion in 2100," United Nations, June 21, 2017, https://www.un.org/develop
ment/desa/en/news/population/world-population-prospects-2017.html.

7. **images of starving children:** World Health Organization (WHO),
"Obesity and Overweight, Fact Sheet," February 16, 2018, http://www.who.
int/mediacentre/factsheets/fs311/en/.

8. **one-third to one-half of food:** FAO, "Food Wastage Footprint Impacts on Natural Resources, Summary Report," 2013, http://www.fao.org/do
crep/018/i3347e/i3347e.pdf; "Waste Not, Want Not," *The Economist*, February 24, 2011, https://www.economist.com/node/18200694.

9. **up to 40 percent is never eaten:** Jean Buzby, Hodan Wells, and Jeff-
rey Hyman, "The Estimated Amount, Value, and Calories of Postharvest
Food Losses at the Retail and Consumer Levels in the United States," Economic Research Service (ERS), EIB-121, February 2014, https://www.ers.usda
.gov/webdocs/publications/43833/43680_eib121.pdf; Dana Gunders, "Wasted:
How America Is Losing Up to 40 Percent of Its Food from Farm to Fork to
Landfill," Natural Resources Defense Council, August 16, 2017, https://assets
.nrdc.org/sites/default/files/wasted-2017-report.pdf.

10. **energy harvested from cropland:** Emily Cassidy et al., "Redefining Agricultural Yields: From Tonnes to People Nourished Per Hectare," *Environ-*

mental Research Letters 8, no. 3 (August 2013): Table 2, http://iopscience.iop.org/article/10.1088/1748-9326/8/3/034015/pdf.

11. **all the energy loses:** Ibid.

12. **global obesity rates:** WHO, "Obesity and Overweight, Fact Sheet."

13. **rates are rising faster in children:** The GBD 2015 Obesity Collaborators, "Health Effects of Overweight and Obesity in 195 Countries over 25 Years," *New England Journal of Medicine* 337, no. 1 (July 6 2017): 13–27, http://www.nejm.org/doi/pdf/10.1056/NEJMoa1614362.

14. **Land used to raise animals:** Jonathan Foley et al., "Solutions for a Cultivated Planet," *Nature* 478 (October 2011): 337–42, http://doi.org/10.1038/nature10452.

15. **world's largest consumer of water:** Ibid.

16. **"Food for Peace":** Randy Schnepf, "U.S. International Food Aid Programs: Background and Issues," Congressional Research Service, September 14, 2016, https://fas.org/sgp/crs/misc/R41072.pdf.

17. **seven in ten farms:** FAO, "The State of Food and Agriculture, Innovation in Family Farming," 2014, xi, http://www.fao.org/3/a-i4040e.pdf.

18. **When a severe drought:** Jeannie Sowers, John Waterbury, and Eckart Woertz, "Did Drought Trigger the Crisis in Syria?" *Footnote*, September 12, 2013, http://footnote.co/did-drought-trigger-the-crisis-in-syria/; John Light, "Drought Helped Spark Syria's Civil War—Is It One of Many Climate Wars to Come?" *Moyers & Company*, September 6, 2013, http://billmoyers.com/2013/09/06/droughthelped-spark-syrias-civil-war-is-it-the-first-of-many-climate-wars-tocome/; Clemens Breisinger, Olivier Ecker, and Jean Francois Trinh Tan, "Conflict and Food Insecurity: How Do We Break the Links?" in *2014–2015 Global Food Policy Report* (Washington, DC, 2015), International Food Policy Research Institute, chap. 7, https://www.ifpri.org/sites/default/files/gfpr/2015/feature_3086.html.

19. **the world's subsistence farmers:** Timothy Snyder, "Hitler's World May Not Be So Far Away," *The Guardian*, September 16, 2015, https://www.theguardian.com/world/2015/sep/16/hitlers-world-may-not-be-so-far-away.

20. **Nine in ten farms:** Robert Hoppe, "America's Diverse Family Farms, 2017 Edition," ERS, EIB-185, December 2017, https://www.ers.usda.gov/webdocs/publications/86198/eib-185.pdf?v=43083.

21. **top 10 percent of family farms:** Ibid.

22. **Seventy percent of farms:** Ibid.

23. **begging door-to-door:** Joel Berg, *All You Can Eat: How Hungry Is America?* (New York: Seven Stories Press, 2008), 60.

24. **until markets realigned themselves:** Ibid., 61–62.

25. **bridge across that chasm:** Food and Nutrition Service (FNS), "A Short History of SNAP," USDA, November 28, 2017, http://www.fns.usda .gov/snap/short-history-snap.

26. **During the Great Depression:** ERS, "Table 7—Food Expenditures by Families and Individuals as a Share of Disposable Personal Income," in "Food Expenditure," last modified January 26, 2016, https://www.ers.usda.gov/data -products/food-expenditures.aspx.

27. **unemployment peaked at 25 percent:** US Census Bureau, "No. HS-29. Employment Status of the Civilian Population: 1929 to 2002," in "Statistical Abstract of the United States: 2003, Mini-Historical Statistics," February 2003, https://www2.census.gov/library/publications/2004/compendia/statab /123ed/hist/hs-29.pdf.

28. **malnutrition from lack of food:** "Too Fat to Fight: Retired Military Leaders Want Junk Food out of America's Schools," Military Leaders for Kids, April 8, 2010, 2, http://cdn.missionreadiness.org/MR_Too_Fat_to_Fight -1.pdf.

29. **National School Lunch Program:** Ibid., 2.

30. **The Food Stamp Act:** FNS, "A Short History of SNAP."

31. **nutritionally adequate diet:** "Chart Book: SNAP Helps Struggling Families Put Food on the Table," Center on Budget and Policy Priorities, February 14, 2018, https://www.cbpp.org/sites/default/files/atoms/files/3-13-12fa -chartbook.pdf; Steven Carlson, Dorothy Rosenbaum, and Brynne Keith-Jennings, "Who Are the Low-Income Childless Adults Facing the Loss of SNAP in 2016?" CBPP, February 8, 2016, https://www.cbpp.org/sites/default /files/atoms/files/2-8-16fa.pdf.

32. **charitable food assistance:** Janet Poppendieck, "Hunger in the United States: Policy Implications," *Nutrition* 16, nos. 7 & 8 (July–August 2000): 651–53, https://doi.org/10.1016/S0899-9007(00)00334-8; Bureau of Labor Statistics, "Volunteering in the United States, 2014," February 2015, http://www.bls .gov/news.release/volun.nr0.htm.

33. **"If virtually nobody wants hunger:** Poppendieck, "Hunger in the United States."

34. **half-*trillion* SNAP dollars:** FNS, "Supplemental Nutrition Assistance Program Participation and Costs, 1969–2017," April 6, 2018, https://fns-prod .azureedge.net/sites/default/files/pd/SNAPsummary.pdf; FNS, "Fiscal Year 2016 at a Glance, Number of Authorized Firms," December 15, 2016, https: //fns-prod.azureedge.net/sites/default/files/snap/2016-SNAP-Retailer-Man agement-Year-End-Summary.pdf.

35. **Walmart takes in:** Heather Haddon and Jesse Newman, "Retailers Worry Food-Stamp Overhaul Will Hit Them Hard," *Wall Street Journal*, last

modified April 6, 2018, https://www.wsj.com/articles/retailers-worry-food
-stamp-overhaul-will-hit-them-hard-1523016003; Dennis Green, "A $13 Bil-
lion Part of Walmart's Business Could Be About to Take a Critical Hit from
Trump," *Business Insider*, April 9, 2018, http://www.businessinsider.com/wal
mart-could-take-hit-from-snap-benefits-reduction-2018-4.

36. **valuation by Wall Street:** Jeff Bukhari, "Amazon Is Worth More
than Walmart, Costco, and Target Combined," *Fortune*, April 5, 2017, http:
//fortune.com/2017/04/05/amazon-walmart-costco-target-market-cap/.

37. **Amazon, whose valuation:** Andrew Sorkin, "What Might Happen
to Amazon's Profit if It Paid Its Workers More?" *New York Times*, April
23, 2018, https://www.nytimes.com/2018/04/23/business/dealbook/walmart
-amazon-flipkart-deal.html. According to the US Department of Health
and Human Services, the poverty threshold for a family of four in 2018 was
$25,100. See: ASPE, accessed October 8, 2018, https://aspe.hhs.gov/poverty
-guidelines.

38. **employees depend on SNAP:** Claire Brown, "Amazon Gets Tax
Breaks while Its Employees Rely on Food Stamps, New Data Shows," *The In-
tercept*, April 19, 2018, https://theintercept.com/2018/04/19/amazon-snap-sub
sidies-warehousing-wages/.

39. **lobbying Congress for food aid:** Shelly Banjo and Annie Gasparro,
"Retailers Brace for Reduction in Food Stamps: Expiration of Added Benefits Will Remove $11 Billion in Aid Over Three Years," *Wall Street Journal*,
last modified November 4, 2013, https://www.wsj.com/articles/grocers-brace
-for-reduction-in-food-stamps-1383168686?mod=djemITP_h&tesla=y#:J7
C9WuNUJo93MA.

40. **The average worker's wages:** Drew Desilver, "For Most U.S. Workers, Real Wages Have Barely Budged for Decades," Pew Research Center,
August 7, 2018, http://www.pewresearch.org/fact-tank/2014/10/09/for-most
-workers-real-wages-have-barely-budged-for-decades/.

41. **three of every five new jobs:** Sylvia Allegretto et al., "Fast Food,
Poverty Wages: The Public Cost of Low-Wages Jobs in the Fast-Food Industry," Center for Labor Research and Education, University of California,
and Department of Urban and Regional Planning, University of Illinois,
October 15, 2013, http://laborcenter.berkeley.edu/pdf/2013/fast_food_poverty
_wages.pdf.

42. **including military households:** Ibid.

43. **one in four in rural America:** ERS, "Rural Child Poverty Chart Gal-
lery," last modified June 7, 2018, https://www.ers.usda.gov/data-products/rural
-child-poverty-chart-gallery/.

44. **fare better as adults:** CBPP, "Chart Book: SNAP Helps."

45. **when seafood in supermarkets:** "MSC Certified 'Fish to Eat,'" Marine Stewardship Council, accessed April 14, 2018, https://www.msc.org/cook-eat-enjoy/fish-to-eat.

46. **farmers enrolled in proprietary programs:** "Land O'Lakes SUSTAIN—What Are Buffer Support Tools," Land O'Lakes, accessed April 14, 2018, https://www.landolakessustain.com/buffer-support-tools.

47. **were never any assurances:** Dan Charles, "Does 'Sustainability' Help the Environment or Just Agriculture's Public Image?" *The Salt*, August 22, 2017, http://www.npr.org/sections/thesalt/2017/08/22/545022259/does-sustainability-help-the-environment-or-just-agricultures-public-image.

48. **no differences were detected:** Susan Selke et al., "Evaluation of Biodegradation-Promoting Additives for Plastics," *Environmental Science & Technology* 49, no. 6 (February 2015): 3769–77, https://pubs.acs.org/doi/pdf/10.1021/es504258u.

49. **world's largest car manufacturer:** Emily Peck, "Here's the Joke of a Sustainability Report That VW Put Out Last Year," *Huffpost*, September 25, 2015, https://www.huffingtonpost.com/entry/volkswagen-sustainability-report-from-last-year-is-a-joke_us_56040f1ae4b0fde8b0d17996.

50. **repeated the same pledge verbatim:** Benjamin Preston, "Volkswagen Scandal Tarnishes Hard-Won US Reputation as Green Company," *The Guardian*, September 25, 2015, https://www.theguardian.com/business/2015/sep/25/volkswagen-scandal-us-reputation-emissions.

51. **expansion was less than 1 percent:** Holly Gibbs et al., "Brazil's Soy Moratorium," *Science* 347, no. 6220 (January 2015): 377–78, http://doi.org/10.1126/science.aaa0181.

52. **public relations triumph:** Kelly Tyrrell, "Study Shows Brazil's Soy Moratorium Still Needed to Preserve Amazon," *News*, University of Wisconsin–Madison, January 22, 2015, https://news.wisc.edu/study-shows-brazils-soy-moratorium-still-needed-to-preserve-amazon/.

53. **a darker picture emerged:** Daniel Nepstad et al., "Slowing Amazon Deforestation through Public Policy and Interventions in Beef and Soy Supply Chains," *Science* 344, no. 6188 (June 2014): 1118–23, http://doi.org/10.1126/science.1248525; Gibbs et al., "Brazil's Soy Moratorium."

54. **acreage planted was misleading:** Sue Branford and Maurício Torres, "Amazon Soy Moratorium: Defeating Deforestation or Greenwash Diversion?" *Mongabay*, March 8, 2017, https://news.mongabay.com/2017/03/amazon-soy-moratorium-defeating-deforestation-or-greenwash-diversion/; Felicity Lawrence and John Vidal, "Food Giants to Boycott Illegal Amazon Soya," *The Guardian*, July 24, 2006, https://www.theguardian.com/world/2006/jul/24/brazil.foodanddrink.

55. **deforestation shot up:** Hiroko Tabuchi, Claire Rigby, and Jeremy White, "Amazon Deforestation, Once Tamed, Comes Roaring Back," *New York Times*, February 24, 2017, https://www.nytimes.com/2017/02/24/business /energy-environment/deforestation-brazil-bolivia-south-america.html.

56. **Over the last several decades:** Philip Pardey, Julian Alston, and Connie Chan-Kang, "Public Food and Agricultural Research in the United States: The Rise and Decline of Public Investments, and Policies for Renewal," AGree—Transforming Food & Ag Policy (April 2013), 2, http://foodandag policy.org/sites/default/files/AGree-Public%20Food%20and%20Ag%20 Research%20in%20US-Apr%202013.pdf.

57. **the answer was also yes:** Ralf Seppelt et al., "Synchronized Peak-Rate Years of Global Resources Use," *Ecology and Society* 19, no. 4 (2014): 50 –63, http://dx.doi.org/10.5751/ES-07039-190450.

58. **But unlike the previous five:** Céline Bellard et al., "Impacts of Climate Change on the Future of Biodiversity," *Ecology Letters* 15, no. 4 (January 2012): 365–77, https://doi.org/10.1111/j.1461-0248.2011.01736.x.

59. **Nutrients like zinc and iron:** Samuel Myers et al., "Increasing CO_2 Threatens Human Nutrition," *Nature* 510 (May 2014): 139–42, https://doi.org /10.1038/nature13179.

60. **already weakened by higher stress:** Bethany Huot et al., "Dual Impact of Elevated Temperature on Plant Defence and Bacterial Virulence in Arabidopsis," *Nature Communications* 8 (November 2017): 1808, https://www .nature.com/articles/s41467-017-01674-2.pdf.

61. **Humans have appropriated:** Roger Hooke, José Martín-Duque, and Javier Pedraza, "Land Transformation by Humans: A Review," *GSA Today* 22, no. 12 (December 2012): 4–10, http://www.geosociety.org/gsatoday/archive/22 /12/pdf/i1052-5173-22-12-4.pdf.

62. **Through our efforts alone:** Ibid.

63. **the "biomass" of mammals:** Justin Smith, "The Great Extinction," *Chronicle of Higher Education*, May 5, 2014, http://chronicle.com/article/The -Great-Extinction/146275.

64. **Cellular agriculture:** Paul Shapiro, "Lab-Made Meat Could Be the Next Food Revolution: Here's What It Tastes Like," *The Guardian*, January 31,2018,https://www.theguardian.com/lifeandstyle/2018/jan/31/eat-it-without -the-guilt-the-story-of-the-worlds-first-clean-foie-gras.

65. **Quantum dots:** Chris Dall, "Small Wonder: Nanoparticles Help Fight Drug-Resistant Bacteria," Center for Infectious Disease Research and Policy, University of Minnesota, October 4, 2017, http://www.cidrap.umn.edu/news -perspective/2017/10/small-wonder-nanoparticles-help-fight-drug-resistant -bacteria.

66. **remembering Amara's law:** "Roy Amara 1925–2007—American Futurologist," in *Oxford Essential Quotations*, 4th edition, ed. Susan Ratcliffe (Oxford, UK: Oxford University Press, 2016).

67. **the peasant sector controlled:** Altieri and Funes-Monzote, "The Paradox of Cuban Agriculture."

68. **higher in Cuba**: "Food Balance—Visualize Data—Food Supply in Cuba 2007—Cuba Food Supply (kcal/capita/day) Grand Total," FAOSTAT, accessed April 15, 2018, http://www.fao.org/faostat/en/#data/FBS/visualize; Altieri and Funes-Monzote, "The Paradox of Cuban Agriculture."

Chapter 12

1. **Borman unexpectedly noticed:** Robert Poole, *Earthrise: How Man First Saw the Earth* (New Haven, CT: Yale University Press, 2010).

2. **astronaut Bill Anders:** Ibid., 2.

3. **Robert Poole later wrote:** Ibid., 8.

4. *Life* **magazine declared:** Ibid., 155.

5. **food has a bigger impact on well-being:** Mark Bittman et al., "How a National Food Policy Could Save Millions of American Lives," *Washington Post*, November 7, 2014, https://www.washingtonpost.com/opinions/how-a-national-food-policy-could-save-millions-of-american-lives/2014/11/07/89c55e16-637f-11e4-836c-83bc4f26eb67_story.html?utm_term=.2b450c74a41d; Institute of Medicine and National Research Council, *A Framework for Assessing Effects of the Food System* (Washington, DC: National Academies Press, 2015), Overview Description, https://www.nap.edu/catalog/18846/a-framework-for-assessing-effects-of-the-food-system.

6. **bread prices rose by 37 percent:** Rami Zurayk, "Use Your Loaf: Why Food Prices Were Crucial in the Arab Spring," *The Guardian*, July 16, 2011, https://www.theguardian.com/lifeandstyle/2011/jul/17/bread-food-arab-spring.

7. **"cheap luxuries.":** George Orwell, *The Road to Wigan Pier* (New York: Mariner Books, 1972), chaps. 5 & 6.

8. **Carl Sagan said it best:** Carl Sagan and Ann Druyan, *The Demon-Haunted World: Science as a Candle in the Dark* (New York: Ballantine Books, 1997), 28.

9. **hurtling through space:** "What Is the Speed of the Earth's Rotation?" Ask the Space Scientist, National Aeronautics and Space Administration, accessed March 19, 2018, https://image.gsfc.nasa.gov/poetry/ask/a10840.html;

Bill Bryson, A Short History of Nearly Everything (New York: Broadway Books, 2003), chap. 2, fn. 2.

10. **Five percent nearer:** Bryson, *"A Short History,"* 247; Michael Hart, "The Evolution of the Atmosphere of the Earth," *Icarus* 33 (1978): 23–39, http://www.tau.ac.il/~colin/courses/CChange/Hart78.pdf; Michael Hart, "Habitable Zones about Main Sequence Stars," *Icarus* 37, no. 1 (January 1979): 351–57, https://www.sciencedirect.com/science/article/pii/0019103579901416. For more information, see: Christopher Palma, "The Habitable Zone," Department of Astronomy & Astrophysics, Penn State University, https://www.e-education.psu.edu/astro801/content/l12_p4.html; Sid Perkins, "Earth Is Only Just within the Sun's Habitable Zone," *Nature*, December 11, 2013, https://www.nature.com/news/earth-is-only-just-within-the-sun-s-habitable-zone-1.14353.

11. **As he put it, "I have lost weight:** David Kessler, *The End of Overeating: Taking Control of the Insatiable American Appetite* (New York: Rodale, 2009), 250.

12. **"the greatest power rests:** Ibid., 248–49.

13. **Year by year, sales of soda:** "U.S. Soda Sales Drops for 12th Straight Year: Trade Publication," Reuters, April 19, 2017, https://www.reuters.com/article/us-soda-sales-study/u-s-soda-sales-drops-for-12th-straight-year-trade-publication-idUSKBN17L2HN.

14. **how foods like apple juice:** Sonya Lunder, "EWG's 2018 Shopper's Guide to Pesticides in Produce," Environmental Working Group, April 10, 2018, https://www.ewg.org/foodnews/summary.php.

Index